Primary and Repeat Arterial Reconstructions

Sachinder Singh Hans • Mitchell R. Weaver
Timothy J. Nypaver
Editors

Primary and Repeat Arterial Reconstructions

Springer

Editors
Sachinder Singh Hans
Vascular and Endovascular Services
Henry Ford Macomb Hospital
Clinton Township, MI, USA

Mitchell R. Weaver
Henry Ford Hospital
Detroit, MI, USA

Timothy J. Nypaver
Henry Ford Hospital
Detroit, MI, USA

ISBN 978-3-031-13896-6 ISBN 978-3-031-13897-3 (eBook)
https://doi.org/10.1007/978-3-031-13897-3

This Springer imprint is published by the registered company Springer Nature Switzerland AG
The registered company address is: Gewerbestrasse 11, 6330 Cham, Switzerland

Foreword

There is no excuse today for the surgeon to learn on the patient.—Dr. William J. Mayo

During the last two decades, the endovascular revolution has transformed treatment of patients with vascular disease. Today, most vascular reconstructions are performed percutaneously, using catheters, guidewires, balloons, stents, and stent-grafts. Open surgery, however, is here to stay, both as a primary and as a redo intervention, performed following failed open or endovascular procedures. Complications of endovascular interventions are frequently dealt with open repair, and there is an increasing number of hybrid procedures where open surgery is combined with an endovascular intervention. Teaching open arterial reconstructions, however, has been challenging, since they are less frequently performed today than just a few years ago and some vascular surgeons who serve as mentors have inadequate experience with complex open surgical operations.

Arterial reconstructions require thorough planning and preparation, knowledge of surgical anatomy and pathology, proper training, appropriate indication, high-quality preoperative imaging studies, perfect surgical technique, and correct postoperative care. To achieve success, this book of Sachinder Singh Hans and colleagues from the Henry Ford Hospital and the University of Michigan offers invaluable help to both a novice and an experienced vascular surgeon.

The 38 chapters of this well-constructed volume cover all major primary and redo open arterial reconstructions performed from the base of the skull to the dorsum of the foot. It focuses on surgical techniques and uses beautiful color illustrations to explain details of the interventions, including dissections, vascular clamping, performance of endarterectomy, placement of grafts, vascular closures and anastomoses, and closure of the wound. Each chapter lists the surgical instruments, suture materials, and vascular grafts or patches used during the procedure.

Read and reread these chapters, keeping in mind that reading is an integral part of the learning process. But also remember what Dr. Will Mayo once said, "see things for yourself; reading alone is not enough." Seize any opportunity to assist or watch your mentor or an experienced surgeon perform these operations and consult collections of the Journal of Vascular Surgery or of your society looking for peer-reviewed surgical videos. In addition, practice your technique at home or in a simulation lab, and learn how to cut tissues, tie knots, and best suture blood vessels. Denton Cooley, one of the most dexterous cardiovascular surgeons, recommended to "get a scalpel and practice just, say, cutting a piece of meat" and "learn how you want to hold your fingers" and "try to become graceful when you operate." The end result will fully justify the time you spent with the learning process.

Few interventions provide a satisfaction that surpasses a beautifully performed and well-functioning arterial reconstruction. With the expert descriptions and detailed illustrations, this practical atlas guides you from the basic to the most sophisticated primary and redo open arterial reconstructions. Use this volume to learn or refresh your memory before an operation and remember what Will Mayo once said: "*There is no excuse today for the surgeon to learn on the patient.*"

Division of Vascular and Endovascular Surgery
Mayo Clinic
Rochester, MN, USA

Peter Gloviczki

Preface

Over the last three decades, the rapid growth of endovascular techniques used in managing patients with both aneurysmal and arterial occlusive disease has led to a significant decline in the number of open arterial reconstructions performed in the United States. Even as endovascular options supplant open arterial procedures, it seems unlikely that open arterial reconstructions will ever disappear. Open arterial reconstructions and operations remain confidently within the domain of the practicing vascular surgeon, and the ability to offer an open therapeutic solution to the patient's problem, often in the setting of failed or complicated prior endovascular procedures, is what sets the vascular surgeon apart from other interventional colleagues. New graduates of vascular surgery training programs may have limited case volume exposure to some open operations and will hopefully find the operative steps detailed in this book essential prior to undertaking a potentially technically challenging open arterial procedure.

We have chosen to highlight the technical steps involved in what we considered as standard open arterial procedures, focusing on the indications for the operation as well as the surgical anatomy, the operative steps, and the recognition and management of potential intraoperative complications. There is purposeful limited discussion involving historical aspects of disease management, disease presentation, methods of diagnosis, results, or alternative surgical or endovascular therapies. This practical and illustrated guide emphasizes the technical steps and potential operative missteps not only for primary arterial reconstructions, but also for those associated with more complex repeat or redo procedures. To preserve uniformity in the approach of patient management, most authors were drawn from Henry Ford Hospital's vascular surgery program. We wish to thank all the contributors for their help in the timely completion of the manuscript. We are also indebted to the publishing staff at Springer—Richard Hruska, Lillie Gaurano, Vijayasankra Gomathy Rajagopal, and Dhanapal Palanisamy—for seeing through to the book's completion.

Bloomfield Hills, MI, USA — Sachinder Singh Hans
Detroit, MI, USA — Mitchell R. Weaver
Detroit, MI, USA — Timothy J. Nypaver

Contents

Contributors

Yunus Ahmed Department of Cardiac Surgery, University of Michigan Medical School, Ann Arbor, MI, USA

Mark F. Conrad Vascular and Endovascular Surgery, St. Elizabeth's Hospital, Brighton, MA, USA

Kaitlyn Dobesh Henry Ford Hospital, Detroit, MI, USA

Sachinder Singh Hans Vascular and Endovascular Services, Henry Ford Macomb Hospital, Clinton Twp, MI, USA

Loay Kabbani Department of Surgery, Henry Ford Hospital, Detroit, MI, USA

Wayne State University, Detroit, MI, USA

Michigan State University, Detroit, MI, USA

Henry Ford Hospital, Heart and Vascular Institute, Detroit, MI, USA

Alice Lee Henry Ford Hospital, Detroit, MI, USA

Srihari K. Lella Vascular and Endovascular Surgery Resident, Massachusetts General Hospital, Harvard Medical School, Boston, MA, USA

Khalil Masabni Division of Vascular Surgery, University of Arizona, Tucson, AZ, USA

Farah Hanif Ali Mohammad Henry Ford Hospital, Detroit, MI, USA

Abdul Kader Natour Division of Vascular Surgery, Henry Ford Hospital, Detroit, MI, USA

Henry Ford Hospital, Detroit, MI, USA

Timothy J. Nypaver Division of Vascular Surgery, Wayne State School of Medicine, Henry Ford Hospital, Detroit, MI, USA

Himanshu J. Patel Department of Cardiac Surgery, University of Michigan Medical School, Ann Arbor, MI, USA

Andi Peshkepija Henry Ford Hospital, Detroit, MI, USA

Wayne State University, Detroit, MI, USA

Iraklis I. Pipinos Department of Surgery, University of Nebraska Medical Center, Omaha, NE, USA

Chinmayee Potti Henry Ford Hospital, Detroit, MI, USA

Alexander D. Shepard Division of Vascular Surgery, Henry Ford Hospital, Detroit, MI, USA

Wayne State University School of Medicine, Detroit, MI, USA

Pieter A. J. van Bakel Department of Cardiac Surgery, University of Michigan Medical School, Ann Arbor, MI, USA

Mitchell R. Weaver Henry Ford Hospital, Detroit, MI, USA

Wayne State University School of Medicine, Detroit, MI, USA

Chapter 1
Basic Arterial Techniques

Sachinder Singh Hans

Arterial Dissection and Mobilization

Anatomically, most arteries and veins often run parallel to each other and are often surrounded by fascial sheath in the extremities. Arterial exposure and mobilization are usually performed by using sharp dissection. After incising the sheath anteriorly over the artery, the artery should be dissected on each side, staying close to the peri-adventitial plane (skeletonizing the artery). The lateral dissection should be extended to involve 50% (one half) of posterior surface of the artery so that there should be either no or very minimal tissue posterior to the artery before a right-angled vascular clamp is passed. Failure to perform satisfactory dissection along the posterior wall of the artery and passing the right-angled clamp blindly can damage the posterior branches resulting in significant bleeding during mobilization of abdominal aorta and iliac arteries. Only anterior and lateral dissection is necessary, as these large vessels can be safely clamped from each side, thus avoiding injury to the surrounding veins (Fig. 1.1). During application of vascular clamps, care should be taken to define the exact location and extent of plaque. The plaque is usually posterior; therefore, the clamp should be applied with the anterior wall approximating the posterior wall (Figs. 1.2 and 1.3). A vascular clamp like a Satinsky or Glover clamp may be selected for arteries with posterior plaque. In patients with circumferential or heavily calcified plaques, a double-looped silastic loop may be applied. In patients with very hard calcified plaques (as in patients with end-stage renal artery disease), either a manual pressure with fingers or with a Kittner ("peanut") dissector is applied proximally and distally. Arterial control is often obtained with the help of application of atraumatic vascular clamps or with the help of endoluminal balloon catheter or Garrett arterial dilators (Fig. 1.4) resulting in significant bleeding during

S. S. Hans (✉)
Vascular and Endovascular Services, Henry Ford Macomb Hospital, Clinton Twp, MI, USA

S. S. Hans et al. (eds.), *Primary and Repeat Arterial Reconstructions*, https://doi.org/10.1007/978-3-031-13897-3_1

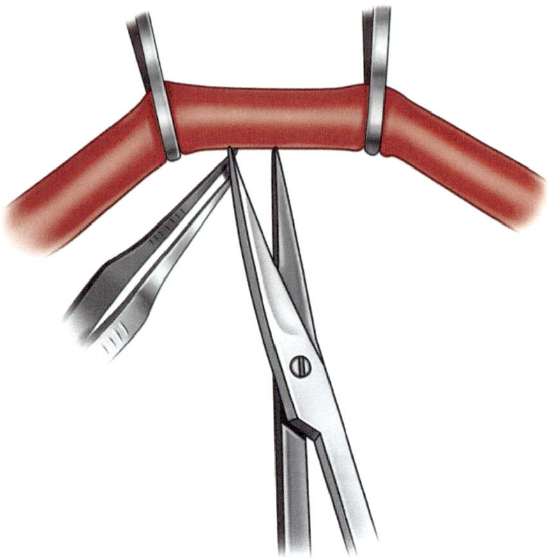

Fig. 1.1 Dissection around each side of an artery using atraumatic forceps (DeBakey or Gerald) and scissors. Silastic vessel loop retraction can aid in mobilization of an artery

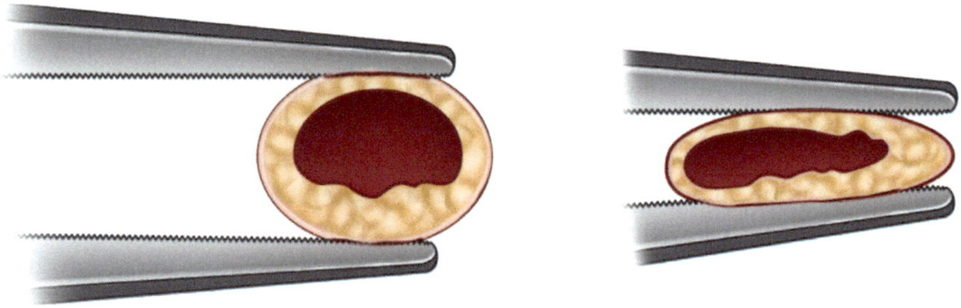

Fig. 1.2 Application of vascular clamp with vessel compressed anteroposteriorly

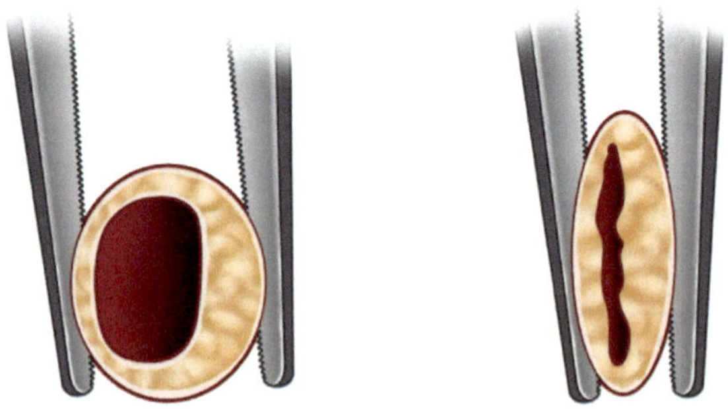

Fig. 1.3 Vessel compressed with a vascular clamp side to side because of plaque location in the lateral wall

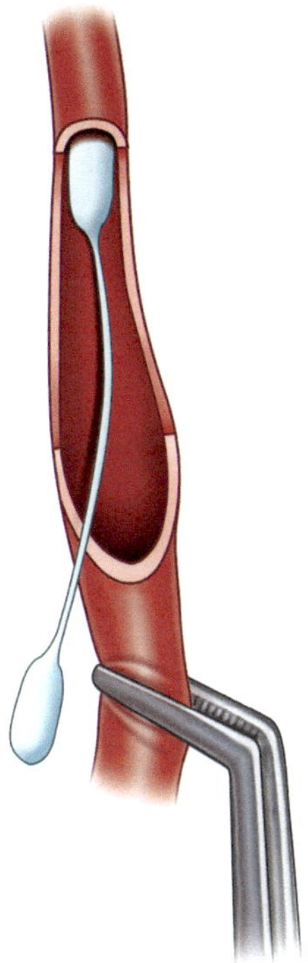

Fig. 1.4 Distal control of the artery obtained by an arterial dilator

mobilization of arteries (Teleflex Inc., Wayne, PA). A longitudinally arteriotomy is performed and calcified plaque is removed with the help of arterial dissector before vascular clamps are applied. Clamps should be applied in such a way that the wall of the blood vessel be approximated to control the bleeding but should not be clamped excessively so as to result in clamp injury or fracture of the plaque. Once a proximal graft to artery anastomosis has been completed, the clamp is removed and a clamp is then applied to the graft just distal to the proximal anastomosis.

Vascular Clamps

Prior to application of vascular clamps, silastic vessel loops doubled on itself are passed proximally and distally in most arteries except around the aorta and iliac arteries as this may cause significant bleeding from the surrounding veins.

Vascular clamps have longitudinal rows of interdigitating or opposing serrations. Clamps despite being atraumatic can cause intimal injury and fracture of the plaque. For small-diameter arteries, clamps like Yasergil, Edward bulldog clamp, or Micro bulldog may be helpful. Endoluminal occlusion can also be useful for calcified

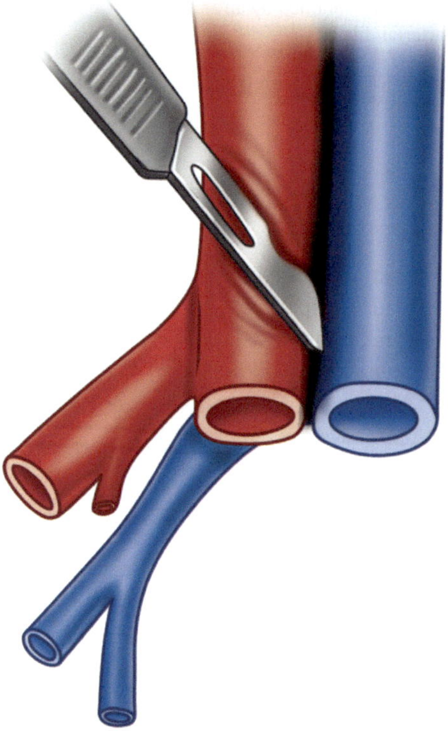

Fig. 1.5 Sharp dissection with a 15-blade scalpel (belly of the cutting edge) separating the adventitia of the artery from the surrounding vein

arteries or in patients with excessive scarring from previous arterial reconstructions. Endoluminal control can be obtained by Fogarty balloon catheter or an angioplasty catheter. In medium- and small-sized arteries, arterial dilators (Garrett), which are available in various sizes (1–10 mm), can help provide hemostatic control especially in patients with arterial trauma. In patients with repeat arterial reconstructions, there is often obliteration of the tissue planes. Once the anterior wall of the artery is exposed, the lateral wall of the artery is dissected from the surrounding veins with the aid of a 15-blade scalpel kept at an angle (not vertical) from the surrounding veins using a sharp dissection with the belly of the scalpel (Fig. 1.5).

Systemic Heparinization

Arterial reconstructions require administration of systemic heparin. In patients with ruptured aneurysm with hypovolemic shock, heparin should not be administered, until proximal anastomosis is completed, and the coagulation profile should be obtained prior to administration of heparin in order to avoid coagulopathy. In most instances, a dose of 100 IU/kg body weight should be administered 5–10 min prior to arterial clamping. Adequate anticoagulation is achieved by keeping the activated clotting time between 250 and 300 s. In most cases, heparin should be reversed with protamine sulfate after the completion of anastomosis and distal flow is confirmed.

Arterial Incision and Closure

In most arterial reconstructions, longitudinal incision is made by an 11-blade or a 15-blade scalpel (Fig. 1.6). In patients undergoing arterial embolectomy (normal arteries), transverse incision is preferred. The arteriotomy opening is extended with the help of angled Potts scissors, keeping the lower blade of the scissors against the anterior wall of the artery in order to avoid damage to the intima of the posterior wall of the artery (Fig. 1.7).

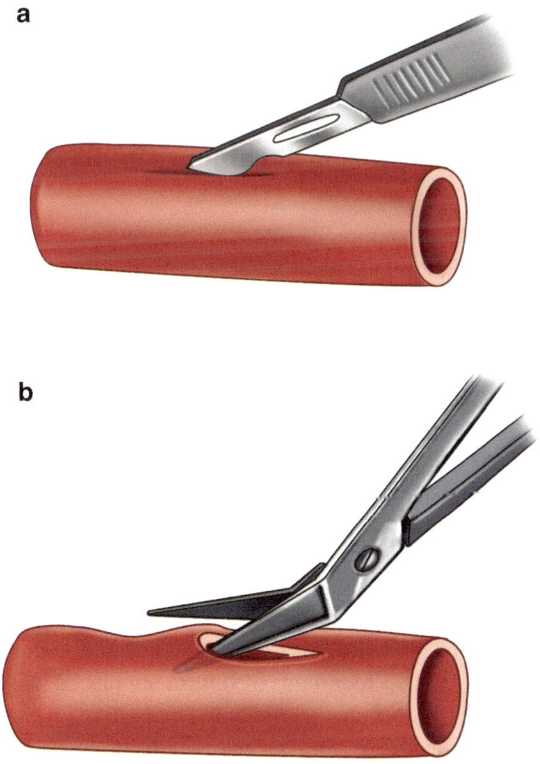

Fig. 1.6 (**a**) Arteriotomy with a 15-blade or an 11-blade scalpel. (**b**) Potts scissors through the arteriotomy and butting the anterior wall extending the arteriotomy

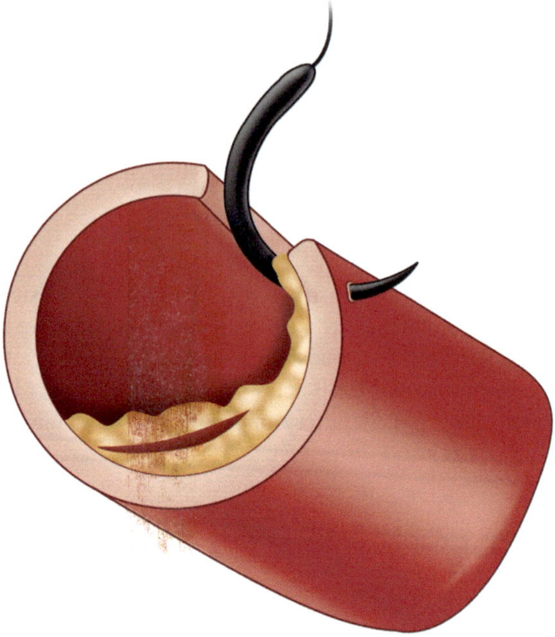

Fig. 1.7 Suturing done from intima with a needle coming out of the adventitia

Arterial Suturing Techniques and Suture Materials

Most often, continuous suturing (over and over) technique is preferred, making certain that intima is taken in the suture line. Interrupted suture is preferred in small-sized arteries like brachial artery closure. In children where subsequent growth is anticipated, interrupted sutures should be performed. Sutures are usually placed 1 mm apart and 1 mm from the edge of the arteriotomy, and the suture loop should lay 1 mm from the previous suture loop and from one end of the arteriotomy and continued till 60–70% of its length has been completed and a second suture has started from the opposite end and the knots are tied about two-thirds/one-third distance from each end. A monofilament vascular suture is preferred, and most vascular surgeons use polypropylene swedged into a half of a circle or three-eight of a circle, round-bodied needles. In suturing graft to the host artery, the suturing is started from the outer wall of the graft to its inner wall, and the needle is subsequently passed into the intima and then to the adventitial layer of the artery. Suturing in deep body cavities or where accuracy is necessary, a parachute technique is preferred. Three or four loops of sutures are placed loosely with sutures parallel to each other as a parachute and tightened by pulling on each side. One must be certain that sutures are not crossing or caught in the previously placed suture as tightening of an

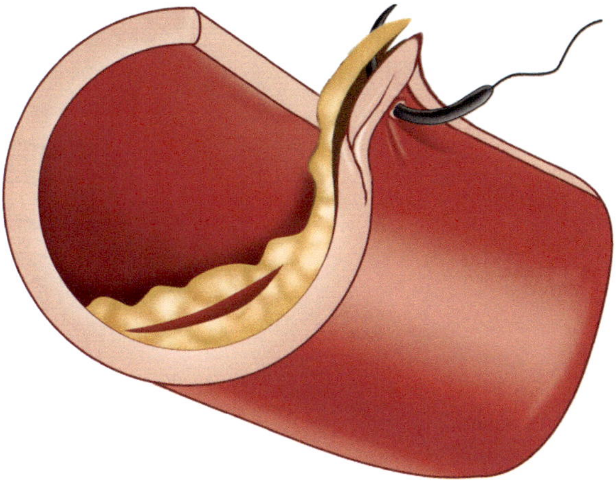

Fig. 1.8 Suturing from adventitia to intima may lift the plaque with the potential of dissection

improperly placed suture may result in laceration of the wall of the artery. The direction of the suturing should be from the intima (arterial lumen) outward so the plaque is not lifted during the application of the suture (Figs. 1.7 and 1.8). The needle and the suture should be brought and be pulled in the direction it was placed. In most cases, a 3-0 cardiovascular polypropylene suture is used for the aorta and a 4-0 cardiovascular polypropylene suture for iliac arteries, a 5-0 or 6-0 for femoral arteries, and a 7-0 for infrapopliteal arteries. Optical magnification (vessel loops) is useful so that arteriotomy and artery-to-graft anastomosis are sutured in a meticulous fashion. Before completion of an anastomosis, suture line is inspected. Any additional reinforcement sutures should be placed before releasing the clamp on large arteries like aorta/iliac arteries once the clamps are released; Gelfoam (Pfizer) soaked in thrombin should be applied using gentle pressure with a gauze. In patients receiving antiplatelet medications, Floseal (Baxter, Deerfield, IL) followed by Gelfoam soaked in thrombin with gentle pressure by dry gauze helps in achieving satisfactory hemostasis. In patients with friable aortic anastomosis, application of BioGlue (CryoLife, Kennesaw, GA) followed by Gelfoam soaked in thrombin and pressure and a laparotomy pad is helpful. These adjuncts are used mainly for patients with diffuse oozing. In situations where there is active pulsatile bleeding between the suture line, vascular clamp should be reapplied, and additional sutures in the form of horizontal mattress using pledgets help in achieving hemostasis. Control of bleeding without application of clamps may result in the increase in the size of needle hole with excessive bleeding due to strong arterial pulsation (Figs. 1.9, 1.10, and 1.11). The pledgets are used to control of bleeding from the suture line can be either synthetic or autogenous by removing a small portion of nearby fascia. Synthetic pledgets are preferred for reinforcement of an aortic suture line and fascial pledgets for arteries like subclavian and femoral arteries.

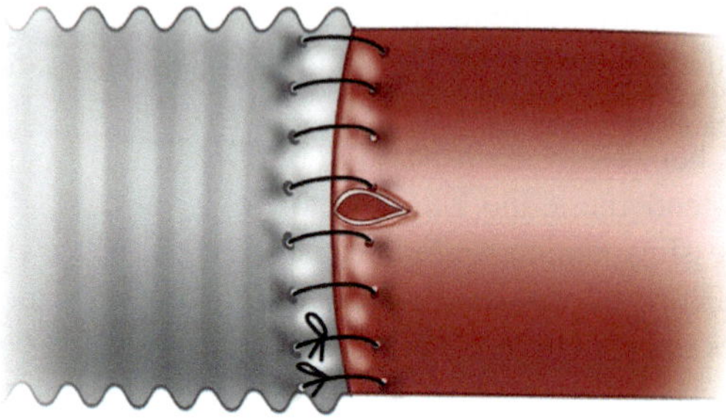

Fig. 1.9 Suture line with a hole in the aorta during anastomosis of the Dacron graft to the aorta

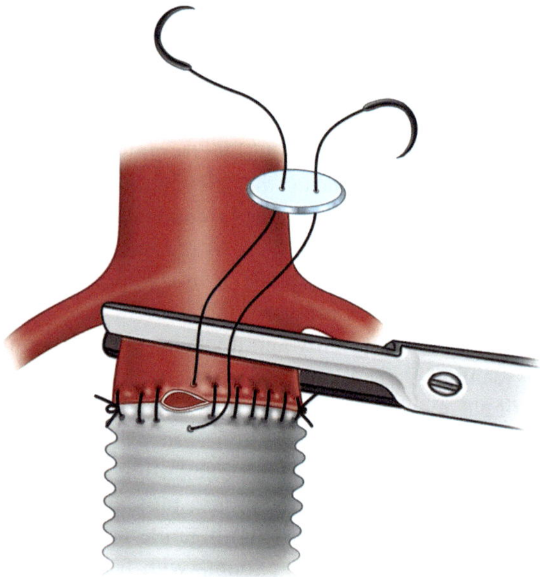

Fig. 1.10 Control of bleeding (the site of leak) as proximal and distal vascular clamps are applied. Horizontal mattress of a 4-0 cardiovascular polypropylene using a Dacron pledget for satisfactory hemostasis

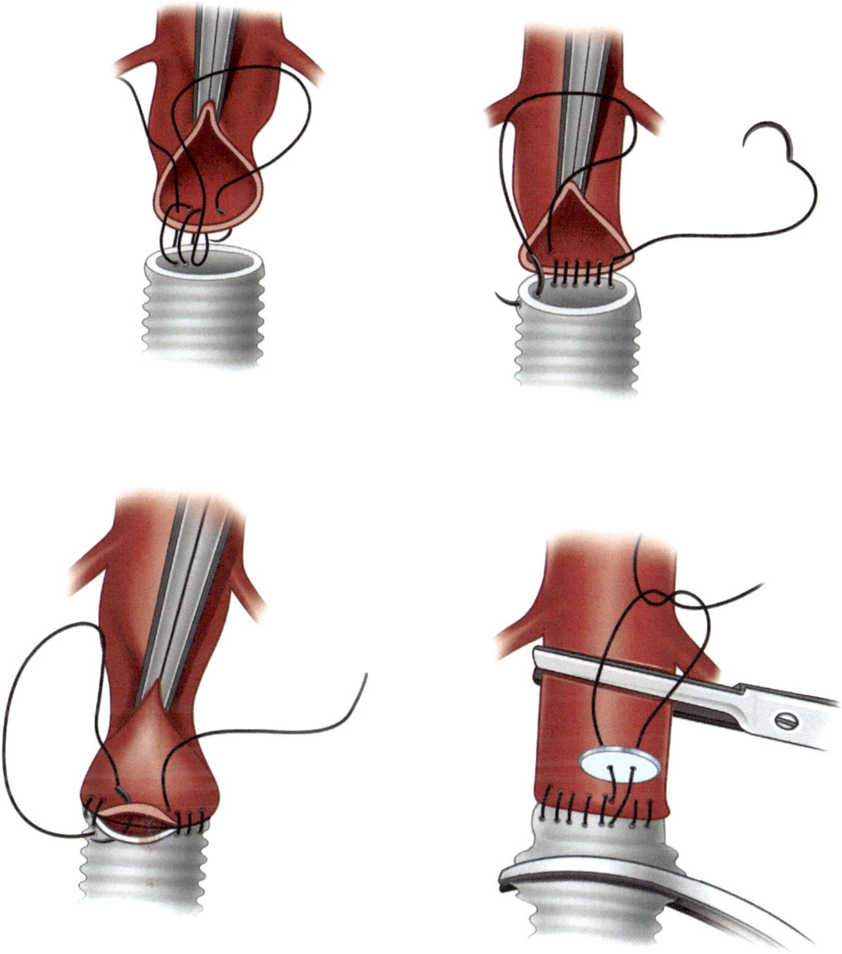

Fig. 1.11 Proximal end-to-end anastomosis between the infrarenal aorta to the Dacron graft. Aortotomy is spatulated anteriorly. Posterior suture line is started first in a continuous manner using both needles, continued on each side, and completed on either side

Types of Grafts to Artery Anastomosis

Two types of anastomosis, end to end and end to side, are most often performed in construction of artery-to-graft anastomosis. Side-to-side anastomosis are occasionally performed for construction of the arteriovenous fistula for hemodialysis access or as an adjunct to infragenicular prosthetic bypass at the site of distal anastomosis to help improve the patency of the synthetic graft.

End-to-End Anastomosis

A typical end-to-end anastomosis of a large vessel is exemplified in the arterial reconstruction following open repair of abdominal aortic aneurysm (AAA). The end of the divided aorta below the renal arteries is anastomosed to a prosthetic graft (Dacron or PTFE). After proximal control is obtained, the anterior wall of the aortic neck is divided, and the posterior wall can be left intact. The posterior wall of the aorta can be used as a double layer to buttress the suture line. In patients with satisfactory thickness of the aortic neck, the continuous suture starting intraluminal at 4 o'clock position is started. A double-armed 3-0 cardiovascular polypropylene suture is started in a continuous fashion with the suture line kept on loops (strings of a parachute) and the needle comes out in about 8 o'clock position. The suture line is then tightened on each side to bring the graft to the aortic neck. To avoid accidental loosening of the suture line, a new suture is tied to the first one on either side at 4 o'clock and at 8 o'clock and continued anteriorly. In patients with tenuous aortic neck or in patients with juxtarenal abdominal aortic aneurysm, a two-layer anastomosis is performed with two techniques. (1) In patients with juxtarenal abdominal aortic aneurysms, the initial suture line is started at 3 o'clock and at 9 o'clock as horizontal mattress suture and continued anteriorly in the same fashion. And a second layer of a continuous over and over suturing is done. (2) In patients with weak and tenuous aortic neck or in patients with juxtarenal AAA, a two-layer anastomosis is performed with two techniques. Technique one is telescoping technique in patients with juxtarenal AAA. Technique two consists of interrupted sutures and a second with continuous suture. In patients with thin-walled and friable aortic neck, the first layer comprises of interrupted horizontal mattress.

End-to-Side Anastomosis

A technique to end-to-side attachment to a prosthetic graft to the artery is shown in Figs. 1.9, 1.10, 1.11, and 1.12. The length of the arteriotomy is about two and a half times the diameter of the graft. After arteriotomy is made, the prosthetic graft is cut in a lazy "S"-shaped manor to produce a wide anastomosis with diminished chance of turbulence and intimal hyperplasia. The anastomosis is started at the heel using a double-armed suture at 11:30' and 12:30'clock position, and suture line continued on each side with suture line stopping around 8 o'clock and then the second suture is continued to complete the suture line (Figs. 1.12, 1.13, and 1.14). Before completing the anastomosis, appropriate flushing maneuvers are performed to prevent distal embolization. In patients with end-to-side saphenous vein anastomosis to the common femoral artery, the hood of the greater saphenous vein (in situ technique) is spatulated, and a parachute technique is used to ensure the accuracy of the placement of all the sutures. In patients undergoing subclavian transposition into the

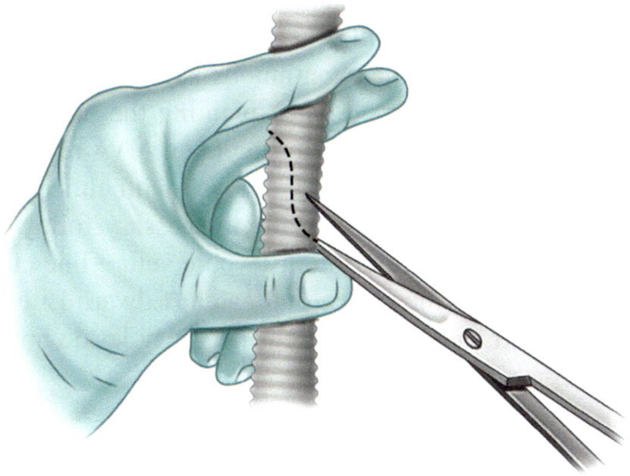

Fig. 1.12 Dacron graft cut with a heavy scissors in a lazy "S" shape for end-to-side femoral anastomosis of the aortofemoral graft

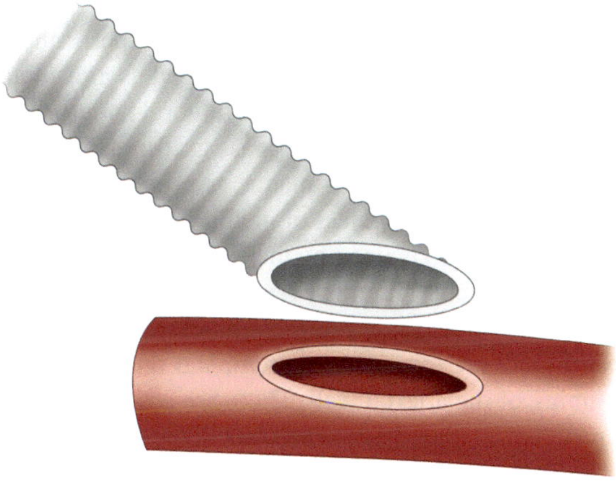

Fig. 1.13 Arteriotomy and cut Dacron graft

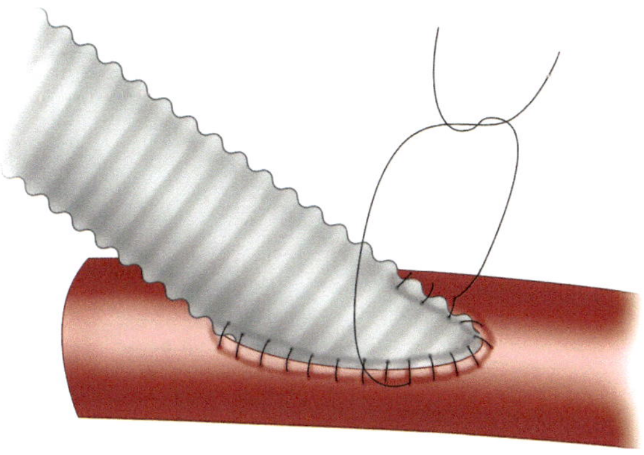

Fig. 1.14 End-to-end anastomosis

common carotid artery, an end-to-side anastomosis is performed with suturing starting on the posterior wall in a continuous fashion using a parachute technique and turning the corners of a continuous suturing on either side of the arteriotomy. A similar technique is used when planting the inferior mesenteric artery as a carrel patch to the prosthetic graft during open AAA repair. In these situations, an ellipse of the recipient artery/graft is removed with either curved Potts scissors or an arterial punch. Patch grafting is often necessary following carotid endarterectomy or performance of any arteriotomy where suture line closure may result in narrowing of the artery. Bovine pericardial patch (Edward Lifesciences) is frequently used as it is quite soft and pliable and the needle holes do not bleed excessively as observed with the use of PTFE patch.

Endarterectomy

Endarterectomy is a common procedure performed for open arterial reconstructions. Endarterectomy can be performed as an isolated procedure such as a carotid endarterectomy or as in common femoral endarterectomy. It can also be performed in conjunction with arterial bypass grafting. The strongest arterial layer is adventitia, and the atheromatous plaque is primarily located in the subintimal plane and involves variable thickness of media. The most satisfactory plane of dissection leaving the adventitia is lined by the external elastic membrane (Fig. 1.15). These circular fibers of media should be removed in patients undergoing carotid endarterectomy. In patients undergoing femoral endarterectomy, circular fibers of the media can be left if there are formerly adherent, and removal of these fibers may result in severe thinning of the arterial wall. There are essentially three methods for used for endarterectomy: (1) open, (2) semi closed, and (3) eversion.

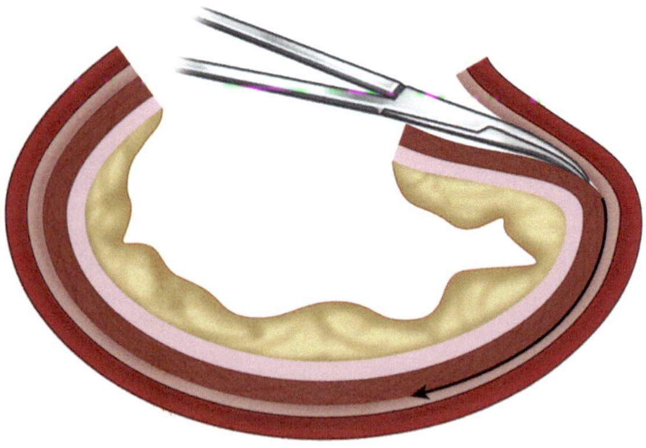

Fig. 1.15 Transverse section of the artery showing the plane of endarterectomy

Open Endarterectomy

The classical example of open endarterectomy is carotid endarterectomy. This procedure is more suitable for short-segmented lesions. The arteries open longitudinally after primary and distal clamping following administration of systemic heparin. A cleavage plane is developed between the thickest part of the plaque and the adventitia with the help of arterial dissector (dural elevator) and continued distally till the plaque ends in a feathery end (Figs. 1.16, 1.17, and 1.18). Tacking sutures at the distal end of the endarterectomy are not necessary unless the intima does not appear to be well adherent to the arterial wall. In those circumstances, two tacking sutures of a 7-0 cardiovascular polypropylene suture at 4 o'clock and at 8 o'clock positions are applied (Fig. 1.19). Proximally, the plaque is usually sharply divided by Potts scissors. In patients with thick atheromatous plaque proximally, the vascular clamp is tightened to intentionally fracture the plaque, and this enables the calcified core to be removed from the proximal end from the jaws of the clamp (Figs. 1.17 and 1.18), thus resulting in approximation of the intima to the wall of the artery. All the debris are irrigated with heparinized saline and removed with a fine pointed pickup. Arteriotomy is generally closed with a bovine patch graft (Fig. 1.20).

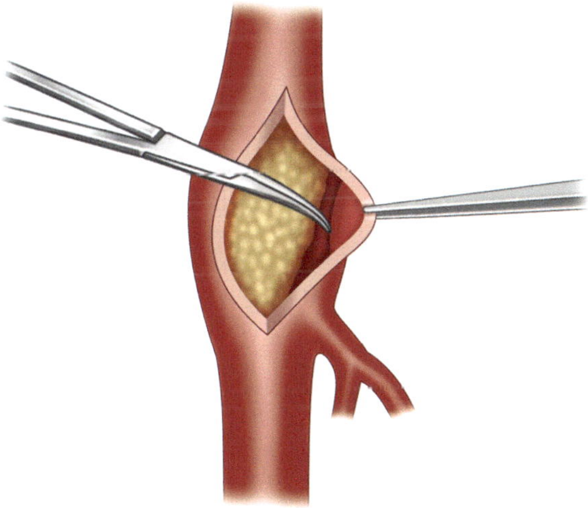

Fig. 1.16 Plaque being separated with a dural elevator (dissector) (Hemostat is shown separating the plaque. It should be Freer also called Penfield dural elevator)

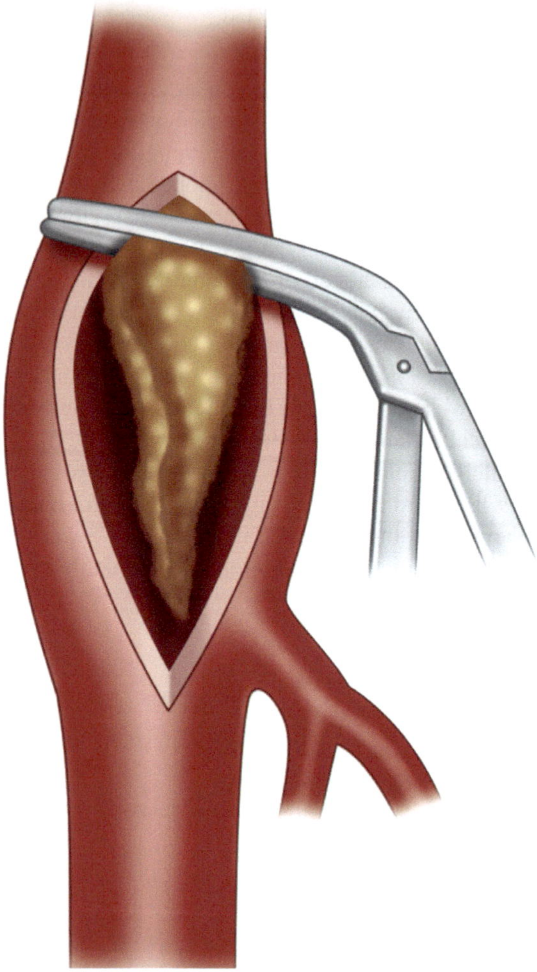

Fig. 1.17 Proximal end of the plaque is divided sharply using a hemostat or a Kelly clamp

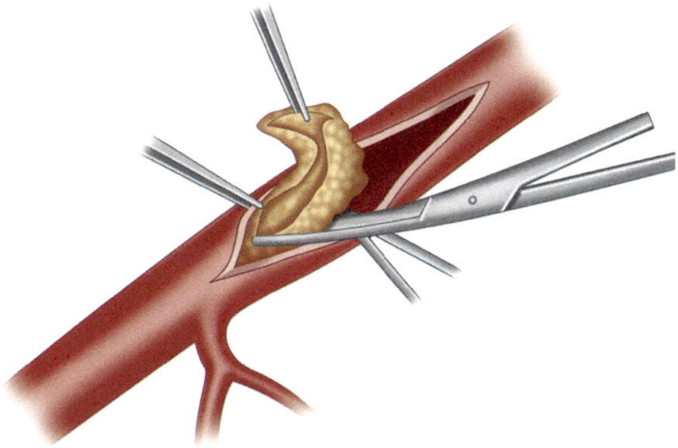

Fig. 1.18 Distally, plaque is divided or separated until it ends as a feathery end

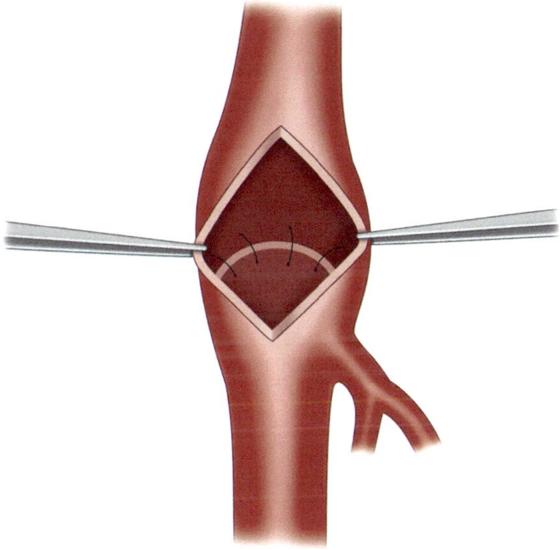

Fig. 1.19 Tacking sutures applied distally from the intima to the adventitia to prevent intimal flap formation

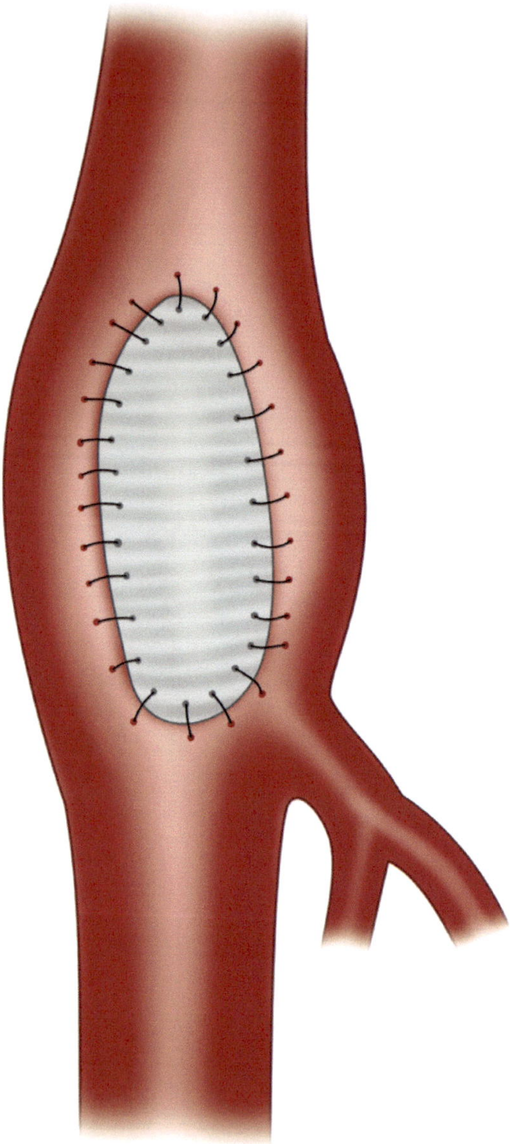

Fig. 1.20 Patch closure following endarterectomy

Semi-Closed Endarterectomy

Semi-closed endarterectomy can be performed where the plaque is considerably longer than carotid or common femoral endarterectomy procedures. In this case, the incision is shorter, and an instrument like a ring stripper or arterial dilators is passed and the core of the plaque is separated from the outer wall with the help of Vollmar ring stripper, which is passed in a spiral fashion while maintaining tension on the artery. The dissected core is divided at the site of proximal arteriotomy and retrieved from the distal end. The proximal and the distal intima are trimmed and secured. This procedure is not commonly performed as there is a risk of perforation, embolization, and arterial thrombosis due to distal intimal flap. With the use of Garrett arterial dilators (increasing size), from 3 to 6 mm passed from proximal arteriotomy to distal arteriotomy and then in a reverse fashion, the plaque is completely removed with two small incisions and the intervening arterial wall is kept intact (Fig. 1.21). Primary closure or patch grafting at the arteriotomy site is performed depending upon the anticipated size of the vessel following closure. This technique is described in detail in the chapter on iliac and femoral endarterectomy.

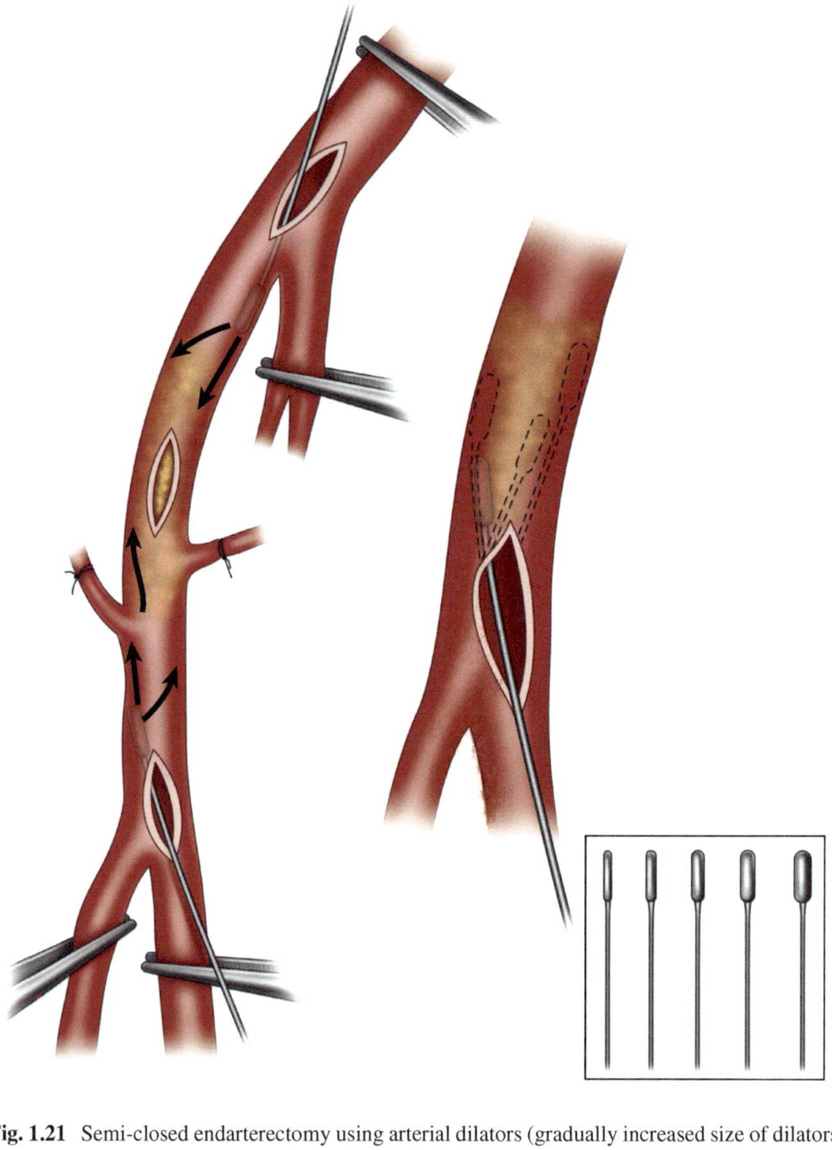

Fig. 1.21 Semi-closed endarterectomy using arterial dilators (gradually increased size of dilators) separating the plaque from the outer wall of the artery

Eversion Endarterectomy

Eversion endarterectomy is performed in patients undergoing carotid endarterectomy with a redundant internal carotid artery. After exposure and mobilization of the distal common carotid artery and the proximal carotid artery, the internal carotid artery at its origin is divided obliquely and is then everted with the removal of the plaque, till the plaque ends in a feathery fashion so that a satisfactory distal end point is achieved. Divided internal carotid artery is pulled downward and anastomosed to the carotid bulb, first as a posterior layer closure, followed by closure of the anterior wall. This helps in removing the redundancy of the internal carotid artery and the procedure avoids patch grafting, which is performed in most patients following carotid endarterectomy. This is described in detail on the chapter on carotid endarterectomy.

Vascular Grafts

As large conduits for large vessels and arteries, a Dacron graft or expanded PTFE graft is generally used. For infrainguinal arterial reconstruction, autogenous saphenous vein graft is preferred. Synthetic grafts are available in different diameters and are marketed as straight grafts or bifurcation grafts. In general, autogenous saphenous vein should be 3 mm or larger in diameter to serve as a suitable conduit for an infrainguinal bypass. If the greater saphenous vein (varicose, thrombophlebitic, or small-diameter vein) is not a satisfactory conduit for arterial bypass, then a PTFE graft can be used as an alternate conduit. Saphenous vein for lower extremity revascularization can be used in an in-situ fashion or in a reverse vein fashion.

Special Suturing Technique in Narrow Deep Spaces

When suturing is necessary for prosthetic graft to the aorta in a deep recess or body cavity such as abdominal aortic anastomosis, a needle should be placed in the top of the holder near the tip in a perpendicular fashion and needle advanced. With the needle holder set in the anterior to posterior position and the needle in the same axis as the needle holder, the handle of the needle holder is depressed posteriorly so that the 3-0 or 4-0 cardiovascular polypropylene suture or the needle comes out of the posterior wall of the aorta and can be retrieved by DeBakey forceps. This technique is very helpful in situations where reinforcement sutures are necessary after completion of proximal anastomosis in the posterior wall of the proximal aortic anastomosis (Fig. 1.22).

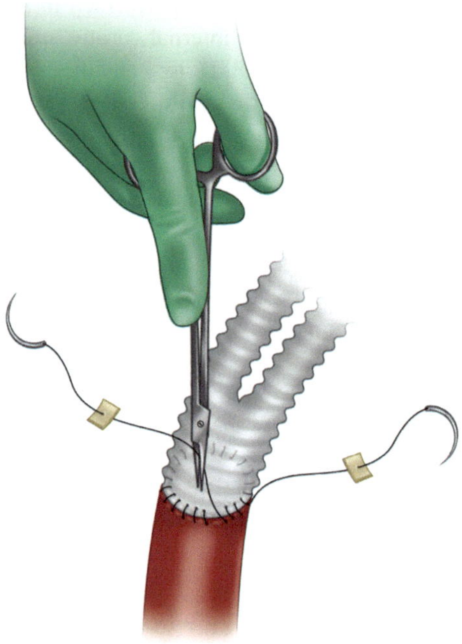

Fig. 1.22 Control of bleeding at the posterior wall of proximal aortic suture line. In normal circumstances, the needle is held vertically perpendicular to the needle holder (transverse to the axis of the needle holder). In case of bleeding at the posterior wall of proximal aortic suture line at 5 o'clock in a deep narrow space, the needle is grasped in the axis of the needle holder with the tip of the needle directed posteriorly toward the lumbar spine. The handle of the needle holder is held at 11 o'clock position and the needle is then thrust from the edge of a Dacron graft (posterior wall) to the posterior wall of the aorta. A horizontal mattress suture of 3-0 or 4-0 cardiovascular polypropylene on a pledget is tied encompassing the "hole" in the aorta. In such situations, the standard technique of passage of the needle in the needle holder may be technically demanding

Part I
Open Repair of Aneurysmal Disease

Chapter 2
Open Repair of Descending Thoracic Aortic Aneurysm

Pieter A. J. van Bakel, Yunus Ahmed, and Himanshu J. Patel

Introduction

Thoracic aortic aneurysms (TAAs) are frequently a silent and indolent disease, with a natural history of slow expansion. Over 95% of descending TAAs remain asymptomatic, and diagnosis often occurs incidentally when imaging is obtained for other reasons [1]. The less frequent presentation is seen when patients develop acute aortic syndromes, such as aortic dissection or aortic rupture. In this latter scenario, the prognosis is usually poor. The International Registry of Acute Aortic Dissection (IRAD) found an overall in-hospital mortality rate for patients presenting with acute type A dissection patients of 32.5%, including 26.6% for patients undergoing surgery and 55.9% for patients receiving medical therapy alone. Patients with acute type B dissection had an in-hospital mortality rate of 13% [2]. In contrast, presentation with thoracic aortic rupture is associated with a mortality rate of 54% in the first 6 h after onset of symptoms [3]. Treatment of these complications can consist of either open aortic repair, thoracic endovascular aortic repair (TEVAR), or a hybrid approach using both open and endovascular techniques.

Indications for Repair

While descending TAA repair can be done by either open repair or TEVAR, recent observational studies have suggested a short-term benefit for the endovascular approach [4]. Current guidelines suggest for patients with degenerative descending

P. A. J. van Bakel · Y. Ahmed · H. J. Patel (✉)
Department of Cardiac Surgery, University of Michigan Medical School, Ann Arbor, MI, USA
e-mail: hjpatel@med.umich.edu

S. S. Hans et al. (eds.), *Primary and Repeat Arterial Reconstructions*,
https://doi.org/10.1007/978-3-031-13897-3_2

TAA that does not involve the visceral segment and anatomy that is suitable for endovascular repair; TEVAR is the intervention of choice. Indications for intervention in the elective setting include size criteria (descending TAA greater than 5.5 cm or a TAA greater than 5.0 cm with a positive family history for TAA or known connective tissue syndrome) and growth criteria (descending TAA with rapid aortic expansion of >0.5 cm/year) or pathologic type (saccular aneurysm or pseudoaneurysm). In the urgent clinical setting, aortic repair is indicated in complicated type B aortic dissection, symptomatic or ruptured descending TAA, or blunt thoracic aortic injury. Recognizing that endovascular repair is the preferred therapy in many clinical settings, contraindications for this approach often include the presence of connective tissue disease, unsuitable vascular access, and lack of an appropriate proximal or distal landing zone. In this setting, open repair becomes the gold standard therapy.

Surgical Anatomy

An understanding of thoracic aortic anatomy is crucial in surgical decision-making and reduction in frequency of postoperative complications (Fig. 2.1). The thoracic aorta originates from the left ventricular outflow tract as the root and ascending segments. The ascending aorta has a typical normal diameter of approximately 3 cm and becomes more oval in shape as it turns into the arch segment. In most patients, there is a leftward arch anterior and lateral to the trachea, and thus, the approach to

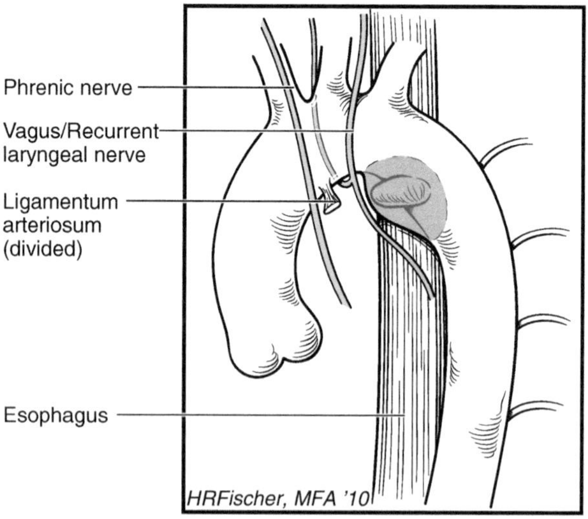

Fig. 2.1 This figure depicts the important surgical anatomy and structures adjacent to the aorta, in the region of the arch. The lesion described in this case is a traumatic injury

the descending aorta is via a left thoracotomy. While the typical branches to the head and upper extremities are the brachiocephalic trunk, left common carotid artery, and left subclavian artery, the prevalence of bovine trunk anatomy and aberrant subclavian artery origins are higher in patients with thoracic aortic disease. Important structures in proximity to the arch and proximal descending aorta include the left phrenic nerve and left vagus nerve laterally and the left mainstem bronchus and esophagus medially. The segment of the arch between the left subclavian artery and the ligamentum arteriosum is known as the aortic isthmus, and this region contains the left recurrent laryngeal nerve. The descending aorta begins at the level of the fourth thoracic vertebra, and the adjacent thoracic duct passes superiorly and posteromedially. It starts on the left side and gradually shifts to the midline. Once it crosses the diaphragm through the posterior aortic hiatus, it becomes the abdominal aorta.

Preoperative Assessment

A complete history and physical with necessary laboratory tests are obtained. In patients actively smoking, we require 2 months completely off tobacco prior to elective repair to reduce the incidence of complications. Our typical workup includes a transesophageal echocardiogram to evaluate cardiac function, but most importantly to ensure no more than mild aortic insufficiency exists. We also obtain a cardiac catheterization and treat any significant stenosis prior to elective repair. Additional testing includes pulmonary function tests to determine ability to function on single lung ventilation and tolerate the operation, carotid duplex scans, and ankle brachial indices. Cross-sectional imaging of the entire aorta and its bifurcation to the femoral heads is necessary, and we prefer computed tomography.

Steps of Operation for Resection of the Entire Descending Thoracic Aorta

The standard operative approach for open surgical repair of descending TAA is as follows [5]. The patient is placed in a right lateral decubitus position with the left chest up on the operating table and is widely prepped and draped. A double-lumen endotracheal tube is placed to permit single-lung ventilation. A transesophageal echocardiography probe is placed both to guide hemodynamic management but also to provide easy identification of the esophagus during dissection of the aorta. A spinal canal drain is used for any resection that involves more than the distal arch and proximal descending aorta to reduce the risk for spinal cord ischemia (SCI).

A standard left posterolateral thoracotomy is made. To reach the arch aorta, usually, entry is required in the third or fourth intercostal space. To access the distal thoracic aorta, the left chest is entered at the seventh or eighth intercostal spaces. When the entire descending aorta requires resection, both intercostal spaces are entered. Proximal control is obtained by dividing the ligamentum arteriosum, avoiding the left recurrent laryngeal nerve and identifying the left subclavian artery. Next, distal control is obtained at the aortic hiatus, where the aorta is mobilized just above the celiac artery. In this region, one must take caution to identify the right pleura, which often is attached to the medical aspect of the aorta. Finally, the last step in dissection is to identify specific intercostal vessels guided by preoperative imaging that will be reimplanted to reduce risk for spinal cord ischemia.

Cardiopulmonary bypass with femoral cannulation and full heparinization with 3 mg/kg is used in all cases. In the event that extensive aortic resection or arch resection is required, we use adjunctive deep hypothermic circulatory arrest (HCA) to reduce neurologic complication frequency. A blood conservation strategy of intraoperative autologous blood donation is also used in all patients who have hemoglobin levels above 10 mg/dL. Typically, with normal blood counts, 2–3 units of autologous blood are removed prior to heparin administration and then transfused after heparin reversal. The femoral venous cannula is inserted with TEE guidance and Seldinger technique. Arterial return is achieved by cannulation of an 8-mm Dacron graft secured to the femoral artery. This maintains left leg perfusion during cardiopulmonary bypass. A left ventricular vent was placed via the left superior pulmonary vein. The patient is placed on cardiopulmonary bypass and cooled to a minimum temperature of 18 °C when using adjunctive HCA. The head is packed in ice. Prior to initiation of HCA, neuro-protective agents consisting of mannitol, methylprednisolone, and pentobarbital are administered.

When the patient reaches a bladder temperature of 18 °C, they are placed in a steep Trendelenburg position. Systemic potassium is given to arrest the heart and a cross-clamp was applied at the T4 level with the flow reduced to a half from the femoral artery to maintain perfusion to the lower body during upper body HCA.

The descending thoracic aorta is incised proximally and the aorta mobilized circumferentially to separate it from adjacent structures, particularly the esophagus (Fig. 2.2). A proximal anastomosis is created with a running 4-0 or 5-0 polypropylene suture to a Dacron graft with a single prefabricated side branch. Following completion of the anastomosis, the prefabricated side branch is cannulated for cardiopulmonary bypass and flow is then reinstituted to the upper body. The aorta is de-aired out through the open distal end of the graft, and the proximal clamps are placed distal to the prefabricated side branch to restore flow to the upper body and heart. Rewarming is then initiated unless a period of lower body HCA is needed for securing the distal anastomosis.

Attention is then focused on the distal thoracic aorta (just proximal to the celiac artery), where the aorta is mobilized and circumferentially encircled (Fig. 2.3). The distal clamp is placed beyond the location of the intended anastomosis. Flow is maintained to the lower body via the left femoral artery cannulation. The Dacron graft is sized to an appropriate length, and the distal anastomosis to the distal

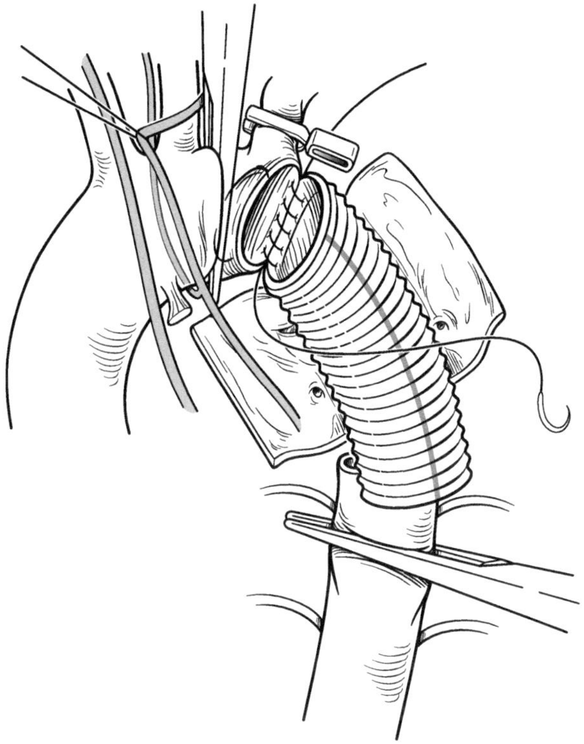

Fig. 2.2 In this case, where a clamp was used (not HCA), note the circumferential division of the proximal aorta for construction of the proximal anastomosis. Note also the placement of the distal aortic clamp, which ensures that distal perfusion is maintained via retrograde femoral artery flow

descending thoracic aorta is constructed, again using a running polypropylene 4-0 or 5-0 suture. The clamps are temporarily released with adequate de-airing maneuvers, and the remainder of the resected descending aorta is completely excised longitudinally. The target intercostal vessels for reimplantation are then sewn onto the posterior aspect of the aortic graft as an island patch or with a Creech reimplantation technique. The clamps are then released after adequate de-airing maneuvers, and the patient is then separated from cardiopulmonary bypass when normothermic. The native aortic sac is ensured to be hemostatic with over-sewing of remaining intercostal vessels. The femoral artery graft is removed and the artery primarily repaired during rewarming. Protamine sulfate and autologous blood are administered after decannulation. At this point, hemostasis is assured in the aneurysm bed and at the anastomoses. The native aorta is closed over the graft, to separate the graft from the visceral organs surrounding it. Two chest tubes (apical and basal positions) are placed and the left chest and left infrainguinal incisions are closed routinely.

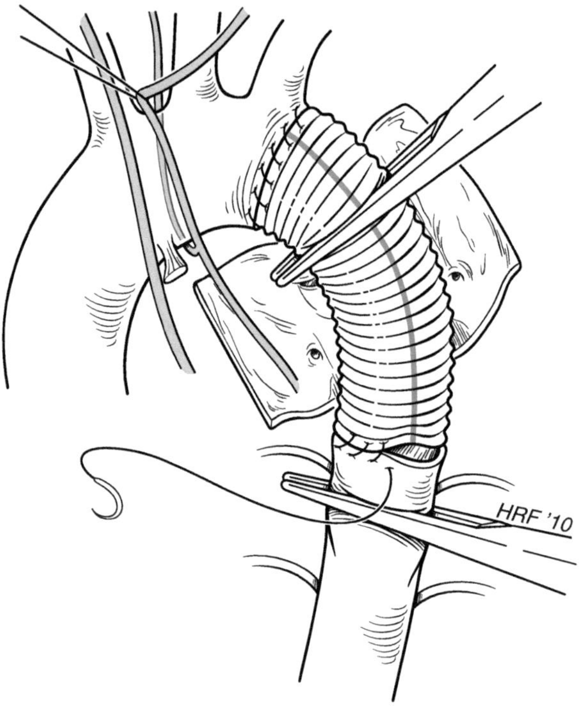

Fig. 2.3 Construction of the distal anastomosis with, again, circumferential aortic dissection to prevent injury to the esophagus

Complications

Advances in surgical techniques have improved the morbidity and mortality of aortic aneurysm surgery. To prevent major complications in the postoperative stage, adequate postoperative management is essential. Important adverse outcomes following aortic surgery include mortality, stroke, spinal cord ischemia, renal failure, chylothorax, and freedom from reoperation. The most common complication after open descending TAA repair is postoperative respiratory failure. Risk factors to develop respiratory failure include active cigarette smoking, COPD, and cardiac, renal, or bleeding complications. To reduce the risk, we stress early ambulation and incentive spirometry, in addition to ensuring tobacco cessation prior to surgery. In recent years, we have used intraoperative intercostal nerve cryoablation to reduce narcotic use and aid in reduction of postoperative pain [6].

Improvements in operative care, in particular, increased care of intercostal artery preservation and implementation of neuro-protective agents, have led to decreased risks for spinal cord ischemia (SCI). Cerebrospinal fluid drainage is recommended in patients at high risk for SCI, and the lumbar drain will be left in situ for 48 to 72 h postoperatively. During open TAA repair, different adjunctive techniques are used to increase the tolerance of the spinal cord to impaired perfusion, such as hypothermic circulatory arrest, distal perfusion, and permissive postoperative hypertension. Neurophysiologic monitoring can be performed to monitor and detect SCI to help guide the preservation of intercostal arteries and the hemodynamic optimization to prevent and treat SCI. Preserving a systemic hypothermia during open repair and the perfusion of the spinal cord have proven to be the most effective in preventing SCI [7–9].

Postoperative renal function impairment can be prevented by preoperative hydration and intraoperative mannitol administration. Postoperative renal complication has been associated with reduced long-term survival and increased postoperative mortality [10–12].

Summary

In conclusion, while thoracic endovascular aortic repair has emerged as the therapy of choice for most clinical scenarios involving the descending aorta, open repair continues to have its place in the treatment strategy for this aortic segment [13]. Successful outcomes for this procedure can be achieved with careful preoperative planning, deep understanding of the anatomy and techniques of cardiopulmonary bypass, meticulous surgical technique, and diligent postoperative care.

Acknowledgments We gratefully acknowledge the support provided by the Joe D. Morris Collegiate Professorship, the David Hamilton Fund, the Phil Jenkins Breakthrough Fund, and the Singh Family Fund in Aortic Research.

References

1. Elefteriades JA, Farkas EA. Thoracic aortic aneurysm. Clinically pertinent controversies and uncertainties. J Am Coll Cardiol. 2010;55(9):841–57. https://doi.org/10.1016/j.jacc.2009.08.084.
2. Tsai TT, Trimarchi S, Nienaber CA. Acute aortic dissection: perspectives from the international registry of acute aortic dissection (IRAD). Eur J Vasc Endovasc Surg. 2009;37(2):149–59. https://doi.org/10.1016/j.ejvs.2008.11.032.
3. Johansson G, Markström U, Swedenborg J. Ruptured thoracic aortic aneurysms: a study of incidence and mortality rates. J Vasc Surg. 1995;21(6):985–8. https://doi.org/10.1016/S0741-5214(95)70227-X.
4. Walsh SR, Tang TY, Sadat U, et al. Endovascular stenting versus open surgery for thoracic aortic disease: Systematic review and meta-analysis of perioperative results. J Vasc Surg. 2008;47(5):1094–1098.e3. https://doi.org/10.1016/j.jvs.2007.09.062.
5. Patel HJ, Shillingford MS, Mihalik S, Proctor MC, Deeb GM. Resection of the descending aorta: outcomes after use of hypothermic circulatory arrest. Ann Thorac Surg. 2006;82:90–6.
6. Clemence J Jr, Malik A, Farhat L, Wu X, Kim KM, Patel H, Yang B. Cryoablation of intercostal nerves decreased narcotic usage after thoracic or thoracoabdominal aortic aneurysm repair. Semin Thorac Cardiovasc Surg. 2020;32:404–12.

7. Coselli JS, LeMaire SA, Miller CC, et al. Mortality and paraplegia after thoracoabdominal aortic aneurysm repair: a risk factor analysis. Ann Thorac Surg. 2000;69(2):409–14. https://doi.org/10.1016/S0003-4975(99)01478-2.
8. Coselli JS, LeMaire SA, Köksoy C, Schmittling ZC, Curling PE. Cerebrospinal fluid drainage reduces paraplegia after thoracoabdominal aortic aneurysm repair: results of a randomized clinical trial. J Vasc Surg. 2002;35(4):631–9. https://doi.org/10.1067/mva.2002.122024.
9. Estrera AL, Miller CC, Chen EP, et al. Descending thoracic aortic aneurysm repair: 12-year experience using distal aortic perfusion and cerebrospinal fluid drainage. Ann Thorac Surg. 2005;80(4):1290–6. https://doi.org/10.1016/j.athoracsur.2005.02.021.
10. Conrad MF, Crawford RS, Davison JK, Cambria RP. Thoracoabdominal aneurysm repair: a 20-year perspective. Ann Thorac Surg. 2007;83(2):S856–61. https://doi.org/10.1016/j.athoracsur.2006.10.096.
11. Di Luozzo G, Geisbüsch S, Lin HM, et al. Open repair of descending and thoracoabdominal aortic aneurysms and dissections in patients aged younger than 60 years: superior to endovascular repair? Ann Thorac Surg. 2013;95(1):12–9. https://doi.org/10.1016/j.athoracsur.2012.05.071.
12. Aftab M, Coselli JS. Renal and visceral protection in thoracoabdominal aortic surgery. J Thorac Cardiovasc Surg. 2014;148(6):2963–6. https://doi.org/10.1016/j.jtcvs.2014.06.072.
13. Patel HJ, Williams DM, Upchurch GR Jr, Dasika NL, Deeb GM. A comparative analysis of open and endovascular repair for the ruptured descending thoracic aorta. J Vasc Surg. 2009;50:1265–70.

Chapter 3
Open Repair of Juxtarenal and Infrarenal Abdominal Aortic Aneurysm

Sachinder Singh Hans

Surgical Anatomy

The abdominal aorta begins as the aorta passes through the median arcuate ligament of the diaphragm at the level of T-12 vertebral body. It descends anterior to the lumbar vertebrae and branches into the left and right common iliac arteries at the level of L4/L5 disc slightly to the left of midline. The main branches of the abdominal aorta are inferior phrenic, celiac trunk, superior mesenteric artery, and inferior mesenteric artery, with most of these branches arising anteriorly. Lateral branches include adrenal, renal, and gonadal arteries. Posterior branches include lumbar (which are paired) and median sacral artery just above the bifurcation of the aorta into common iliac arteries (Fig. 3.1).

S. S. Hans (✉)
Vascular and Endovascular Services, Henry Ford Macomb Hospital,
Clinton Twp, MI, USA

S. S. Hans et al. (eds.), *Primary and Repeat Arterial Reconstructions*,
https://doi.org/10.1007/978-3-031-13897-3_3

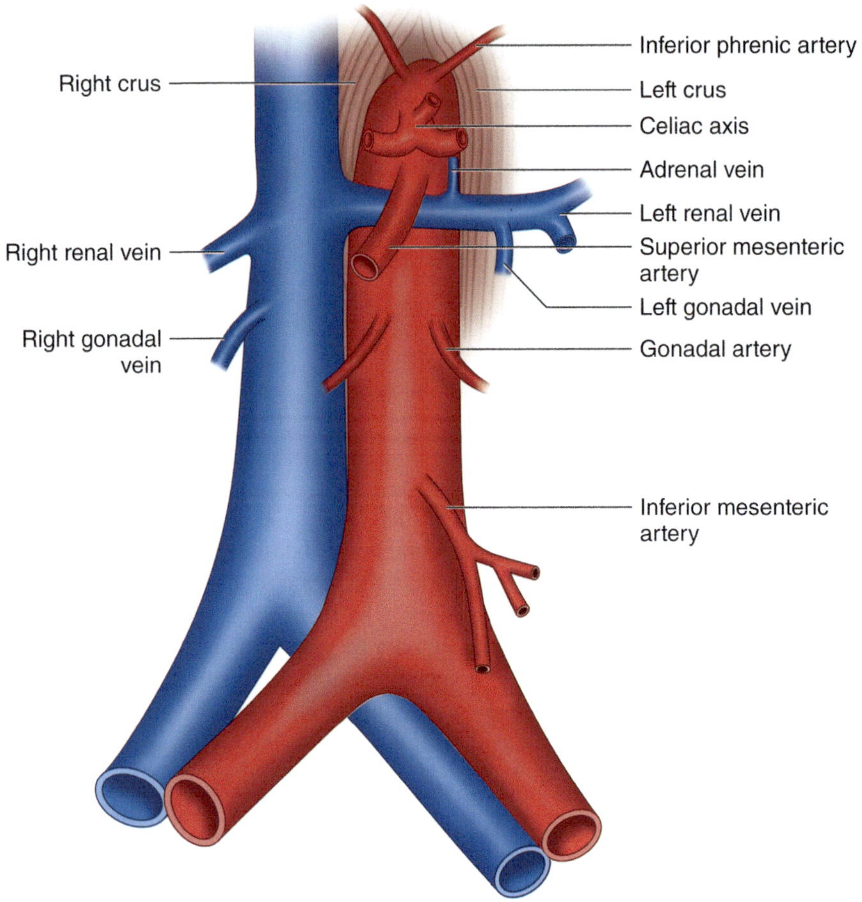

Fig. 3.1 Surgical anatomy of the abdominal aorta. (*1A*) Inferior phrenic artery. (*2A*) Celiac axis. (*3A*) Superior mesenteric artery. (*4A*). Gonadal artery. (*5A*). Inferior mesenteric artery. (*1V*) Adrenal vein. (*2V*). Left renal vein. (*3V*). Left gonadal vein. (*4V*) Right renal vein. (*5V*) Right gonadal vein. (*1C*) Right crus. (*2C*) Left crus

Anatomical Relations

On the right side, the abdominal aorta is related superiorly to the cisterna chyli and thoracic duct, the azygos vein, and the right crus of the diaphragm. The right crus separates it from the inferior vena cava. On the left, the aorta is related superiorly to the left crus, and at the level of L2 vertebral body, the structures on the left of the aorta are the fourth portion of the duodenum and inferior mesenteric vein.

Indications for Repair

The number of patients undergoing open repair of infrarenal abdominal aortic aneurysm (AAA) and juxtarenal AAA is diminishing due to the adaptation of endovascular repair and with further availability of fenestrated grafts and branched grafts. However, there remain a small number of patients with complex anatomy, who are not suitable for endovascular repair, and for them, open repair may be the only option. Generally, in men, abdominal aortic repair is recommended for 5.5 cm (AP/Tr) aneurysm and in women with 5 cm AP/transverse diameter. For common iliac artery (CIA) aneurysm, the 3.5 cm is generally the agreed diameter for open repair and for hypogastric aneurysm 3.0 cm. Prior to consideration for open repair, other factors such as expected life expectancy, diameter of the aorta at the level of the renal arteries, as compared to the size of the aneurysm, and growth of the aneurysm during the past year and morphology of the aneurysm (saccular vs. fusiform) needed to be taken into account prior to recommending open repair.

Operative Steps

Transperitoneal Approach

A midline incision is commonly used from the xiphoid process to just above the symphysis pubis. A supraumbilical transverse incision should be considered if concomitant distal renal artery reconstruction is planned. Infraumbilical transverse incision is useful in patients with large associated common iliac and hypogastric aneurysm (Fig. 3.2). A left flank retroperitoneal approach is useful for juxtarenal or pararenal AAA with main limitation of poor visualization of the distal right CIA. This approach is advantageous in patients undergoing redo aortic surgery and AAA repair in the presence of a horseshoe kidney and inflammatory AAA in patients with prior multiple abdominal operations, in patients with associated COPD and in patients who are morbidly obese.

Preoperative medical assessment and cardiac risk should be evaluated. Patient should undergo thin-section CTA of the abdomen and pelvis to identify venous anomaly such as retro left renal vein, assessment of clamp sites, and type of reconstruction. In addition, concomitant intra-abdominal pathology such as carcinoma of the kidney if present can be diagnosed and decisions made for planning treatment of associated pathology. Large bore IV line (central line), Foley catheter, and nasogastric tube (intraoperatively) are inserted and cell saver and body warmers are necessary. In patients with juxtarenal AAA, the superior end of the incision extends to the xiphoid process, and in patients with associated iliac artery aneurysm, the incision should be extended to the symphysis pubis.

Mechanical retractors such as Integra Omnitract (Integra LifeSciences Co, Plainsboro, NJ USA), Thompson retractors (Thompson Surgical Instruments,

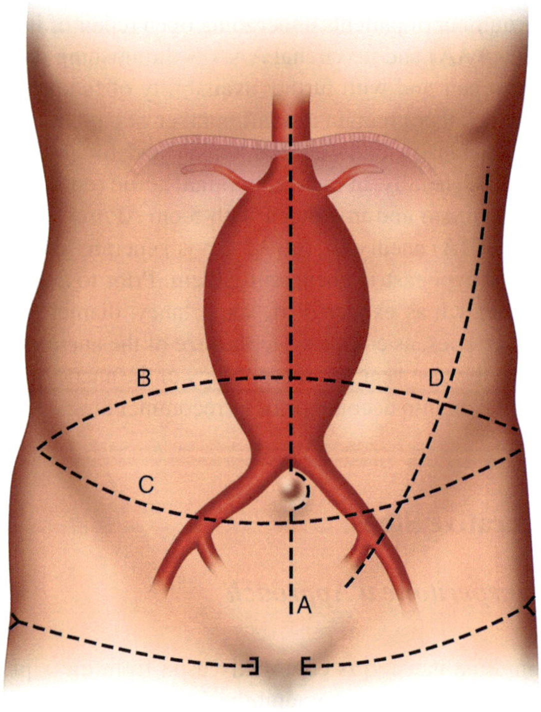

Fig. 3.2 Outline of the various incision for the repair of AAA. (**a**) Vertical midline. (**b**) Supraumbilical transverse incision. (**c**) Infraumbilical transverse incision. (**d**) Left retroperitoneal flank incision

retroaortic

Traverse City, MI), and Bookwalter 3 Systems (Symmetry Surgical, Antioch, TN, USA) are helpful in achieving satisfactory exposure. The aneurysm exposed via inframesocolic approach, the fourth portion of duodenum, and the ligaments of Treitz are mobilized and divided. Inferior mesenteric vein if crossing toward the right can be ligated and divided. The transverse colon stomach and greater omentum are packed with wet towels and retracted superiorly with the blades of the retractor. Small bowel is retracted to the right and the descending colon is retracted to the left, and sigmoid colon retracted downward.

The retroperitoneal tissue in the midline overlying the aneurysm is divided, and in patients with thick retroperitoneum, it is preferable to tie the tissues with 2-0 silk free ties on each side before the division. In patients with relatively thin retroperitoneum and loose tissue with lymphatics, the division can be performed with electrocautery. Then inferiorly, the dissection in the posterior peritoneum is continued between small bowel mesentery and sigmoid mesocolon. The left renal vein is

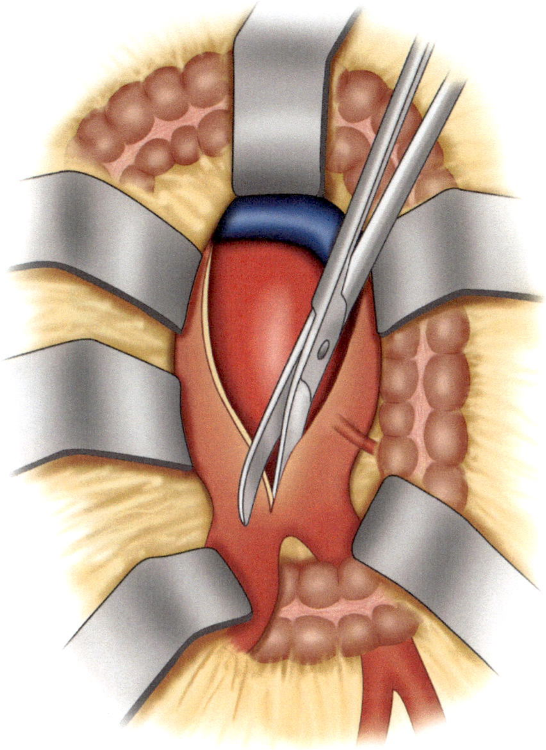

Fig. 3.3 Exposure of AAA via midline transperitoneal incision. Left renal vein seen superiorly. Retroperitoneal tissue of the aortic bifurcations is being dissected. Bookwalter with retractor blades applied over the wet towels. Retraction of the abdominal viscera away from the AAA

cleared of lymphatic and loose areolar tissue anteriorly, inferiorly, and superiorly, exposing the gonadal and the left adrenal vein (Fig. 3.3).

Lymphatic tissue should be ligated with silk ties to prevent postoperative chylous ascites. In the contemporary practice, AAA repair is done primarily for juxtarenal aneurysms; therefore, a silastic loop should be passed around the left renal vein between the inferior vena cava and the adrenal vein. Aorta is carefully dissected and mobilized. One usually encounters gonadal arteries on each side just below the renal arteries, and they should be suture ligated with 5-0 cardiovascular polypropylene proximally and silver clips applied distally before division. At this point, one should also pay attention to any posterior collar renal vein. Circumferential dissection of the pararenal aorta in order to pass a silastic loop or a tape is unnecessary.

In patients with juxtarenal AAA, ligation of either the adrenal vein or the gonadal vein should be performed so that the left renal vein can be retracted cephalad. But it is far more convenient to divide the left renal vein close to the inferior vena cava and preserve the venous outflow via the adrenal vein and gonadal vein (Fig. 3.4). The decision to either preserve or ligate the left renal vein should be made early as ligation of the gonadal vein and adrenal vein will mandate preservation of the left renal

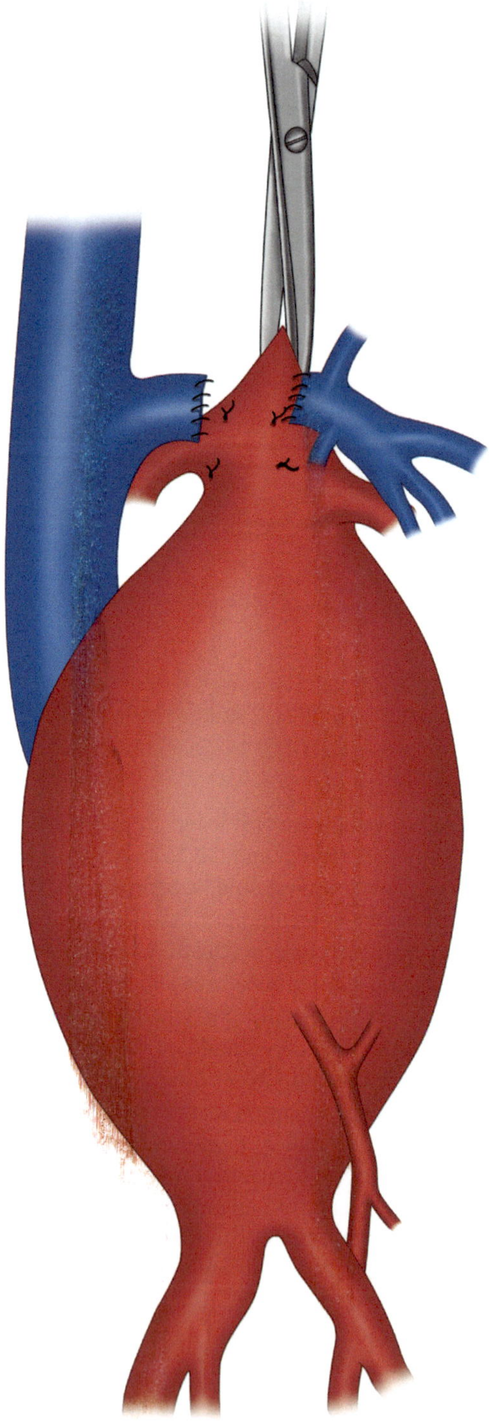

Fig. 3.4 Division and ligation of the left renal vein medial to the gonadal and adrenal vein with suprarenal aortic control

vein. After mobilization of the left renal vein and downward traction and division of the periaortic fatty tissue, the fibers of the crus of the diaphragm as a tight fibromuscular band are divided. At this time, adrenal arteries can be suture ligated proximally near the aortic wall with a 5-0 CV polypropylene suture and a silver clip is applied distally prior to their division. Digital dissection cephalad from this point will elevate the pancreas, thus enabling the clamp to be placed above the superior mesenteric artery if necessary. For ligation of the left renal vein, a 4-0 cardiovascular polypropylene stick tie should be used, and its division should proceed close to the inferior vena cava. Following this, the dissection proceeds caudally and the origin of the inferior mesenteric is exposed and dissected. There are usually small veins adherent to the origin and proximal centimeter or so of the inferior mesenteric artery, which may require suture ligation with a 5-0 cardiovascular polypropylene suture. The parasympathetic nerve plexus passing on the anterolateral aspect on the left side of the AAA and over the origin of the left CIA should be preserved whenever it is feasible.

If exposure of the distal CIA is necessary, the sigmoid colon is mobilized following incision along the white line of Toldt. Extensive dissection of the distal aorta and the proximal CIA should be avoided in patients in whom aorto-bi-iliac reconstruction is to be performed. Due to dense inflammatory adherence of the CIA to the caval confluence, there is danger of excessive venous bleeding should a small tear of a communicating vein may extend to the iliac veins or inferior vena cava.

In most instances, distal anastomosis to the femoral artery should be avoided unless there is associated severe iliac arterial occlusive disease. Femoral artery anastomosis increases early wound complication and late development of anastomotic aneurysms.

Prior to aortic clamping, 100 units/kg of heparin is administered by anesthesia team to keep the activating clotting time between 250 and 300 s. Distally CIA is clamped first before the aorta is clamped to prevent distal embolization. To prevent distal embolization, heparin should circulate for 5–10 min following administration before iliac and aortic clamps are applied.

In patients with juxtarenal AAA, adrenal arteries located just above the renal arteries are suture ligated with 5-0 cardiovascular polypropylene and divided. Both the right and left crus of the diaphragm are divided on each side of the suprarenal aorta for placement of suprarenal aortic clamp (Fig. 3.5). In some patients, one renal artery may be inferior to the other renal artery, and if the aorta is relatively "soft," interrenal aortic clamping may be sufficient.

Prior to aortic clamping, infusion of mannitol is started. The type of graft and the graft size are selected. A Dacron graft or expanded PTFE graft can be used for arterial reconstruction. Author prefers a Dacron graft for aortic reconstruction in patients with associated iliac arterial occlusive disease; an expanded PTFE graft or Dacron graft is equally suitable for arterial reconstruction. Following clamping, the aneurysm sac is opened longitudinally 3 cm below the origin of the renal arteries and extending inferiorly to the right of the origin of the mesenteric artery avoiding sympathetic nerves crossing the origin of the left CIA and distal aorta. The intraluminal thrombus is bluntly removed and, if large, can be "scooped" out by the hand.

Fig. 3.5 Division of the right and left crus

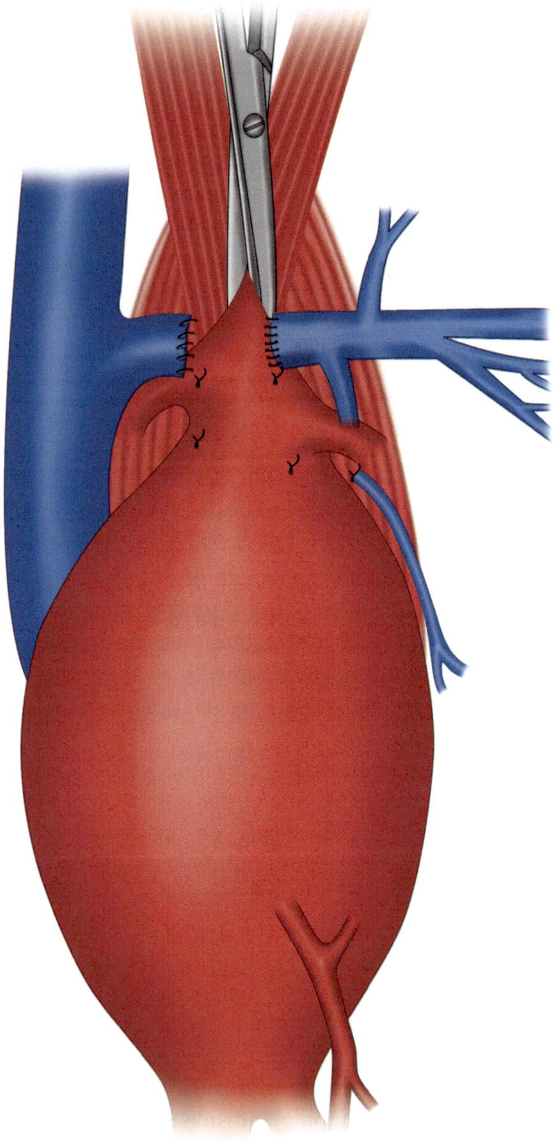

The back bleeding from the lumbar arteries can be brisk, and their origin should be oversewn with a figure of eight 2-0 "silk" suture. As one lumbar artery is being sutured, the other can be temporarily controlled by a Kittner sponge. If there is a calcified plaque surrounding the origin of the lumbar artery, it should be removed with Russian forceps before applying figure of 8 silk suture. If the inferior mesenteric artery has good back bleeding, it can be suture ligated close to its origin. Otherwise, silastic loop doubled on itself or a small bulldog clamp is applied.

Reconstruction then can either proceed with a tube graft or a bifurcated graft. A tube graft is preferred if CIA is not aneurysmal or there is no associated occlusive disease involving the common or the external iliac arteries. The proximal anastomosis is started by making a transverse incision across the previously placed longitudinal incision a few centimeters below the renal artery (T-type of incision) and dividing the lateral wall of the aorta. The posterior wall of the neck of the aorta is not divided. In patients undergoing reconstruction with bifurcated graft, the main shaft of the graft is divided 3–4 cm above its bifurcation to prevent kinking of its limbs. The proximal anastomosis started at 4 o'clock position, using a 3-0 or 4-0 cardiovascular polypropylene suture, incorporating the double thickness of the aorta till the suture line reaches the 8 o'clock position in a continuous manner using a parachute technique. Another row of continuous sutures starts at 4 o'clock and at 8 o'clock with suture tied to the previous suture line. With suture tied to the initial suture and continued laterally and anteriorly (Figs. 3.6, 3.7, 3.8, and 3.9). A distal aortic sewing ring is created by dividing the aorta just above the bifurcation and keeping the posterior wall intact, and on the right lateral wall, the inferior vena cava should be carefully visualized and protected from injury.

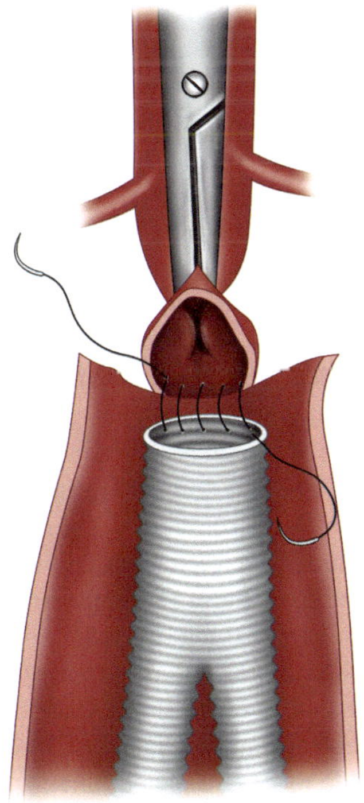

Fig. 3.6 Proximal aortic anastomosis. Posterior wall of the aorta is not divided and can be used as a double layer for reinforcement of a continuous suture line

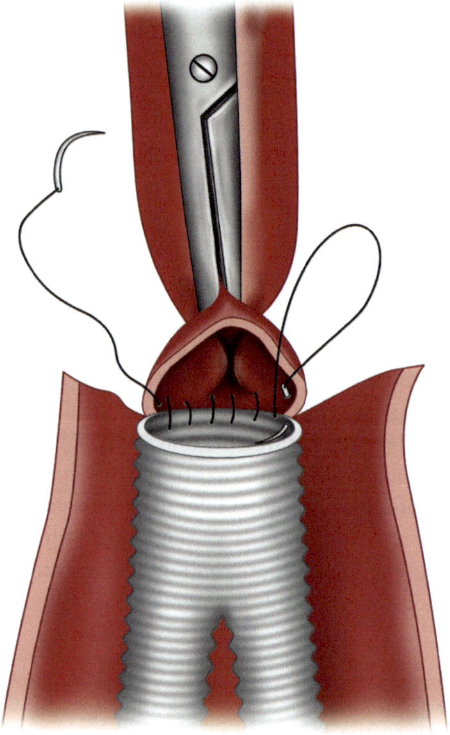

Fig. 3.7 Suture line continued on each side and the suture is tightened

In patients with weakened aortic wall near the neck, it is preferable to divide the posterior wall aortic neck completely (transection). One may encounter adherent lumbar veins at this juncture. In such cases, the graft and aortic neck are sutured using all interrupted mattress sutures starting from the posterior wall, and pledgets are used to buttress the suture line. A second layer of continuous suturing is done starting posteriorly and then laterally and completing it anteriorly.

In patients with juxtarenal AAA, a suture technique (two layers) telescoping the Dacron graft into the aortic neck is taking bites almost near the orifices of the renal arteries (Figs. 3.10, 3.11, 3.12, 3.13, 3.14, 3.15, 3.16, and 3.17). After the completion of proximal anastomosis, the retractors should be released to prevent injury to the SMA as forceful retraction can lead to dissection of the SMA due to intimal damage. Even before the proximal anastomosis is started, the blades of the self-retaining retractors should be applied in such a manner that adequate exposure is obtained, but a forceful retraction is not necessary as it may cause injury to surrounding structures and compression of the inferior vena cava resulting in diminished venous return and hypotension. Common iliac anastomosis is constructed in an end-to-end fashion. Common iliac artery should be divided completely and dissected from the iliac vein. Two sutures are started posteriorly and continued in each side to be completed anteriorly. Antegrade flow to at least one hypogastric artery should be preserved to prevent pelvic ischemia. If the origin of the external iliac and

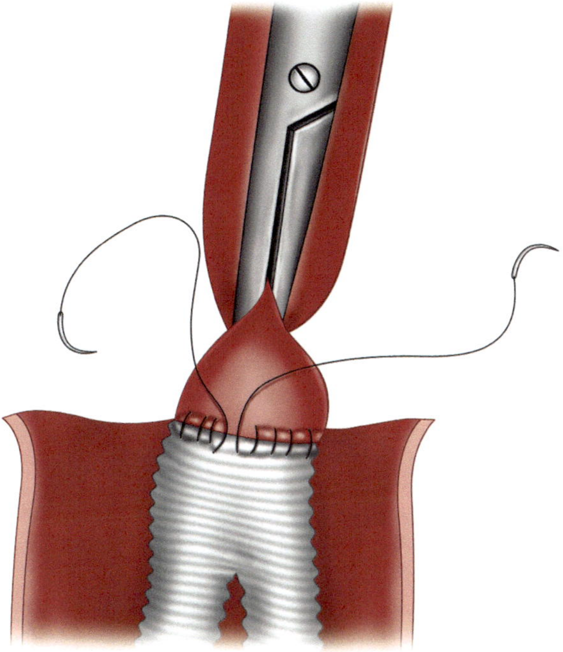

Fig. 3.8 Anterior suture line continued

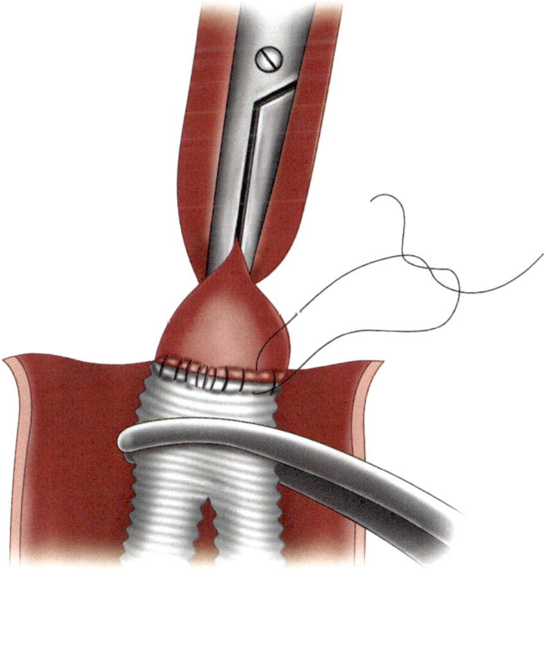

Fig. 3.9 Anterior suture line is almost completed

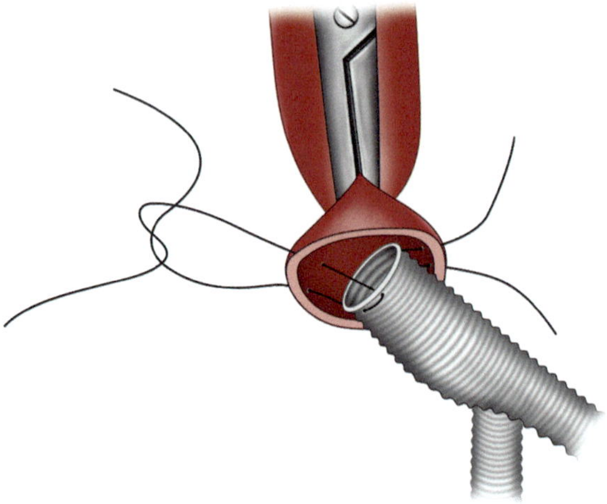

Fig. 3.10 A telescopic proximal anastomosis (all upper case) for repair of juxtarenal AAA. In first layer of horizontal mattress sutures between the Dacron graft and juxtarenal aorta at 9 o'clock position

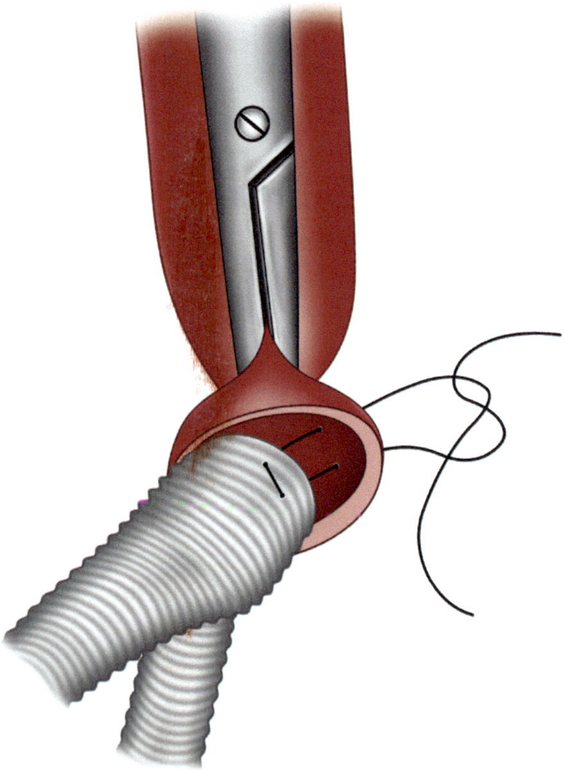

Fig. 3.11 Another suture started at 3 o'clock position in a similar fashion

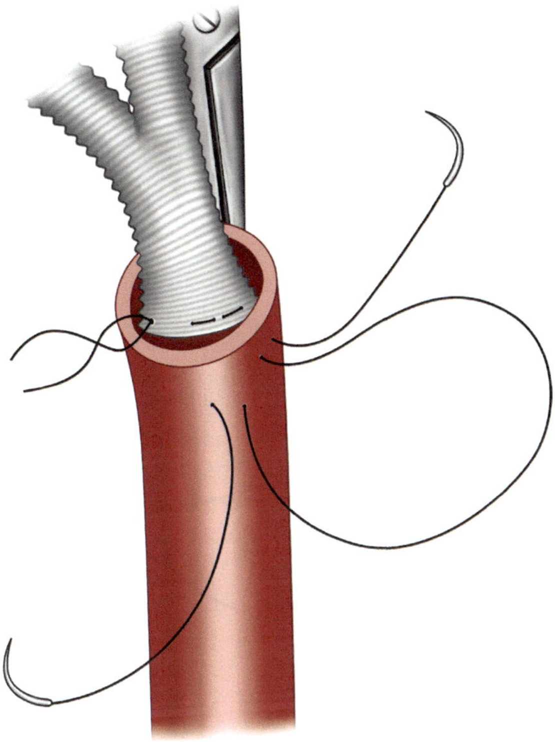

Fig. 3.12 Horizontal mattress suture technique is continued posteriorly taking wider bites in the aorta as compared to the Dacron graft

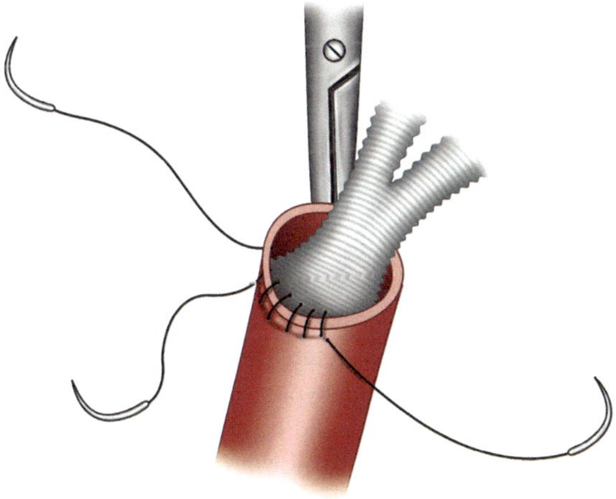

Fig. 3.13 Second layer of continuous suture is performed posteriorly

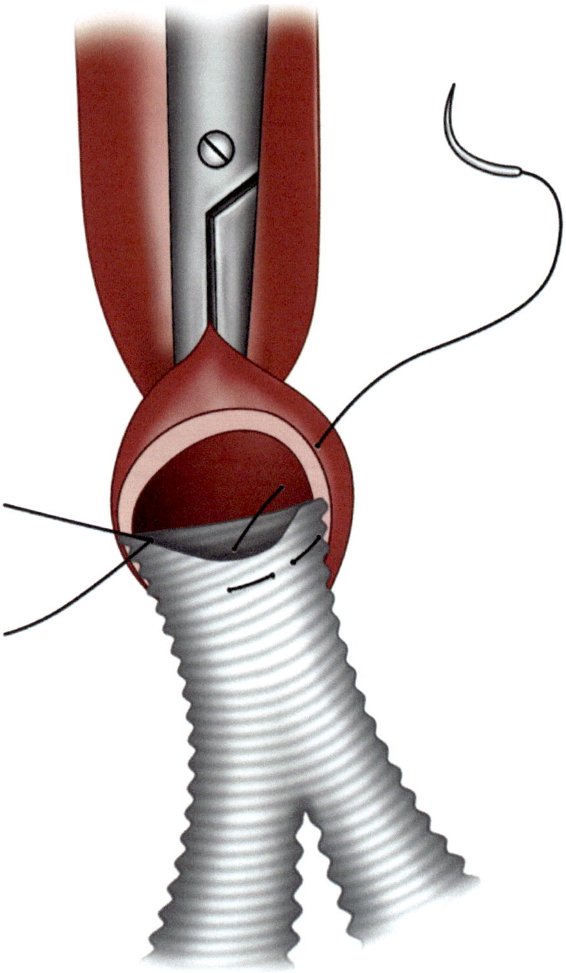
Fig. 3.14 Graft is laid in its bed and the first layer of horizontal mattress suture is started at 3 o'clock and continued anteriorly toward 12 o'clock

the hypogastric is quite apart due to the presence of common iliac aneurysm, it is preferable to anastomose the graft limb to the hypogastric artery, and anastomoses of external iliac artery end to side to the iliac limb of the graft if it is redundant is performed; otherwise, an interposition graft between the external iliac artery and the anastomosed limb to the hypogastric artery is preferred. Before completion of distal anastomosis, clamps should be released in such a manner to prevent atheromatous debris embolizing into the lower extremities. Following completion of distal anastomosis, the clamps are released gradually to prevent declamping shock. The anesthesia team should be informed so that the administration of intravenous fluids is increased. Arterial Blood gasses should be obtained. Usually, there is a 15–20 mmHg drop in blood pressure when the graft limb is opened, and failure of the drop in blood pressure usually indicates inadequate perfusion of the extremity. After completion of iliac anastomosis on one side, there is a distinct possiblity of fresh

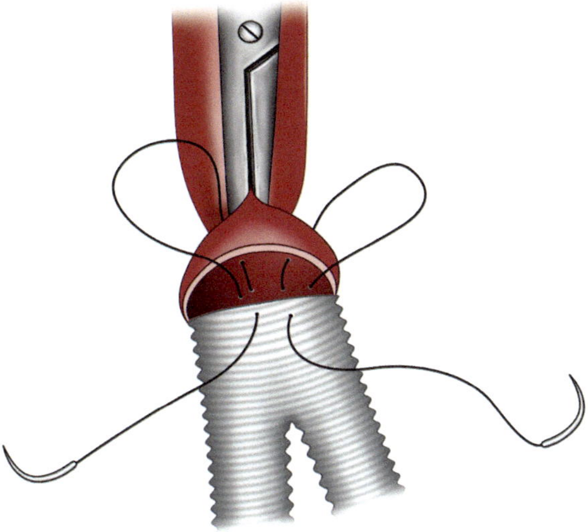

Fig. 3.15 Near completion of the first layer of horizontal mattress suture line

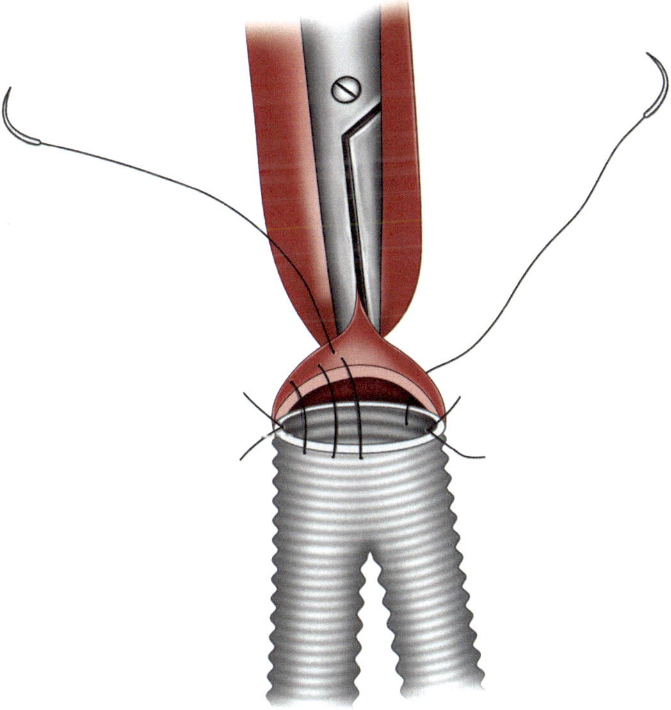

Fig. 3.16 Second layer of continuous suture line (over and over)

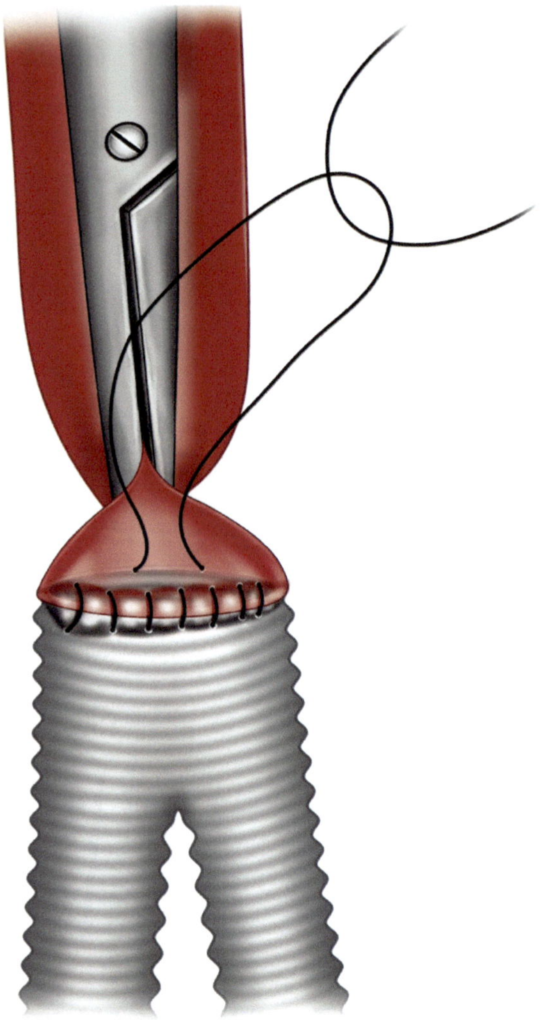

Fig. 3.17 A completed two-layer telescoping anastomosis between the Dacron graft and the juxtarenal aorta

bleeding from the lumbar artery or arteries in the posterior wall of aneurysm sac which demands immediate attention.

In patients with tube graft clamp, release should be extremely gradual, as declamping shock can be much more severe as compared to patients undergoing aortic bi-iliac reconstruction. Doppler signals in posterior tibial and dorsalis pedis arteries on both sides should be checked and if distal pulses are not palpable. The inferior mesenteric artery should be reimplanted as Carrel patch in patients with large IMA with poor back bleeding in patients with associated SMA or celiac artery occlusive disease (Fig. 3.18). Retroperitoneum is sutured by approximately small bowel mesentery to the sigmoid mesocolon inferiorly and tissue in dividing the right wall of the aneurysm and descending mesocolon superiorly so that the graft is not in contact with the small bowel and the abdomen is closed in layers with the peritoneum and linear abdomen as a single layer with number one PDS suture.

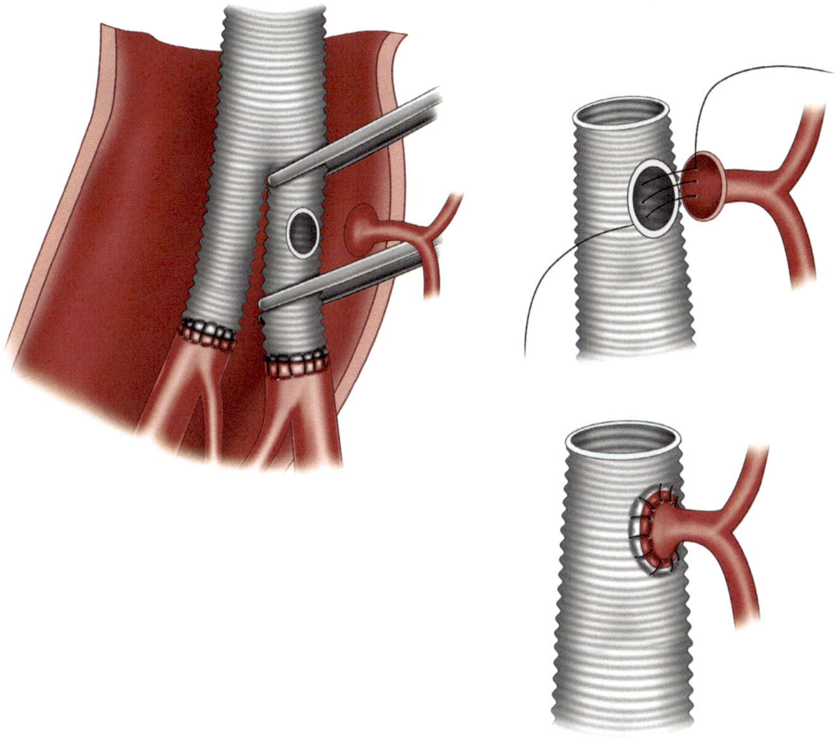

Fig. 3.18 Reimplantation of the inferior mesenteric artery with a disc of aortic wall ready to be implanted into the left limb of the aortoiliac graft as Carrel patch

Retroperitoneal Approach

Patient Position

Patient is placed in a modified right lateral decubitus position with the shoulders at 70 degrees to the operating table and the hips more posteriorly. This is helpful if groin incisions become necessary. Patient is also placed in a jackknife position in a vacuum "beanbag" to open the left flank. The table is tilted toward the right. The mid-point between the patient's right costal margin and right iliac crest is centered over the break of the table (jackknife position). For infrarenal aneurysm repair, the incision extends from the lateral margin of the left rectus sheath from a point midway between the symphysis pubis and umbilicus extending laterally and upward into the eleventh intercostal space for 10–12 cm. In patients undergoing a repair for juxtarenal or pararenal aortic aneurysm, the incision extended into the tenth intercostal space (Fig. 3.19). The muscles of the abdominal wall and intercostal muscles are divided in the line of the incision, and extraperitoneal space is entered at the tip of the 12th rib. The peritoneum along with the transversalis fascia is separated from the abdominal wall muscles anteriorly. In the inferior part of the dissection, the peritoneal sac and its contents are retracted anteriorly and medially (Fig. 3.20). In

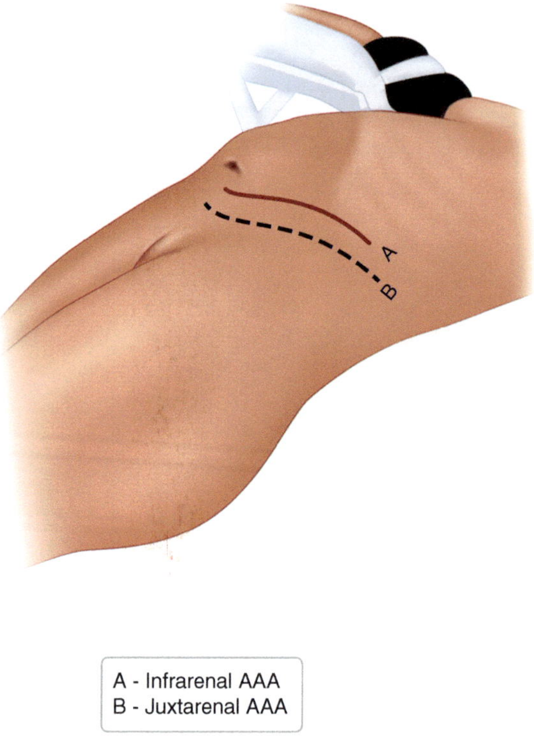

Fig. 3.19 Left flank incision for retroperitoneal incision. (**a**) Infrarenal AAA. (**b**) Juxtarenal AAA

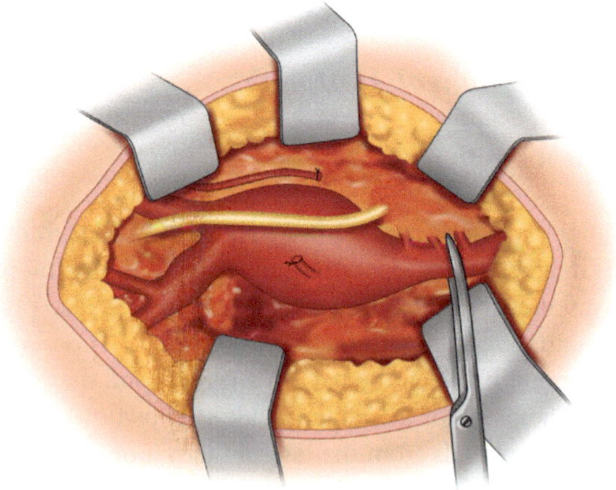

Fig. 3.20 Retroperitoneal exposure of AAA. The plane of dissection is behind the left kidney. Proximal aortic clamp is above the superior mesenteric artery for repair of pararenal AAA

patients with infrarenal AAA, dissection can be performed anterior to the left kidney and kidney left in its bed (Fig. 3.21). In patients with juxtarenal or pararenal aortic aneurysms, the dissection plane is developed behind the kidney. The left kidney and ureter are reflected medially and anteriorly. Inferiorly, distal abdominal aorta and left CIA are dissected. The left renal artery is exposed. The posterior

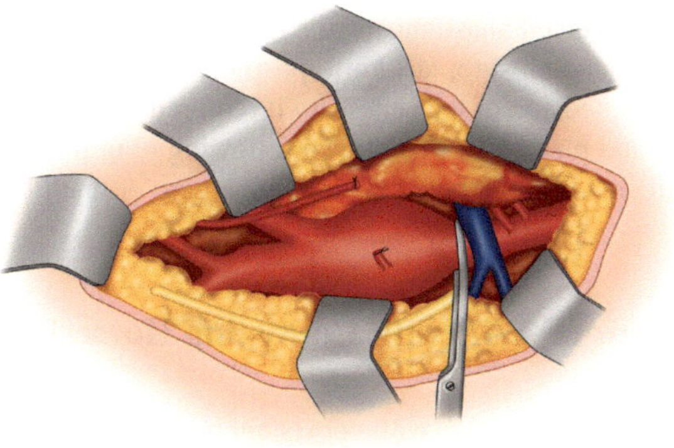

Fig. 3.21 Retroperitoneal exposure with the left kidney in a bed. This technique is necessary in patients with retroaortic left renal vein

lumbar branch of the left renal vein is present just below the origin of the left renal artery and aids in its identification. In patients with retroaortic left renal vein, as determined on preoperative CTA images, the dissection should be performed anterior to the left kidney. The periaortic fascia and lymphatics around the neck of the aorta are ligated and divided exposing the posterior and lateral wall of the aneurysm. Heparin is adminstered by the anesthesia team with monitoring of ACT. Placement of the aortic cross-clamp is the next step as in transperitoneal exposure. Like in transperitoneal exposure, circumferential dissection of the aorta is not necessary.

For exposure of the suprarenal aorta, the dissection proceeds cephalad dividing the left crus, identified as a firm tendinous band crossing the aorta just proximal to the origin of the left renal artery. The origin of the left renal artery is exposed with a Kittner dissector or with a gentle finger dissection, anterior and posterior to the aorta. Silver clips are applied to the lumbar arteries at this time. Fibers of the left crus will need to be divided for another 5 cm proximally and the fascia around the aorta is carefully divided to expose the supraceliac aorta, which is often a better site for proximal aortic clamping than placing the clamp at the suprarenal level. In patients necessitating supraceliac control, incision should be made in the tenth intercostal space, and the peritoneal sac is reflected medially from the left iliac forceps carefully mobilizing the ureter and peritoneal sac. Exposure of the left CIA and its bifurcation is excellent from the left flank approach, but the right CIA can only be exposed in its proximal one third. Division of the IMA and further mobilization of the peritoneal sac medially improve the exposure of the right CIA. If a vascular clamp cannot be safely applied to the right CIA, then endoluminal control with a large Fogarty catheter or a Pruitt occlusion baloon catheter or a large Garrett dilator (Teleflex) can help control retrograde bleeding. Distal right CIA can be exposed by extending the left flank incision to the midline, but this may result in inadvertent entry into the peritoneum. Though challenging, the right lower quadrant incision, 3–4 cm above the right inguinal ligament with rotation of the table to the left, can help in extraperitoneal exposure of the right CIA bifurcation and proximal right external iliac artery. For femoral anastomosis (in patients with associated occlusive disease), groin incisions can be made by rotating the table. Exposure of the right renal artery is inadequate with this approach. Further steps for aortic graft reconstruction are similar to transperitoneal repair. After completion of the proximal and distal anastomosis, the aneurysm sac is closed around the prosthetic graft. For wound closure, jackknife position is discontinued, and the table made supine. Partial division of the necessary if required is oversewn over a temporary 16 F catheter and pleural air is removed following lung inflation. Muscles of the abdominal wall are closed in layers with number zero or one PDS suture.

Repair of AAA with Coexisting Horseshoe and Pelvic Kidney

Open repair of AAA with coexistent horseshoe and pelvic kidney should be undertaken after complete evaluation of renal arterial supply. In patients with horseshoe kidney, thickness of the isthmus should be evaluated. Thin-section CTA of the abdomen and pelvis is mandatory in preoperative planning. Renal arteries measuring greater than 2 mm in diameter supplying the horseshoe kidney should be preserved and reimplanted into the prosthetic graft as Carrel patch (similar to IMA reimplant). Both transperitoneal and retroperitoneal approaches have been used for open repair of AAA with horseshoe kidney. If the transperitoneal approach is selected, the wide isthmus of the horseshoe kidney if present should be persevered with the main body of prosthetic graft brought behind the isthmus. During retroperitoneal approach, isthmus and the fused kidney mass are mobilized anteriorly, and the graft remains behind the horseshoe kidney. For patients with associated pelvic kidney, transperitoneal approach with preservation and reimplantation of renal blood supply, should be performed.

Take-Home Points

1. The dissection of the aortic neck and bilateral common iliac arteries should be performed anteriorly and on each side, and passage of vessel loop should be avoided in order to prevent injury to the posterior lumbar vein (joining the left renal vein) and injury to the common iliac veins.
2. In patients undergoing left retroperitoneal approach for repair of the AAA with associated retroaortic left renal vein, the kidney should be left in its bed and should not be mobilized anteriorly. Injury to the left ureter should be avoided by keeping the dissection close to the aortic neck and anterolateral wall of the aneurysm. If venous injury occurs, proximal control and distal control distal to the injury site are obtained with a Kittner sponge. Commonly, the vascular clamps, which are used to control bleeding from arteries, should not be applied to the veins as the tear in the veins may extend. Following distal and proximal compression, complete mobilization of the overlying CIA or even transection of the CIA may be necessary to perform lateral venorraphy for repair of the injured iliac vein using 5-0 cardiovascular polypropylene running suture. Patients undergoing common iliac vein repair should have a follow-up duplex venous imaging as the incidence of deep venous thrombosis is increased in such circumstances.

Chapter 4
Paravisceral Abdominal Aortic Aneurysm Repair

Alexander D. Shepard

The paravisceral (PV) aorta is defined as the aorta running from the aortic hiatus to the renal arteries. Abdominal aortic aneurysms (AAAs) involving this segment of the aorta represent a unique challenge for open repair. The required operative exposure is unfamiliar to many surgeons and is much more extensive than that used for infrarenal (IR) AAAs. Clamping of the aorta at this level produces obligatory periods of renal/visceral ischemia, and the reconstruction techniques used are much more involved than the simple end-to-end anastomoses of IR repair. Careful preoperative assessment is mandatory with particular attention to cardiac, pulmonary, and renal function. Undoubtedly, the most important preoperative test is a thin-cut, high-quality computed tomographic angiogram (CTA), which allows careful planning for operative approach, aortic clamp sites, and reconstruction techniques.

The indications for repair are the same as for any AAA and are determined primarily by size, configuration, and the presence of symptoms. Given the risk of these procedures, our size threshold for intervention is usually a bit higher than the 5.5 cm diameter (for males) and 5.0 cm (for females) that we use for IR AAA.

Anesthetic Considerations

Intraoperative monitoring with arterial line, central line, and Foley catheter is routine, supplemented by transesophageal echocardiography as needed. For repairs where a prolonged period (>30 min) of supraceliac (SC) aortic clamping is

A. D. Shepard (✉)
Division of Vascular Surgery, Henry Ford Hospital, Detroit, MI, USA
e-mail: ASHEPAR2@hfhs.org

S. S. Hans et al. (eds.), *Primary and Repeat Arterial Reconstructions*,
https://doi.org/10.1007/978-3-031-13897-3_4

anticipated, a lumbar catheter is placed preoperatively to drain cerebrospinal fluid (CSF) to reduce the risk of spinal cord ischemia. An epidural catheter helps with postoperative pain management.

Operative Approach

Although juxtarenal AAA can be repaired through a midline, inframesocolic approach, more proximal aneurysms require retroperitoneal (RP) exposure with rotation of the abdominal viscera medially. This exposure is most easily accomplished through a left flank (thoracoretroperitoneal or thoracoabdominal) approach utilizing an oblique incision in the tenth or ninth (rarely the eighth) intercostal spaces depending on the amount of aortic exposure needed and the level of clamping planned. We use the tenth interspace for suprarenal (SR) aneurysms and the ninth for most PV AAA. The patient is positioned on a vacuum beanbag in a modified left thoracotomy position with the shoulders at 70–80° to the table. Depending on the level of distal exposure required, we leave the patient in an almost pure lateral position (when sewing a tube graft to the bifurcation) or rotate the hips posteriorly (when iliac/femoral anastomoses are anticipated).

The incision is begun at the umbilicus at the lateral margin of the left rectus sheath and carried posteriorly into the appropriate intercostal space for 10–15 cm. Taking the incision even further posteriorly (as far as the paraspinous muscles if necessary) allows more proximal aortic exposure, while extending the incision to the midline facilitates more distal exposure. The musculature of the abdominal wall and intercostal space is divided with no effort to avoid entry into the left chest. The retroperitoneal (RP) space is entered at the tip of the tenth rib. A pure RP approach can be utilized (our preference) by dissecting the peritoneum away from the transversalis fascia anteriorly, as far as the rectus sheath, and from the lumbodorsal fascia (the posterior extension of the transversalis fascia) posterolaterally. If one chooses to use a transperitoneal approach, then it will be necessary to divide the peritoneal reflection of the descending colon laterally after entering the peritoneal cavity. This peritoneal incision is carried superiorly along the spleen before curving medially to the aortic hiatus. Great care must be taken to avoid splenic injury with this maneuver.

Division of the diaphragm is performed circumferentially 2–3 cm from its lateral attachments to avoid injury to phrenic nerve branches with the attendant risk for postoperative respiratory morbidity [1]. This division begins at the costal margin and is carried posteriorly as far as necessary to avoid tearing the diaphragm during subsequent rib retraction. A mechanical retraction system (e.g., Thompson or Omni-Tract) provides excellent exposure. In most situations, an exposure plane posterior to the left kidney is created. After blunt dissection through loose areolar tissue, the left kidney and peritoneal sac with its contents are retracted to the patient's right. One needs to avoid a deeper plane that can result in stripping the lumbodorsal fascia off the flank musculature.

At this juncture, the aorta and aneurysm should be palpable in the base of the wound. Initial dissection is focused on identification of the left renal artery (RA); this is the only important structure that can be injured during the initial dissection of the aorta and serves as a good landmark for identification of other vessels. In thin patients, this artery is usually visible originating from the left lateral wall of the aorta/aneurysm, coursing anteriorly to the retracted left kidney; in more obese patients, some dissection is necessary to find it. This artery is mobilized back to its origin off the aorta. In most patients, a lumbar branch of the left renal vein (RV) is reliably present, crossing over the aorta just below the left RA. Inadvertent transection of this vein can lead to troublesome bleeding, and it should always be sought and ligated and divided when found. If this venous branch is much larger than normal, concern for a retro-aortic left renal vein (RV) (2% incidence) should prompt review of the preop CTA. In this setting, exposure of the aorta anterior to the kidney is necessary to avoid interrupting the venous drainage of the left kidney.

The left posterolateral wall of the aorta/aneurysm is exposed by dividing overlying periaortic fat and lymphatics using an ultrasonic scalpel. This dissection is carried both cephalad and caudal. Immediately above the origin of the left RA, the left diaphragmatic crus is identified as a firm tendinous band crossing the aorta. Crural fibers are divided several cm along the axis of the aorta and the underlying aortic wall exposed. In most situations, normal-caliber SC aorta is encountered at this level; fascia investing the aorta is incised allowing index finger passage anterior and posterior to the aorta to establish a plane for cross-clamp placement. Lumbar arteries at this level should be avoided. Circumferential dissection of the SC aorta is unnecessary if the clamp arms pass beyond its far wall. Caval injury is not a concern at this level.

Suprarenal control is only slightly harder to obtain because of more lymphatic structures and the proximity of the RAs to the superior mesenteric artery (SMA). When the SMA originates close to the two RAs ($\leq$ 1.5 cm), we avoid SR clamping because of the risk of damage to the SMA. Supramesenteric clamping is occasionally possible for some SR AAA but is much more involved than SC clamping because of the presence of more dense lymphatics at this level and the peri-celiac neural plexus. Dissection of the SMA origin usually requires careful ligation of these structures to avoid a postop chyle leak. Only the first 2–3 cm of the SMA can be dissected out from a retro renal approach because more distal exposure is precluded by the crossing left RA. In the unlikely event that more distal SMA exposure is necessary, the kidney is left in its normal anatomic location and the aorta is approached anterior to the left kidney as with a retro-aortic left renal vein.

After obtaining proximal aortic control, the origins of the left RA, SMA, and celiac trunk are exposed as needed. During aortic reconstruction, we favor extraluminal control of the celiac and SMA with small vascular clamps or doubled-up vessel loops. We find this less unwieldy than intraluminal control with balloon occlusion catheters. The distal AAA sac is next exposed by dividing overlying tissues with an ultrasonic scalpel taking care that the left ureter is retracted medially along with the peritoneal sac. The left iliac is identified distally and circumferentially mobilized. The right iliac can be more difficult to control because of its adherence to the caval confluence. Dissecting this vessel out a few cm distal to the aortic bifurcation and avoiding circumferential mobilization can minimize the risk of venous injury. Easily accessible lumbar arteries arising from the aneurysm sac are ligated to reduce bleeding after opening the sac. Lumbars at the level of the proximal neck should be preserved if possible (Fig. 4.1).

Aortic clamp level: The level of proximal aortic clamping is dependent on the anatomy of the aneurysm and the presence of aortic plaque burden as defined by the preoperative CTA. Clamping a diseased aorta can result in renal/visceral and lower extremity atheroembolism. The more proximally the aorta is clamped, the greater both the renal/visceral ischemic burden and cardiac strain so the most distal feasible clamp site is preferred. When SR clamping is not possible, we have preferred SC over SM clamping because it is less cumbersome, and the SC aorta is reliably the least diseased segment of the abdominal aorta. SM clamping maintains some visceral perfusion through the celiac and is associated with less cardiac strain; however, the SMA must be controlled to prevent significant backbleeding. Mannitol (25 g) is always administered 20 min prior to aortic clamping to enhance renal protection. A bicarbonate drip (0.05 mEq/kg/min) is also started prior to SC clamping to minimize the associated acidosis. With some PV AAA, it is sometimes possible to clamp the IR aorta first, if the neck is not too aneurysmal or diseased; this maneuver allows control of backbleeding lumbars in the AAA sac without extending precious visceral/renal ischemia time. When using SC clamping to perform a juxta–/suprarenal aneurysm repair, backbleeding from uncontrolled visceral and segmental branches can be controlled by inflating a 10 cc Foley balloon catheter in the paravisceral aorta. We routinely heparinize prior to clamping regardless of clamp level to reduce the risk of both large vessel and microvascular thrombosis, a cause of multiorgan failure, which can complicate these procedures [2]. Careful

Fig. 4.1 Exposure of a paravisceral AAA through a left flank retroperitoneal approach

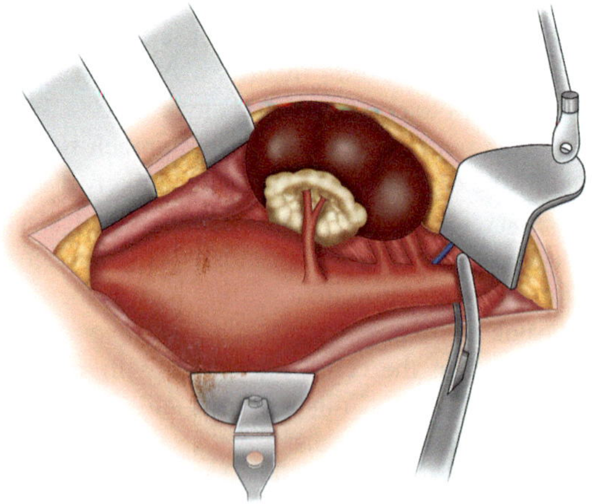

communication with anesthesia is necessary during clamping/unclamping. Blood should be in the room and an autotransfusion device available when opening the aneurysm sac.

Vital organ ischemia protection: Proximal aortic clamping is accompanied by obligatory renal +/− visceral ischemia). Acute kidney injury (AKI) is a common complication of these repairs. Keeping clamp times to a minimum and optimizing renal hemodynamics prior to clamping are important. When coming from the left flank, the right RA is in a dependent position and cannot be clamped prior to aortic clamping. Mural thrombus or other sac debris can "drop" into this artery when/after opening the aneurysm sac; for this reason, we often insert a small balloon-tipped occlusion catheter into the origin of this vessel soon after the aneurysm is opened. When anticipating >30 min of renal ischemia or in patients with chronic kidney disease, cold renal perfusion is routinely performed to reduce renal metabolic demands. Balloon-tipped Pruitt perfusion catheters (9 Fr for large RAs or 5 Fr for smaller or diseased RAs) are inserted, and 250 mL of 1 °C Ringer's lactate solution (plus heparin, mannitol, and methylprednisolone) is infused into each kidney followed by 50 mL q 15 min for the duration of clamping. The value of this adjunct in the prevention of AKI is well described [3]. We have also cold perfused the SMA (500 mL followed by 75 mL q 15 min) during SC clamping for visceral protection noting less coagulopathy and hemodynamic changes with unclamping. Although spinal cord ischemia is rare with PAAA repair, we undertake a spinal cord protection protocol whenever we anticipate an SC clamp time more than 30 min. A preop lumbar drain is placed and 50–75 cc of CSF drained following which the drain is set to maintain an intrathecal pressure $\leq$ 10 cmH_2O. We avoid high-dose vasodilators during cross-clamp and employ moderate passive hypothermia to 34 °C.

Aortic reconstruction Techniques: Albumin impregnated Dacron grafts are preferred for these reconstructions to avoid the needle hole bleeding and perigraft seromas associated with PTFE. The overwhelming majority of repairs can be accomplished with a 20 or 22 mm diameter graft. The type of proximal anastomosis performed is dependent on the proximity of the renal and visceral arteries to each other and normal aortic caliber. For JR AAA (defined as an aneurysm without an IR neck suitable for clamping/anastomosis), an end-to-end anastomosis is performed to the aorta immediately below/adjacent to the RAs frequently taking stitches through the lower borders of the RA ostia (Fig. 4.2). More proximal aneurysms require some type of beveled anastomosis incorporating the origins of the renal/visceral arteries. There are several options that depend on the relationship of the RAs to the aneurysm. The simplest option leaves the RAs on an anterior tongue of the aorta (along with the SMA and celiac as needed) using a graft with a posterior bevel (Fig. 4.3). This approach is only possible when most of the aneurysm is located posteriorly and the two RAs originate close to each other anteriorly. Far more commonly, the RAs are separated by aneurysmal aorta and it is necessary to use a lateral bevel. With this reconstruction, the right RA, SMA, and celiac are left on the aorta medially and the left RA and its origin excised from the aortic wall. The graft is trimmed with a lateral bevel and sewn in place with 3-0 polypropylene

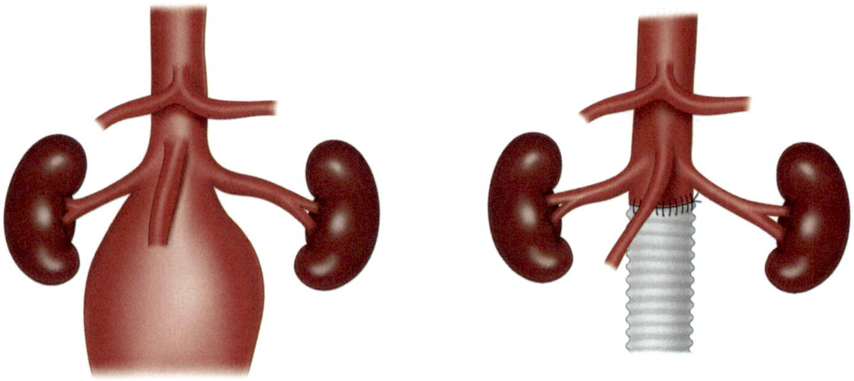

Fig. 4.2 Construction of proximal aortic anastomosis immediately below the RA (and incorporating the RA ostia into the suture line as needed) during JR AAA repair

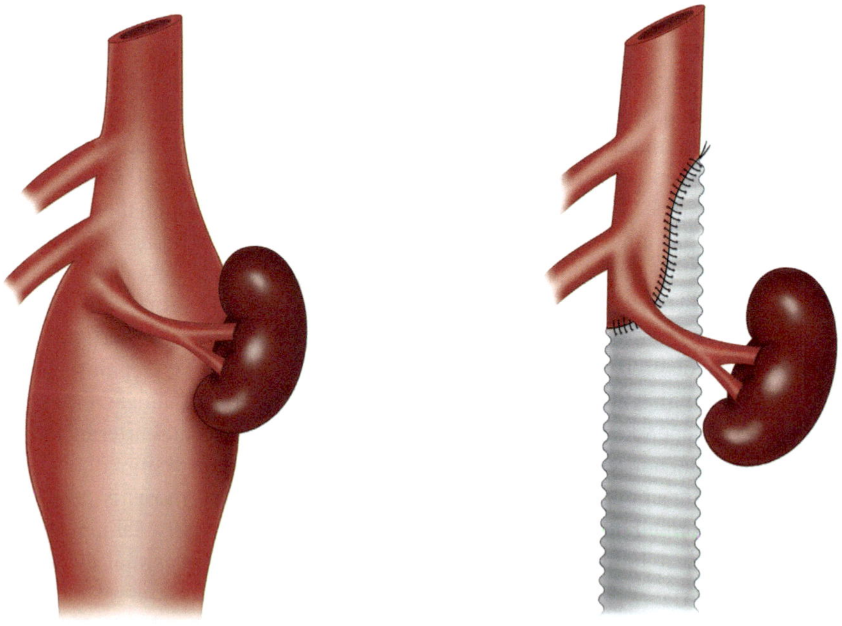

Fig. 4.3 Proximal aortic reconstruction with a posterior beveled anastomosis, leaving the celiac, SMA, and both RAs on an anterior segment of the aorta. To utilize this type of reconstruction, both RAs need to arise anteriorly off the aorta in close proximity to each other

(48 cm length) using the inclusion technique (Fig. 4.4). This anastomosis is started at the level of the dependent right RA and runs along the posterior wall taking double-thickness bites (Creech technique) (Fig. 4.5). At the edge of the trimmed aortic wall, the suture line is transitioned to single-thickness bites. The other end of

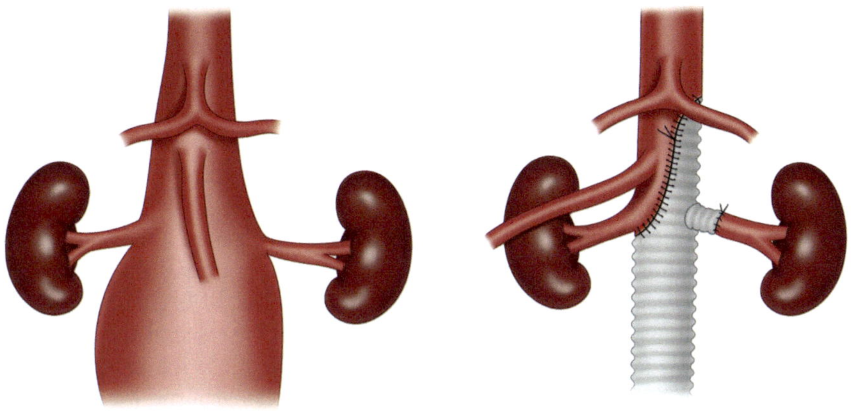

Fig. 4.4 Proximal aortic reconstruction with a laterally beveled anastomosis, incorporating the celiac, SMA, and right RA on a segment of the aorta and either bypassing or reimplanting the left RA. This is more commonly utilized than the reconstruction shown in Fig. 4.3

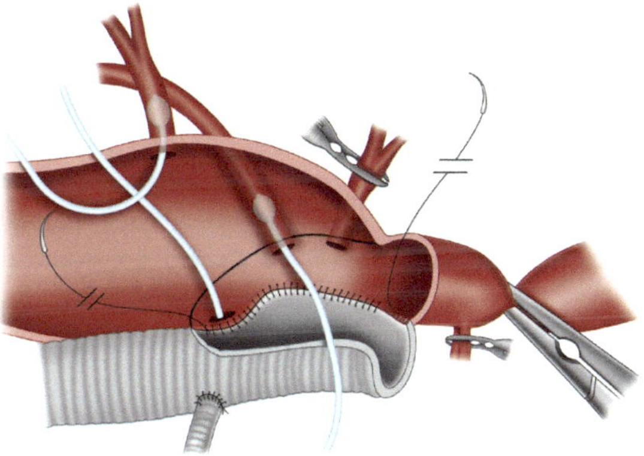

Fig. 4.5 Laterally beveled proximal anastomosis with perfusion catheters in SMA and both RAs and construction of posterior wall suture line. Small clamp is on the celiac artery

the suture is carried around the right RA anteriorly until the two stitches meet near the SMA. When utilizing the inclusion technique, it is important to leave behind as little aorta as possible to minimize the risk of recurrent aneurysm formation from degeneration of the remaining aortic wall. Following aortic flushing, the perfusion catheters are removed, the suture line is secured, and flow is restored first to the right RA and then the viscera after careful communication with the anesthesia team.

At this point, one can proceed with revascularization of either the lower extremities or the left RA. We usually go with the distal aorta first (or at least one iliac) to both unload the heart *and* to restore hypogastric flow to improve spinal cord perfusion. Continued cold perfusion of the left RA protects the kidney during distal aortic reconstruction, or alternatively, a small Pruitt carotid shunt can be used to provide flow from a sidearm graft off the aorta. The left RA can either be reimplanted directly on to the prosthetic aortic graft, utilizing a small button of aortic wall, or it can be bypassed with a previously constructed sidearm graft. If a sidearm graft is used (our preference), it is imperative that this conduit (usually slightly oversized at 7 or 8 mm in diameter) be appropriately positioned on the aortic graft to avoid subsequent kinking (2 o'clock position with the SMA at 12 o'clock). The graft to RA anastomosis should always be performed under a fair amount of tension since there is invariably graft/artery redundancy when the kidney is returned to its normal location, which can lead to kinking.

With aneurysms originating well above the celiac (true extent 4 thoracoabdominal aneurysm), an end-to-end anastomosis between the graft and the descending thoracic aorta is necessary with reimplantation of the celiac, SMA, and right RA as a separate inclusion patch (Fig. 4.6). When the origins of the visceral and right renal arteries are widely spaced apart, it may not be possible to use the inclusion technique without leaving an unacceptable amount of aneurysmal aortic wall behind. A prefabricated graft with four sidearms—celiac, SMA, and both RAs (Vascutek® Coselli thoracoabdominal graft)—is useful in this situation as it is in patients with suspected connective tissue abnormalities (Fig. 4.7). Great care is needed when using this graft to ensure that the sidearms line up with their respective branches. After performing the proximal aortic anastomosis, we move to the right RA anastomosis, which must be done prior to the others or risk losing exposure to this vessel. Following reperfusion of the right kidney, we connect the perfusion catheters present in the SMA and left RA to their respective limbs and restore flow to these organs. This approach reduces renal/visceral ischemia and allows an unhurried distal aortic/iliac anastomosis. After lower-extremity revascularization, the SMA, celiac, and finally the left RA grafts are performed sequentially. It is important to do the left RA last to maintain exposure for the visceral anastomoses and reduce the risk of tearing

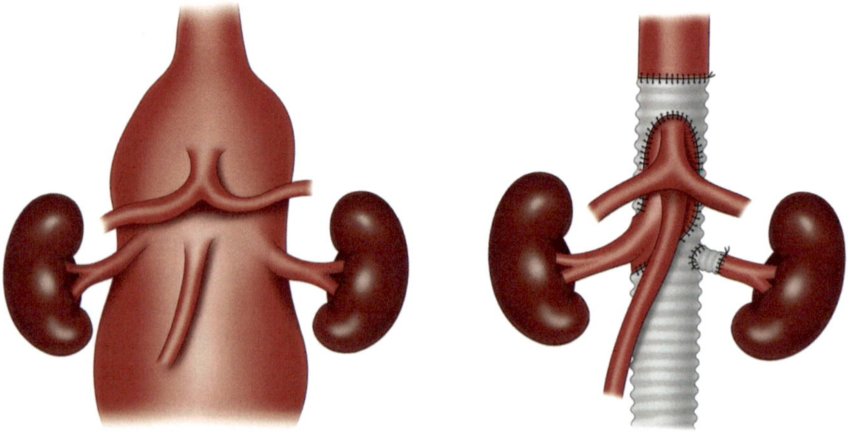

Fig. 4.6 Extent 4 TAAA repair showing end-to-end proximal aortic anastomosis and Carell patch reimplantation of the celiac, SMA, and right RA on a small island of the aorta. The left RA is reconstructed with a short sidearm graft

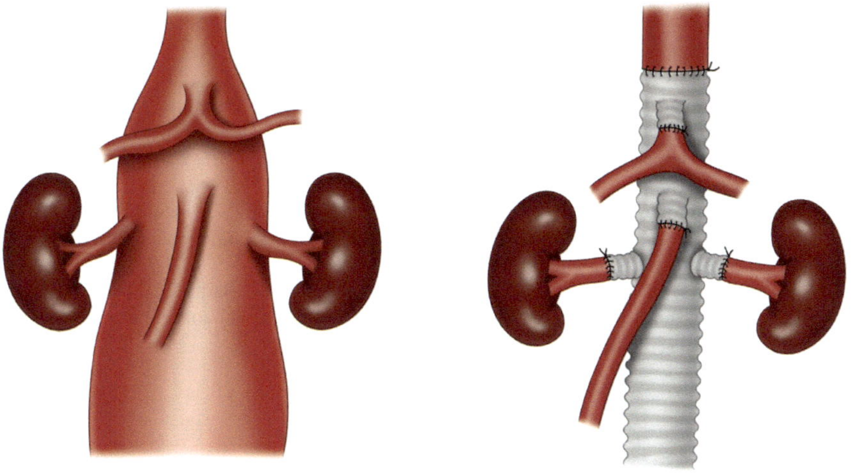

Fig. 4.7 Extent 4 TAAA repair with a preconstructed 4-branched (Coselli) graft. Sidearm grafts are individually sewn to the celiac, SMA, right RA, and left RA. This graft must be carefully measured/trimmed and aligned rotationally prior to proximal anastomotic construction. *AAA* abdominal aortic aneurysm, *JR* juxtarenal, *SMA* superior mesenteric artery, *RA* renal artery, *TAAA* thoracoabdominal aortic aneurysm

this bypass during visceral reconstruction. To avoid kinking, the Coselli graft limbs are left very short (10–15 mm).

Following completion of all anastomoses, patency of reconstructed vessels is checked by Doppler probe auscultation and the hemostatic profile corrected with protamine/clotting factors as necessary. We have found point-of-care thromboelastography very useful. Closure is performed after placement of #19 Fr postero-basal channeled pleural tube; 2-0 or 0 Prolene is used on the diaphragm, looped #1 PDS for rib approximation, and layered 0 or 2-0 PDS for the wound. A spinal cord protection protocol is maintained for 24 h in all patients with a lumbar drain.

Conclusions

Aneurysms of the PV aorta can be repaired with morbidity and mortality approaching that of open IR AAA repair in experienced hands [4]. There are several keys to success: First, careful operative planning based on high-quality preoperative imaging. This is not an operation where one "opens up the hood" and figures out things on the fly. A second key is to reduce blood loss by avoiding venous injuries, ligating/clamping lumbar arteries prior to opening the sac, and controlling backbleeding branches. Minimizing vital organ ischemia by keeping clamp times low and utilizing adjuncts to extend ischemic tolerance (cold renal/visceral perfusion, CSF drainage) is also critical. And finally, technical precision as opposed to speed will assure the best possible outcome.

References

1. Anagnostopolous PV, Shepard AD, Pipinos II, Nypaver TJ, Cho JS, Reddy DJ. Factors affecting outcome in proximal abdominal aortic aneurysm repair. Ann Vasc Surg. 2001;15:511–9.
2. Anagnostopoulos PV, Shepard AD, Pipinos II, Raman SBK, Chaudhry PA, Mishima T, Morita H, Suzuki G. Hemostatic alterations associated with supraceliac aortic cross-clamping. J Vasc Surg. 2001;35:100–8.
3. Koksoy C, LeMaire SA, Curling PE, Raskin SA, Schmittling ZC, Conklin LD, Coselli JS. Renal perfusion during thoracoabdominal aortic operations: cold crystalloid is superior to normothermic blood. Ann Thorac Surg. 2002;73:730–8.
4. Kabbani LS, West CA, Viau D, Nypaver TJ, Weaver MW, Barth C, Lin JC, Shepard AD. Survival after repair of pararenal and paravisceral abdominal aortic aneurysms. J Vasc Surg. 2014;59:1488–94.

Chapter 5
Open Thoracoabdominal Aortic Aneurysm Repair

Mark F. Conrad and Srihari K. Lella

Introduction

Aneurysms that simultaneously involve the thoracic and abdominal aorta and/or those that extend through the visceral aortic segment are referred to as thoracoabdominal aortic aneurysms (TAA). These are uncommon when compared to isolated infrarenal aortic aneurysms and comprise no more than 2–5% of the total spectrum of degenerative aortic aneurysms. However, the tendency toward aortic enlargement is strong in this population as up to 30% of the said patients will also develop an abdominal aortic aneurysm in their lifetime. The modern era of open surgical management of TAA has seen a shift from a straight clamp-and-sew approach to the addition of adjunctive measures aimed at reducing ischemia to the spinal cord, visceral vessels, and lower extremities and the potential for significant morbidity. Indeed, a number of surgical and non-surgical adjuncts (many discussed herein) intended to minimize distal ischemia and improve outcomes have been investigated, and our approach to these complex aneurysms has evolved over time. Despite improvements in operative strategies, open repair of TAA still carries a 5–10% risk of perioperative morbidity and mortality in the form of renal, respiratory, and spinal cord ischemic complications. Endovascular repair of TAA using modular grafts with branched and fenestrated technologies has been successful but is limited by anatomic considerations, and a lack of general availability as the procedure is only performed in select centers with individual device exemption protocols. Indeed,

M. F. Conrad (✉)
Vascular and Endovascular Surgery, St. Elizabeth's Hospital, Brighton, MA, USA
e-mail: Mark.conrad2@steward.org

S. K. Lella
Vascular and Endovascular Surgery Resident, Massachusetts General Hospital, Harvard Medical School, Boston, MA, USA

S. S. Hans et al. (eds.), *Primary and Repeat Arterial Reconstructions*,
https://doi.org/10.1007/978-3-031-13897-3_5

despite advances in endovascular devices and techniques, there remains a cohort of patients with TAA who will require open repair, and this is unlikely to change in the foreseeable future.

Initial Evaluation

Anatomic Classification

TAA are classified according to the scheme originally devised by Crawford, which in the most basic terms considers whether the lesion is primarily a caudal extension of a descending thoracic aneurysm or a cephalad extension of a total abdominal aortic aneurysm (Fig. 5.1). This classification is especially useful in patients requiring operative repair since it has direct implications for both the technical conduct of operation and the incidence of operative complications, in particular, ischemic spinal cord injury (SCI). There is considerable variation in the operative approach required to manage different TAA lesions. For example, a type IV TAA can be repaired with the clamp-and-sew approach and should be accomplished with an expected morbidity and mortality that is similar to that of on open AAA repair. But the same cannot be said for the more extensive type II TAA lesions where the entire descending thoracic aorta is involved and repair is accomplished using distal aortic perfusion with atrial–femoral bypass.

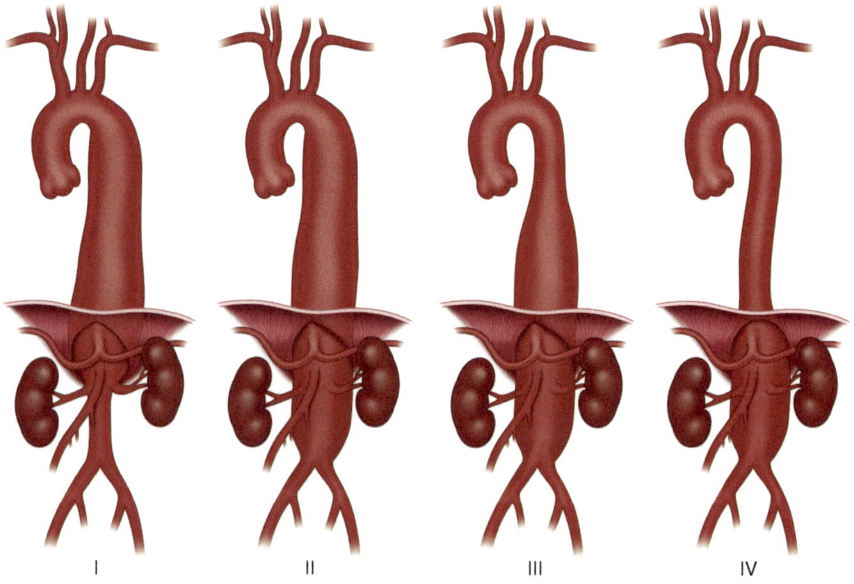

Fig. 5.1 Crawford classification of the extent of thoracoabdominal aortic aneurysms

Natural History

The expected natural history of TAA is progressive enlargement and eventual rupture regardless of etiology or location. Since thoracic aneurysms are uncommon when compared to AAA, fewer natural history studies are available. The general consensus is that the expected mean rate of growth for TAA is around 0.2 cm per year. This is accelerated in patients with dissections and connective tissue disorders such as Marfan syndrome. The size of the aorta at initial diagnosis has been shown to be an important predictor of future dilation, but there still remains substantial variation in individual aneurysm growth rates making prediction of future aortic size difficult. Population-based studies place the incidence of TAA at 5–6 per 100,000 people with a 5-year actuarial survival of 13% if left untreated and aneurysm rupture is identified as the cause of death in nearly 75% of untreated patients. Factors associated with increased risk of rupture include increasing aneurysm diameter, a rapid rate of expansion, the presence of chronic obstructive pulmonary disease (COPD), steroid use, female gender, advanced age, and the presence of renal insufficiency. Contemporary series indicate that the rupture risk is negligible in TAA less than 5 cm, equivalent to the risk of surgical morbidity in the 5–6 cm range, and it increases substantially at aneurysm diameters larger than 6 cm and/or growth rates of ≥10 mm per year. To wit, 6 cm is the surgical threshold for consideration of intervention in patients with degenerative TAA. For patients with TAA secondary to chronic dissection and/or those with Marfan syndrome, a 5.0–5.5 cm threshold is often used.

Clinical Presentation

Although patients commonly present in an asymptomatic fashion with incidental detection during radiologic surveillance for other disease processes, symptoms referable to TAA do occur and should be evaluated in a timely manner. In addition to the acute onset of severe pain, which may be associated with aneurysm expansion, rupture, and/or acute dissection, large thoracic aneurysms may produce symptoms of back, epigastric, or flank pain related to either compression of local structures or chronic inflammatory changes of the mediastinal pleura. Unlike AAA where back pain usually indicates an acute event, the pain associated with thoracic aneurysms may be atypical or chronic in nature and the presence of even uncharacteristic pain is an independent risk factor of rupture and should be taken seriously. When the aneurysm erodes into the thoracolumbar spine or chest wall, complaints of chest and back pain can be prominent and, again, may be present for weeks or even months. The new onset of hoarseness can be related to a left recurrent laryngeal nerve palsy, while compression or erosion of the tracheobronchial tree or pulmonary parenchyma will produce a chronic cough, hemoptysis, dyspnea, or dysphagia lusoria. Perhaps related to reluctance to recommend operation because of the threat of surgical morbidity, up to 40% of thoracic aortic aneurysm patients will present with symptoms. This explains the higher incidence of patients treated for rupture when compared to AAA series. Our results are consistent with those available from a review of the literature indicating that some 25% of patients will be treated under urgent or emergent circumstances with approximately half of these presenting with a frank rupture. Unfortunately, we and others have demonstrated that such non-elective operations are associated with a significant increase in morbidity.

Diagnostic Imaging

Accurate and complete radiographic evaluation is essential for precise operative planning with no equivocation in the surgeon's mind as to the proximal and distal extent of aortic resection. In contemporary practice, a dynamic, fine-cut, contrast-enhanced CT angiogram with or without helical reconstruction provides the physician with important information. This includes the qualitative assessment of the aorta at the proposed site of proximal cross-clamp, the location and patency of the visceral vessels, and the topography and location of the origins of the renal arteries and the adequacy of renal perfusion. Imaging will also identify the distal extent of the aneurysm and the status of the iliac vessels including the presence of occlusive disease in the pelvis that could decrease the efficacy of distal aortic perfusion.

Accurate assessment of the size of thoracic aortic aneurysms is contingent upon measurement in the appropriate perpendicular plane. When imaging a tortuous aorta or evaluating sections through the aortic arch or lower descending aorta, it is important to understand that individual axial images may section the aorta in a plane that is off axis. Such measurements result in an erroneous overestimation of aortic diameter and underscore the importance of personally viewing CT scans prior to initiation of therapy. One way to avoid this error is through three-dimensional reconstruction of the thoracic aorta with determination of the centerline of axis that ensures that any cross-sectional measurement will be perpendicular to the aortic axis. The quality of current CT scanners with three-dimensional reconstruction is exceptional, and in our practice, this has become the image modality of choice for the evaluation and treatment of thoracic aortic aneurysms.

Preoperative Evaluation

The majority of patients who undergo TAA resection will have degenerative aneurysms, and as such, most will be around 70 years of age with a history of hypertension. A history of cigarette smoking with some form of COPD is common, and up to 25% of patients have severe disease with an FEV1 < 50% predicted.

Cerebrovascular disease is also common, and up to 30% of patients will have some degree of associated visceral or renovascular disease, which could add complexity to the visceral portion of the repair. Indeed, the presence of extreme preoperative azotemia (GFR <30) constitutes a relative contraindication to elective repair unless preoperative studies show that there is some potential for recovery of function with renal artery reconstruction as the mere presence of renal disease is a predictor of increased mortality.

Despite the firm literature base against routine preoperative cardiac testing, all patients should be evaluated with physiologic testing to assess perioperative myocardial ischemic potential. In addition, patients with a history or symptoms suggestive of heart failure should have an assessment of left ventricular function. While patients with significant impairments of pulmonary reserve can usually be detected on a historical basis alone, we routinely obtain preoperative pulmonary function studies. Preoperative consultation with a pulmonologist for optimization of bronchodilator therapy and pulmonary toilet is an important component in the management of patients with significant COPD. However, institution of preoperative steroid therapy with the intent of improving respiratory function is contraindicated since we have observed this maneuver to precipitate aneurysm rupture. Finally, advanced age is an important component only in as much as it is accompanied by overall fragility and impaired functional status.

Surgical Treatment

Treatment Options

Graft replacement by direct surgical approach is the current standard of care for TAA. Total endovascular repair continues to evolve but remains limited by a lack of commercial availability of branched/fenestrated grafts and anatomic considerations. The hybrid approach that combines visceral artery debranching with endovascular exclusion of the TAA has allowed surgeons who lack the resources to perform distal perfusion to offer TAA repair to their complex patients, but the reported results compare poorly with open repair at high-volume centers. Medical therapy is appropriate in patients who are frail and have prohibitive associated comorbid conditions or small aneurysms. This consists of aggressive blood pressure control with beta-blockade, which has been shown to decrease the rate of aortic dilation. The goal of antihypertensive therapy is to keep the systolic pressure at a low-normal range of 105–120 mmHg, and this often requires additional medications to maintain. Risk factor modification is another important aspect of patient education regarding TAA. Patients should be counseled regarding smoking cessation and given appropriate support to achieve this goal as elective open TAA repair should not be offered to someone who is actively smoking.

Renal and Spinal Cord Protection

Outcomes of TAA repair are closely correlated with renal and spinal cord complications; accordingly, operative adjuncts to minimize these complications have been principal drivers of the technical conduct of the operation. Consistent with a firm literature base supporting regional hypothermic protection of the kidneys, our approach involves direct installation of renal preservation fluid (lactated Ringer's with 25 g of mannitol/L and 1 g/L methylprednisolone at 4 °C) into the renal ostium during ischemia. In type IV TAA, the left renal artery is transected prior to placing the proximal aortic clamp, and 250 mL of the renal cold solution is instilled into the artery followed by a continuous drip through a six French perfusion balloon-tipped catheter. Once the aorta is opened, renal cold is infused in the right renal artery through the ostium, which should be coursing down and away from the surgeon. In more complex TAA (type I–III), where distal perfusion is used, renal cold is given prior to the start of the visceral reconstruction. Experience has shown that such an infusion will result in a rapid decline of renal parenchymal temperature to 15 °C after the bolus infusion. During the continuous infusion, renal core temperatures remain in the 25 °C range as monitored by direct temperature probes in the renal cortex.

It is evident that most of the nuances, which drive the technical conduct of TAA repair, are directed toward the prevention of SCI, to wit, the abundance of adjuncts, which have been championed to minimize this dreaded complication. To date, only cerebrospinal fluid drainage is appropriately evidence based and used by most surgeons. Other adjuncts aimed at preserving spinal cord blood flow such as intercostal (IC) vessel reconstruction have been championed and/or routinely practiced despite its empiric nature and evidence base limited to retrospective studies including our own. The alternative position with specific respect to IC vessel reconstruction is that it is unnecessary (related to the collateral network) and expends cross-clamp time and blood turnover. Distal aortic perfusion via left atrial–femoral bypass used in conjunction with intraoperative motor-evoked potential (MEP) monitoring to dynamically assess spinal cord ischemia during the operation has replaced epidural cooling as our principal cord protective strategy in patients with more extensive TAA (type I–III). This is based upon a series of studies that used magnetic resonance imaging combined with intraoperative MEP to show that individual intercostal vessels were typically not critical for cord preservation and most collaterals that support the cord originated from the pelvis (i.e., hypogastric arteries); thus, preservation of continuous perfusion of the pelvis is logical and prudent. The addition of MEP monitoring affords the surgeon objective criteria to direct selective IC vessel reconstruction and thus replaces the subjective application of or routine posture toward intercostal vessel reimplantation. The use of MEP monitoring does mandate a departure from anesthetic techniques typically used in North America, and the technical requirements of such monitoring can only be satisfied by a dedicated team specialized in neurophysiology.

Technical Components

Operative Exposure

Irrespective of individual preferences concerning the technical components of the operation, the key to operative success remains the provision of broad, continuous exposure of the entire left posterolateral aspect of the thoracoabdominal aorta (Fig. 5.2). The patient is positioned on the table in the right lateral decubitus position. The location and extent of the thoracic portion of the incision are determined by the proximal extent of the aneurysm as the posterior portion of a standard posterolateral thoracotomy incision is only necessary for type I and type II aneurysms. We keep the thoracic portion of the incision low and have found that the fifth or sixth interspace with posterior division of the sixth or seventh rib provides adequate exposure for even the more proximal aneurysms (Fig. 5.3). The costal margin is divided at the level of the sixth interspace, and a self-retaining retractor system is placed in order to ensure continuous exposure of the entire operative field. A thoracoabdominal incision at the eighth interspace will usually provide adequate exposure for a type IV TAA, and a double lumen tube for deflation of the left lung is generally not necessary in these cases. The abdominal portion of the incision is not extended to the midline; rather, it is kept well lateral on the abdominal wall along

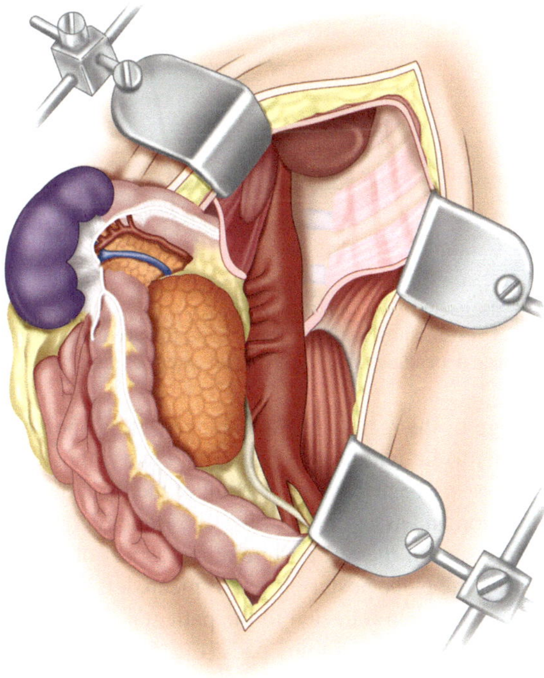

Fig. 5.2 Exposure for TAA repair. Exposure of the left chest and abdomen through a thoracoabdominal incision with the left kidney, spleen, pancreas, and left colon reflected up. This exposes the entire left posterolateral aspect of the TAA

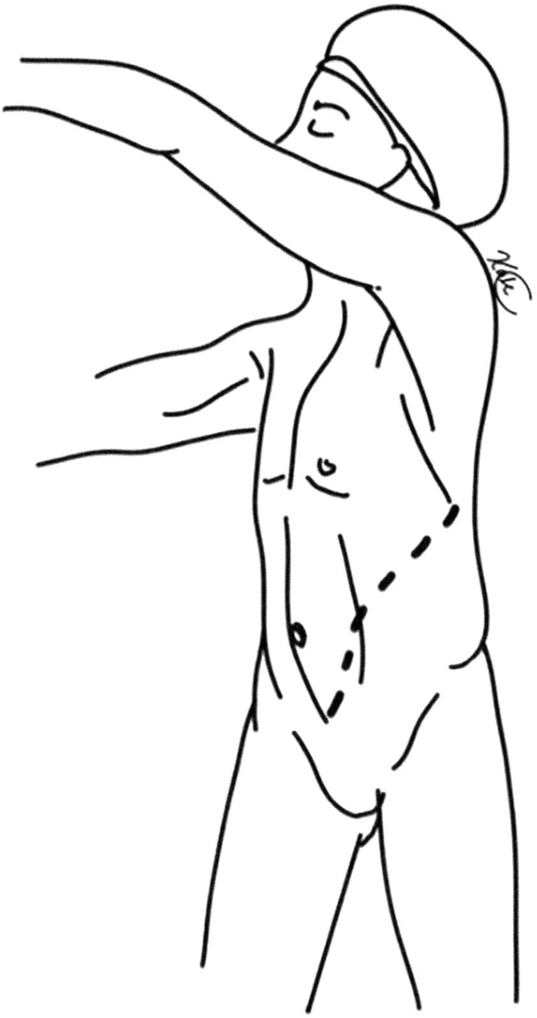

Fig. 5.3 Positioning for TAA repair. The thoracoabdominal incision is made in the ninth–fifth interspace depending upon the proximal extent of dissection

the edge of the rectus. The advantage of this approach is that it allows the visceral contents to lie within the abdominal cavity, thus decreasing evaporative fluid and heat losses. The abdominal portion of the incision is transperitoneal allowing direct inspection and assessment of the visceral circulation when the case is completed.

Exposure of the left posterolateral aspect of the abdominal aorta is obtained by entering the plane posterior to the spleen, left kidney, and left colon. The abdominal contents are then reflected to the patient's right and the left ureter is identified and preserved under laparotomy pads (Fig. 5.4). The retroperitoneal fatty and lymphatic tissues overlying the aorta are transected with electrocautery, and the renal–lumbar vein that courses across the aorta is identified and divided. Located topographically

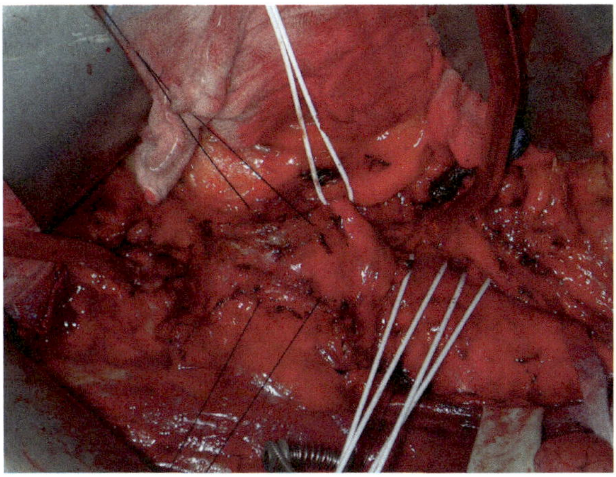

Fig. 5.4 Operative photo of exposure of the visceral segment. The vessel loop at 12 o'clock is around the left renal artery and the two loops at 6 o'clock are around the superior mesenteric and celiac arteries

close to this vein is the left renal artery. Once identified, the left renal artery is dissected toward its origin on the aorta. This serves as a suitable point to initiate the cephalad and caudal division of the retroperitoneal tissues over the aorta inferiorly and division of the median arcuate ligament and diaphragmatic crura superiorly.

There are several methods by which the incision in the diaphragm may be managed. The quickest and simplest method that affords excellent exposure is direct radial division of the diaphragm from underneath the costal margin to the aortic hiatus. This approach, however, will irrevocably paralyze the left hemidiaphragm and ultimately contribute to postoperative respiratory embarrassment. A second approach involves the circumferential division of the diaphragm through its muscular portion leaving a few centimeters attached laterally to the chest wall. There is benefit to preserving the phrenic innervation to the left hemidiaphragm by dividing only a portion lateral to the phrenic nerve insertion and then taking down the muscular fibers of the aortic hiatus. A large Penrose drain can be passed around the diaphragm pedicle and used to retract superiorly and inferiorly as needed during the reconstruction. We have applied this method liberally, particularly in patients with evidence of preoperative pulmonary compromise (Fig. 5.5).

Dissection of Left Pleural Space

After deflation of the left lung, the thoracic component of the dissection is typically straightforward. Electrocautery is used to divide the mediastinal pleura over the aneurysm and proximal aorta. For type I and type II aneurysms, proximal control of the aorta in the region of the left subclavian artery origin is necessary. Further mobility of the vagus nerve is gained by dividing it distal to the origin of the left

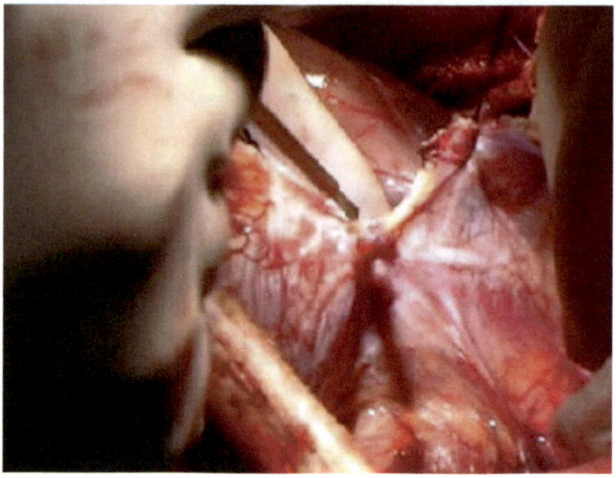

Fig. 5.5 Diaphragm management during extensive thoracoabdominal repair. Radial division provides rapid, direct, and uncompromised aortic exposure but causes left hemidiaphragm paralysis

recurrent nerve, which should be identified and preserved. Should more proximal control be necessary, the ligamentum arteriosum is divided on the underside of the aortic arch. Care must be taken to keep the dissection directly on the aortic arch in order to avoid injuring the left main pulmonary artery. When degenerative aneurysm is the underlying pathology, dissection in this area is usually straightforward. However, in patients with chronic dissection, the prior inflammation from the dissecting process makes exposure more difficult. The aorta is surrounded with a vessel tape on either side of the left subclavian artery depending on the proximal extent of the aneurysm. Blunt dissection on the posterior aspect of the aorta is used to clear sufficient normal aorta to allow placement of the cross-clamp while maintaining adequate length of the aorta for an accurate proximal aortic anastomosis. External control of the left subclavian artery is desirable but not mandatory as intraluminal balloon control can be obtained if the aortic clamp is placed proximal to the left subclavian artery. During the thoracic portion of the dissection, the left inferior pulmonary vein is isolated in cases where atrial–femoral bypass is used; a 4-0 Prolene purse-string suture is used to introduce the venous cannula, which in our experience need not be larger than 19 French.

Clamp and Sew Versus Atrial–Femoral Bypass

In contemporary practice, the clamp-and-sew technique with adjuncts to minimize warm ischemic time is the best way to approach type IV TAA. The technique of distal perfusion through atrial–femoral bypass via a centripetal, motorized pump is the simplest form of distal perfusion and requires no or low doses of systemic heparin to function. Conversely, cardiopulmonary bypass using a femoral vein to femoral artery technique requires an in-line oxygenator and full pump doses of heparin making it less desirable given the extensive dissection required to complete TAA repair. Most surgeons have adopted the liberal use of atrial–femoral bypass for extent I–III TAA. We prefer to continuously perfuse the mesenteric circulation during reconstruction of the visceral aortic segment. This can be accomplished with either a Y-connection from the atrial–femoral bypass circuit or in-line mesenteric shunting from the proximal graft after completion of the proximal anastomosis (Fig. 5.6).

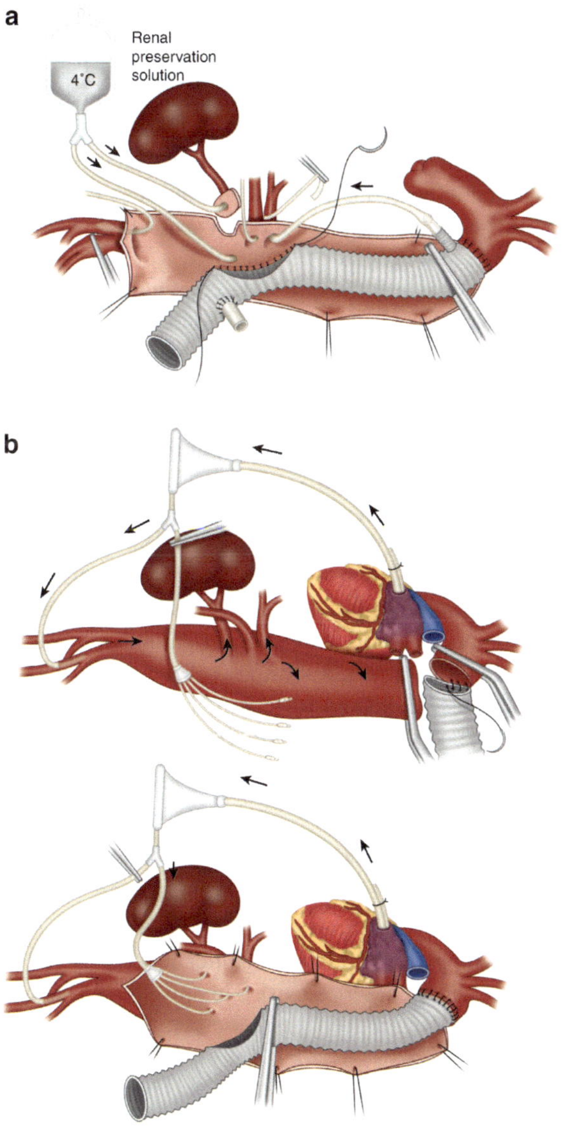

Fig. 5.6 Approaches to operative conduct of thoracoabdominal aneurysm repair. (**a**) Clamp-and-sew technique with associated adjuncts of mesenteric shunting, renal cold perfusion, and epidural cooling (not shown). (**b**) Distal perfusion (left heart bypass) using the heparin-impregnated Bio-Medicus pump where perfusion distal to the proximal cross-clamp is initially maintained via the femoral artery and then by multiple perfusion catheters once reconstruction proceeds distally

Clamping Sequence and Proximal Anastomosis

Next, the aortic prosthesis is prepared by attaching a 6 mm polytetrafluoroethylene (PTFE) sidearm graft that will serve as the conduit for left renal artery reconstruction. An additional sidearm graft of 10 mm PTFE may be placed proximally to provide inflow for the in-line mesenteric shunt. For most aneurysms, a Dacron prosthesis is the preferred conduit. However, a PTFE conduit is used to repair mycotic aneurysms because of its decreased susceptibility to infection.

Atrial–femoral bypass is initiated by cannulation of the left atrium through the left inferior pulmonary vein and the arterial return is via the left common femoral artery. Flows are initially adjusted to maintain distal mean perfusion pressures of at least 60–70 mmHg; any deterioration in MEP should prompt either an increase in the stimulus intensity or an increase in distal perfusion pressures. A sudden drop in MEP amplitude (occurring within 2–10 min) or a sustained progressive drop (within 10–40 min) of >75% from baseline is considered significant and should be addressed. The clamping sequence is begun in close cooperation with the anesthesia team. Efforts are made to place the first sequential clamp so as to allow lower intercostal and visceral retrograde perfusion.

In cases where the entire descending thoracic aorta is resected, proximal intercostal vessel orifices between T_4 and T_8 typically vigorously backbleed and those are rapidly oversewn. Intercostal vessels in the critical T_9 to L_1 aortic segment are evaluated for potential reimplantation, usually guided by changes in MEP signals. These vessels are controlled with balloon occlusion catheters to prevent ongoing backbleeding and also to prevent the negative "sump" effect on net spinal cord perfusion that can result from these vessel orifices when exposed only to atmospheric pressure. Unless there are prompt, significant changes in MEP, we defer any intercostal reconstruction to later stages of the operation. Next, the proximal aortic neck is prepared for reconstruction. Circumferential division of the aorta avoids the late complication of suture line esophageal erosion and permits the use of circumferential Teflon felt wrap if the aorta is particularly fragile and or/dissected. After completion of the proximal anastomosis, a clamp is placed on the main aortic graft distal to the mesenteric shunt sidearm (if present). The clamp is moved to the distal sequential clamp position and the visceral aortic segment is opened.

Renal/Visceral Artery Reconstruction

Visceral and renal artery reconstruction is carried out next. Orificial endarterectomy should be performed when significant occlusive lesions of the right renal and superior mesenteric arteries exist. This involves incising the diseased intima and media and developing a proper endarterectomy plane that can be verified by noting the pinkish color of the inner adventitia. In cases where aortic endarterectomy is required, the superior mesenteric and celiac arteries should be dissected sufficiently to facilitate countertraction from the external side of the vessel if necessary. This, however, is not possible with the right renal artery. In the event that the calcified end of the obstructing plaque does not feather nicely, sharp excision under direct vision is the best way to end the endarterectomy plane.

The most common method of visceral and renal artery reconstruction that has been employed in the majority of our cases is a single inclusion button that encompasses the origins of the celiac, superior mesenteric, and right renal arteries. If the aneurysm is excessively large in the visceral aortic segment, the wide separation of the visceral/renal ostia may necessitate individual inclusion button anastomoses for each vessel. Alternatively, the superior mesenteric artery and right renal artery can be reimplanted as a single inclusion while reconstruction of the celiac trunk is deferred until later. The aortic graft is placed under tension and an elliptical side island is excised from the main aortic graft. This ellipse usually begins on the lateral aspect of the graft and spirals posteriorly in the region of the right renal artery reconstruction. With the graft under tension, it is possible to complete the posterior portion of the anastomosis using single bites of the suture passing through both the aorta and the Dacron graft. Suture bites are taken close to the origin of the visceral vessels in order to avoid leaving excess aneurysmal aortic wall. As the posterior aspect of this suture line continues around the inferior border of the right renal artery, it is important to ensure that the lumen is not compromised. This can be accomplished by placing a 12F perfusion catheter in the artery and gently agitating it up and down, or more recently, we have used a 6 × 15 or 6 × 18 balloon expandable stent to ensure that the suture line does not compromise right renal artery flow. The stent is placed under direct vision after the proximal suture line is beyond the orifice of the artery (Fig. 5.7). Just prior to completion of this suture line, backbleeding and patency of the celiac, superior mesenteric, and right renal arteries are verified and the in-line mesenteric shunt is clamped and removed. A single flush of the proximal aortic cross-clamp is performed in order to ensure that no clot or debris has built up in the graft.

Reconstruction of the left renal artery is now accomplished with a separate sidearm graft of a 6 mm PTFE. This provides a direct deliberate anastomosis in end-to-end fashion while allowing flexibility to deal with the spectrum of occlusive lesions, multiple renal arteries, and other wrinkles that may be encountered. It is important to orient this sidearm graft so that it will not kink when the left renal artery is returned to its anatomic position. Some surgeons advocate the use of a single inclusion button that contains the renal arteries and the visceral vessels. This often requires the inclusion of too great an area of the native, aneurysmal aorta, unless the aneurysm is small in the visceral artery segment. A single, pristine left renal artery and orifice may be directly reimplanted, and the clamp is then advanced to a position inferior to the origin of the left renal artery graft prior to completing the distal aortic anastomosis.

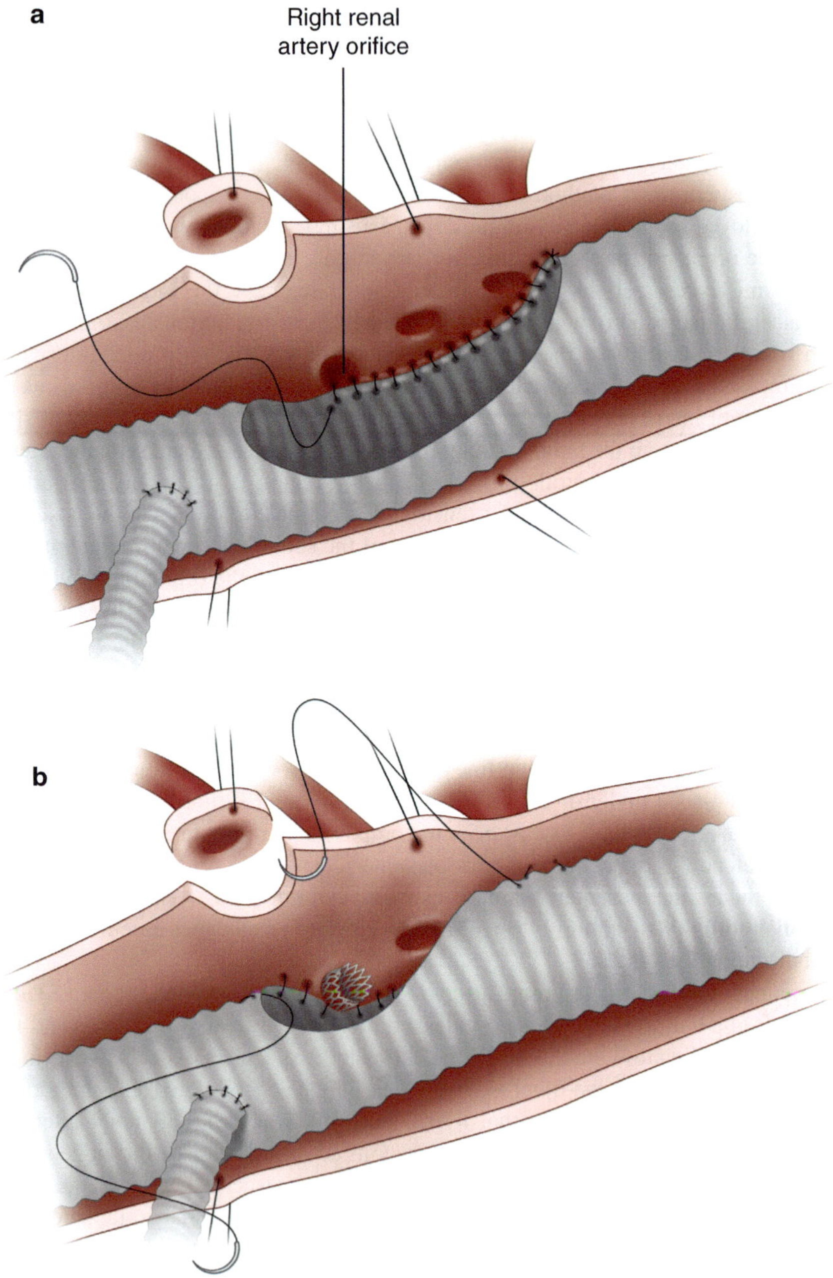

Fig. 5.7 (**a**) Creation of visceral button inclusion anastomosis of the celiac axis, SMA, and right renal artery and 6 mm PTFE sidearm bypass for left renal artery reconstruction. When performing this, we use a 12F perfusion catheter as a stent of sorts in the right renal artery to prevent compromise of its orifice as the anastomosis is carried around these arterial origins. (**b**) Deployment of balloon-expandable stent into the right renal orifice to either treat occlusive lesions or prevent encroachment by the suture line, which should be placed immediately at or into the vessel ostia

Reconstruction of Intercostal Vessels

The next step in the operation involves the intercostal vessels in the T_9 to L_1 segment. If there have been no MEP changes during the operation, the occlusion balloons are removed and the remaining intercostals are oversewn with silk sutures. If, however, reconstruction is desired, it can usually be accomplished through an inclusion button anastomosis. Other methods of intercostal vessel revascularization include the attachment of additional short sidearm grafts to the main aortic graft, or in cases where the vessel origin is rotated superiorly and to the patient's left side, implantation to the main aortic graft using Carrel patches of the aorta that contain the intercostal vessels may be feasible (Fig. 5.8).

Distal Anastomosis

We make every effort to perform tube type of reconstructions to the aortic bifurcation unless there is gross aneurysmal disease of the proximal common iliac arteries. Extending the reconstruction to separate iliac artery reconstructions or, indeed, tunneling to an aortofemoral graft configuration is only performed when no other

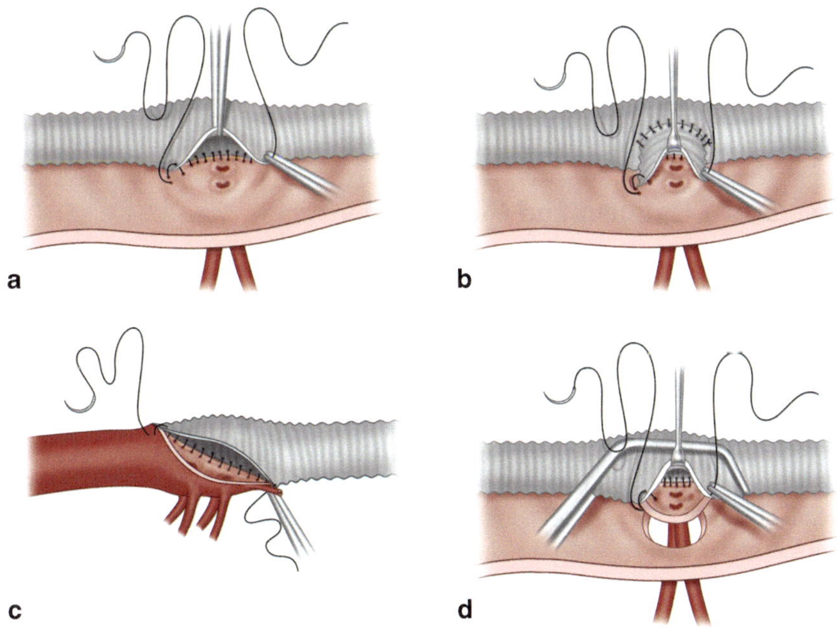

Fig. 5.8 Methods of management of critical intercostal arteries. (**a**) Inclusion button anastomosis. (**b**) Separate sidearm graft. (**c**) Beveled anastomosis preservation when possible. (**d**) Carrell patch mobilization and direct reimplantation into the graft

technical alternative exists. After reestablishment of flow to the lower extremities and verification of adequate lower extremity perfusion by intraoperative pulse volume recordings, Doppler signals in the left renal, celiac, and superior mesenteric vessels are checked in addition to palpation of the superior mesenteric artery pulse in the root of the mesentery.

Postoperative Care

Postoperatively, patients should be monitored in an intensive care unit (ICU) setting. It is important to limit hemodynamic shifts as these can contribute to complications such as renal failure and spinal cord ischemia. Blood pressure parameters should be tailored to the patient with the goal of maintaining adequate perfusion to preserve urine output, cardiac function, and spinal cord perfusion. Oxygen delivery is important in the early phase of recovery, and we rarely extubate patients in the early postoperative period. It they have stabilized overnight, we will pull the tube in the morning. It is important to monitor the hematocrit for signs of ongoing bleeding and all coagulation disorders should be aggressively corrected with the appropriate products. We typically support intravascular volume with fresh frozen plasma (FFP) infusions for the initial 12 h after the operation. CSF drainage is arbitrarily continued for 48 h postoperatively, and the drain is then capped for 24 h of observation prior to removal. Discontinuation of some preoperative antihypertensive medications may be necessary to maintain the relative hypertension necessary to avoid delayed SCI.

Results of Treatment and Complications

Operative Mortality

The operative mortality after TAA ranges from 8% to 16% in large clinical series. Preoperative patient characteristics influence the patient's outcome regardless of the conduct of the operation. In a recent update of our experience with type I–III TAA, a 30-day mortality was 4.4% for elective TAA repaired with atrial–femoral bypass and MEP monitoring. As the number of co-morbid conditions increases so does the overall operative risk, and individual series have reported that preoperative coronary artery disease, COPD, and renal insufficiency contribute to postoperative organ-specific complications and increased mortality. The influence of TAA extent is often (and appropriately) emphasized as having a dominant effect on, in particular, spinal cord ischemia. In particular, perioperative death after type IV TAA repair should mirror that of infrarenal repair. To wit, in our recent published experience, the 30-day mortality for type IV TAA repaired with the clamp-and-sew method was 2.8%.

Renal Failure

We have traditionally defined postoperative renal failure as a doubling of the baseline serum creatinine level or an absolute postoperative creatinine level of >3.0 mg/dL. Minimizing renal ischemic times, the use of cold perfusate, avoidance of intraoperative hypotension, and a posture of aggressive treatment of stenotic lesions with either bypass or open stent placement are all strategies used to avoid postoperative renal insufficiency. Most cases are self-limited. We reserve dialysis for patients that need it for specific clinic indications such as volume overload, hyperkalemia, or acidosis. When needed, continuous venovenous hemodialysis is our preferred method as it provides for a smoother hemodynamic course than conventional hemodialysis. For those patients who continue to require dialysis, conventional hemodialysis is instituted once the patient is out of the intensive care unit and out of the window of risk for spinal cord ischemia. In our experience, and that of others, preoperative renal insufficiency is the most powerful predictor for the development of postoperative renal failure, and postoperative renal dysfunction remains independently associated with short- and long-term survival.

Respiratory Complications

Although most clinical series emphasize spinal cord and renal complications, respiratory failure is the single most common complication after TAA repair. Indeed, if strict criteria are used, up to 40% of patients will suffer some type of respiratory complication. Contributing factors include paralysis of the left hemidiaphragm and the pain associated with an extensive chest wall incision that impedes pulmonary toilet. Accordingly, a diaphragm-sparing technique is applied when possible in contemporary practice. For patients that fail extubation, we favor early placement of a tracheostomy, although this procedure has been needed in less than 10% of patients. A slow wean from ventilatory support, often planned to proceed over several days, is appropriate management in patients with extensive TAA resection, particularly those with bascline pulmonary insufficiency.

Spinal Cord Ischemia

Since the first descriptions of TAA repair, SCI has been the most feared and devastating nonfatal complication associated with TAA reconstruction. The pathogenesis of spinal cord injury after aortic replacement is likely multifactorial but ultimately results from an ischemic insult caused by temporary or permanent interruption of the spinal cord blood supply. SCI manifests along a clinical spectrum from complete flaccid paraplegia to varying degrees of temporary or permanent paraparesis, and the degree of SCI directly predicts long-term survival after TAA repair. Patients with incomplete deficits typically made a reasonable or complete functional outcome and have a long-term survival that is similar to those without SCI. However, patients with an SCID I score (flaccid paralysis) rarely live beyond the first year. The most common predictors of SCI after TAA repair include extent I and II aneurysms and urgency of operation. While a majority of cases of SCI are detected in the immediate postoperative period, there is a trend toward an increase in delayed paralysis in recent series.

Late Outcomes

While some studies report significant continued mortality throughout the first year after operation (up to 30%), these reports include centers where the perioperative mortality approached 19%. It is, therefore, difficult to put these data into context with data from centers where the perioperative mortality is 5–8%. We found the late survival in our patients was identical to that from a population-based study of patients who underwent elective AAA. In addition, late aortic events occur in about 10% of patients, but few of these are graft related. Graft-related complications include occlusion of visceral vessel reconstructions, graft infections (including aortoesophageal fistulas), and the appearance of inclusion patch aneurysms and are rare in our experience. Most late aortic events are the result of native aneurysmal disease in remote (or noncontiguous) aortic segments. These data indicate that the substantial resource investment required to bring these patients through successful operation and recovery is an appropriate expenditure of such resources. With improvement of perioperative outcomes, the focus of long-term follow-up has shifted to examination of the impact of TAA repair on functional outcome. Several reports have emerged validating that a majority of operative survivors return to their preoperative independent living status.

Further Reading

Acher CW, Wynn M. A modern theory of paraplegia in the treatment of aneurysms of the thoracoabdominal aorta: an analysis of technique specific observed/expected ratios for paralysis. J Vasc Surg. 2009;49:1117–24.

Bischoff MS, Di Luozzo G, Griepp EB, et al. Spinal cord preservation in thoracoabdominal aneurysm repair. Perspect Vasc Surg Endovasc Ther. 2011;23(3):214–22.

Conrad MF, Ergul E, Patel VI, et al. Evolution of operative strategies in open thoracoabdominal aneurysm repair (TAA). J Vasc Surg. 2011;53:1195–201.

Conrad MF, Ye JY, Chung TK, et al. Spinal cord complications after thoracic aortic surgery: long-term survival and functional status varies with deficit severity. J Vasc Surg. 2008;48:47–53.

Coselli JS, Bozinowski J, LeMaire SA. Open surgical repair of 2286 thoracoabdominal aortic aneurysms. Ann Thorac Surg. 2007;83:S862–4.

Crawford RS, Pedraza JD, Chung TK, et al. Functional outcome after thoracoabdominal aneurysm repair. J Vasc Surg. 2008;48:828–35.
Lancaster RT, Conrad MF, Patel VI, et al. Further experience with distal aortic perfusion and motor-evoked potential monitoring in the management of extent I-III thoracoabdominal aortic aneurysms. J Vasc Surg. 2013;58:283–90.
Mohebali J, Latz CA, Cambria RP, Lancaster RT, Conrad MF, Clouse WD. The long-term fate of renal and visceral vessel reconstruction after open thoracoabdominal aortic aneurysm repair. J Vasc Surg. 2021;74(6):1825–32.
Patel VI, Ergul E, Conrad MF, et al. Continued favorable results with open surgical repair of Type IV thoracoabdominal aortic aneurysms. J Vasc Surg. 2011;53:1492–8.

Chapter 6
Inflammatory Abdominal Aortic Aneurysm

Sachinder Singh Hans

Inflammatory abdominal aortic aneurysms (AAA) have a defining triad of thickened aneurysmal wall, extensive perianeurysmal fibrosis, and dense adhesions to the ureter and duodenum. In most patients, a diagnosis of inflammatory AAA can be suspected by a CTA of the abdomen and pelvis. Laparotomy findings reveal that the aneurysm is encased in a thick, shining dense fibrotic tissue. The fibrotic tissue is contiguous with the surrounding structures. This fibrotic tissue starts near the renal arteries and usually extends to the bifurcation of the common iliac arteries (CIA) on both sides. Certain modifications in the surgical treatment of inflammatory AAA are necessary to obtain satisfactory outcome. Proximal aortic control is obtained with minimal dissection.

1. The fourth portion of the duodenum is carefully dissected to the right, but the third portion of the duodenum should not be dissected from the aneurysmal wall (Fig. 6.1).
2. Common iliac artery bifurcation is then dissected carefully, and on the left side, the incision is made in the white line of Toldt to expose the left common iliac bifurcation with exposure of the ureter. Similarly, on the right side, the common iliac bifurcation is exposed under the small bowel mesentery with exposure of the ureter. In most patients, the distal anastomosis can be performed to CIA above the bifurcation, but in some instances, both CIA may have to be divided and sutured and anastomosis performed to the proximal external iliac arteries (EIA). Rarely, if the diameter of the EIA is small, distal reconstruction with femoral anastomosis may become necessary.

S. S. Hans (✉)
Vascular and Endovascular Services, Henry Ford Macomb Hospital,
Clinton Twp, MI, USA

S. S. Hans et al. (eds.), *Primary and Repeat Arterial Reconstructions*,
https://doi.org/10.1007/978-3-031-13897-3_6

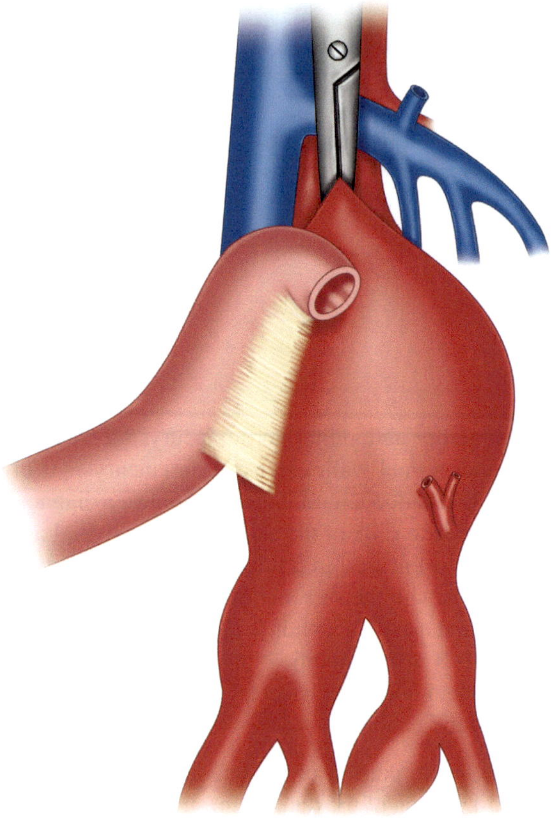

Fig. 6.1 Appearance of inflammatory AAA. The duodenum firmly adherent to the anterolateral wall of AAA. Proximal clamp applied to the aorta just below the renal arteries with the retraction of the left renal vein superiorly

3. After distal iliac and proximal aortic clamps are applied, the incision is made in the aneurysmal wall toward the left of the duodenum, and the wall of the aneurysm is retracted together as one structure toward the right using blade of a self-retaining retractor as described in chapter on infrarenal AAA (Fig. 6.2). Occasionally in patients with lumbar scoliosis, the neck of the AAA may need to be exposed through a right subhepatic approach. In such circumstances, aneurysm with adherent duodenum is exposed on the right side, as the aneurysmal wall is divided along with the attached duodenum to the right of the second and third portions of the duodenum exposing the lumen of the aneurysm (Fig. 6.3). The remaining steps of the operation are like those outlined in Chap. 2.

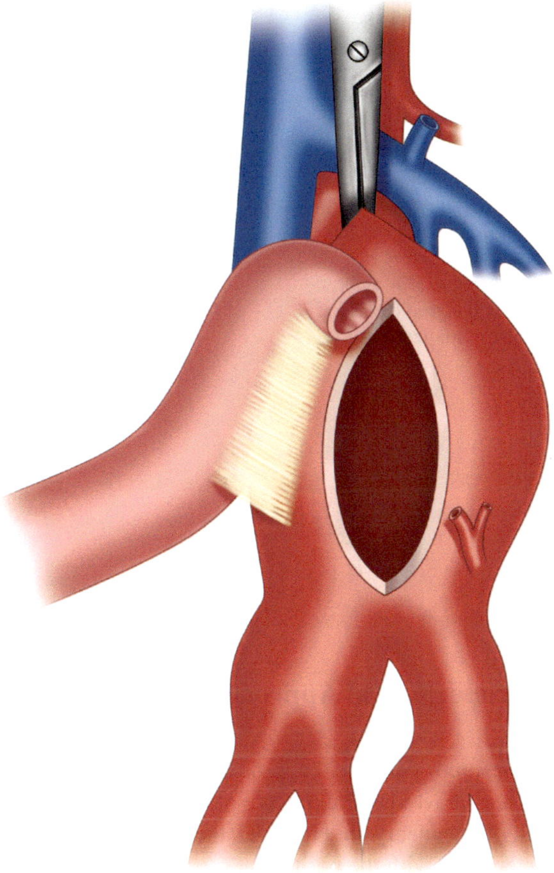

Fig. 6.2 Aneurysm is opened but the duodenum is left attached to the aneurysmal wall. Aortic and iliac anastomosis is carried out in a standard fashion

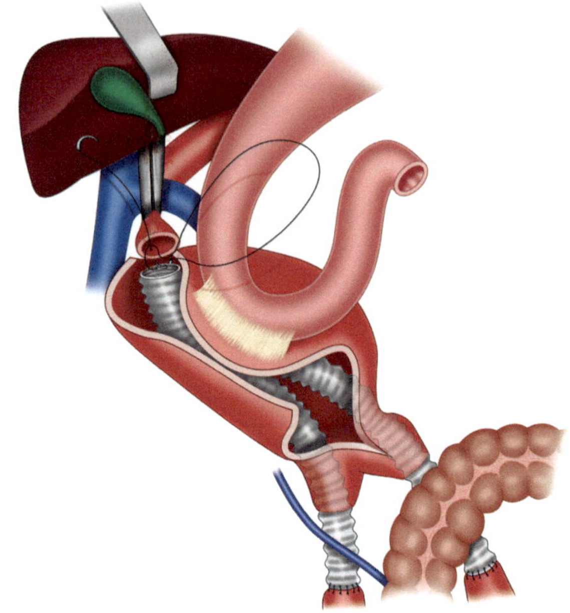

Fig. 6.3 In a patient with scoliosis, there may be extreme angulation of the aortic neck. An inflammatory AAA is shown with the duodenum firmly adherent to the aneurysmal wall. A subhepatic approach is useful for exposure of the aortic neck in these circumstances. The right ureter and sigmoid colon are also visualized

Retroperitoneal Approach

The left retroperitoneal approach is extremely useful for the repair of inflammatory AAA as it avoids the exposure of the duodenum, which is intimately adherent to the wall of the aneurysm. However, the left ureter should be carefully reflected forwards (anteriorly) with the peritoneal sac.

Complications

Venous bleeding from the posterior renal lumbar vein (collar vein) and iliac vein should be carefully avoided as they are more prone to injury because of the inflammatory process. Ureters are also involved in the inflammatory process and should be carefully exposed and protected near the CIA bifurcation.

Take-Home Points

1. Proximal dissection should be limited to the exposure of the left renal vein and renal arteries, and no attempt should be made to separate the duodenum from the wall of the AAA.

Chapter 7
Repair of Aortoenteric Fistula

Timothy J. Nypaver

Aortoenteric Fistula: Operative Management with in-Line Replacement

An aortoenteric fistula (AEF), whether primary or secondary, represents one of the most challenging and dreaded of vascular surgical complications. Secondary AEFs are related to a prior aortic reconstruction and are the most common type of AEF. Secondary AEFs occur because of communication between a previously placed aortic graft or endograft and the bowel, typically located in the third or fourth portions of the duodenum. The communication between the gastrointestinal (GI) tract and the graft material can involve either the anastomosis, a true AEF (Fig. 7.1), or the graft body or limb, a prosthetic enteric erosion. This chapter will outline steps involved in a management of a hemodynamically stable patient diagnosed with an AEF in which aortic graft excision with in-line aortic graft replacement is being considered, typically with a replacement conduit, which is resistant to infection. This mandates familiarity and experience with either harvesting of femoral vein or the use of cryopreserved allografts or, finally, Rifampin-soaked Dacron grafts. This review will concentrate on graft excision with in-line placement with either cryopreserved arterial allografts or Rifampin-impregnated Dacron grafts when the former is not available. Due to the presence of infection with associated inflammation and the recurrent nature of the operative procedure, in-line repair of a secondary AEF is a technically difficult operation, even for the most experienced of vascular surgeons.

Caveats of the operation include the administration of broad-spectrum antibiotics and importantly the necessity of acquiring a cryopreserved allograft prior to the

T. J. Nypaver (✉)
Division of Vascular Surgery, Henry Ford Hospital, Detroit, MI, USA
e-mail: TNYPAVE1@hfhs.org

S. S. Hans et al. (eds.), *Primary and Repeat Arterial Reconstructions*, https://doi.org/10.1007/978-3-031-13897-3_7

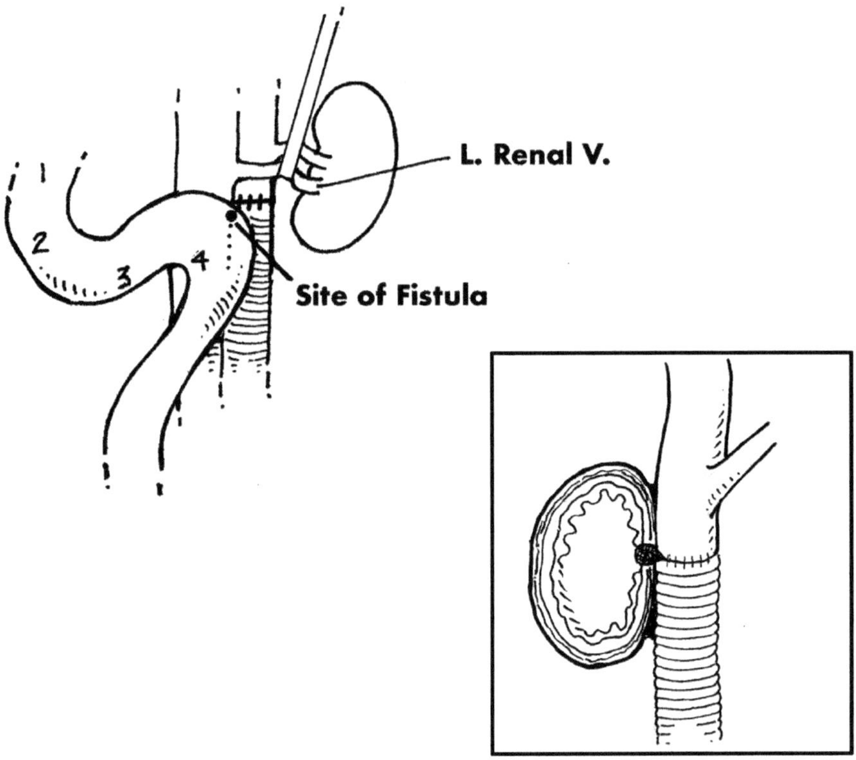

Fig. 7.1 Schematic representing an aortoenteric fistula with involvement of the proximal anastomosis and the fourth portion of the duodenum. Insert: cross-sectional view of anastomotic involvement

aortic procedure. One needs to obtain proximal control above the area of the anastomosis of the previously placed graft or endograft. Extensive debridement of any aortic wall and/or inflammatory tissue associated with the periaortic tissue and tissue around the entire course of the graft must be undertaken. Finally, the duodenal or bowel defect has to be appropriately and expertly closed along with omental coverage of the newly placed in-line conduit, separating the allograft or Dacron graft from the bowel repair and providing a milieu where antibiotic therapy will be the most effective.

The conduct of the operation involves a series of sequential steps, which culminate in the performance of repair of the AEF with in-line graft replacement. This includes (1) initial midline incision and with lysis of adhesion, (2) mobilization of the supraceliac aorta with supraceliac aortic control, (3) distal arterial exposure either at the level of the iliac vessels or at the femoral vessel level, (4) preparation of the conduit of choice: Rifampin-soaked Dacron or cryopreserved graft, (5) dissection into the inflammatory process with mobilization of the graft and exposure of the aortoenteric fistula with exposure of the suprarenal aorta to allow for suprarenal clamping, (6) excision of the proximal portion of the graft and debridement of the proximal infrarenal aorta with subsequent performance of a circumferential proximal anastomosis, (7) reestablishment of renal perfusion (or visceral perfusion if a supraceliac clamp is in place), (8) extensive and complete debridement of the graft and the aortic tissue/wall in proximity to the previously placed graft, and (9) reconstruction of the distal anastomosis at the iliac or femoral level. After performance of the proximal anastomosis and prior to a complete debridement, some form of temporary restoration of distal flow would be advisable and can be accomplished with graft (either a limb of the Rifampin-soaked graft or the iliac branch of the cryopreserved allograft) to distal arterial shunting.

Procedure

The patient is positioned supine and prepped from the neck to the knees. A long midline incision is preferred with proximal control obtained initially at the supraceliac aorta. This is accomplished via mobilization of the left lobe of the liver via dissection in the gastrohepatic ligament and retraction of the gastroesophageal junction to the left. The diaphragmatic crus muscle fibers are exposed and then retracted parallel with their orientation directly onto the aortic pulsation (Fig. 7.2). Blunt finger dissection through the diaphragmatic crus exposes the anterior surface of the aorta, which is then dissected free of the surrounding tissue (anteriorly), and then, one proceeds with exposure on each lateral side, using a combination of blunt finger dissection and instrument dissection (Fig. 7.3). It is important not to extend the exposure to the posterior aorta as one can easily injure the intercostal vessels, which would result in troublesome bleeding. Mobilization is performed with allowance,

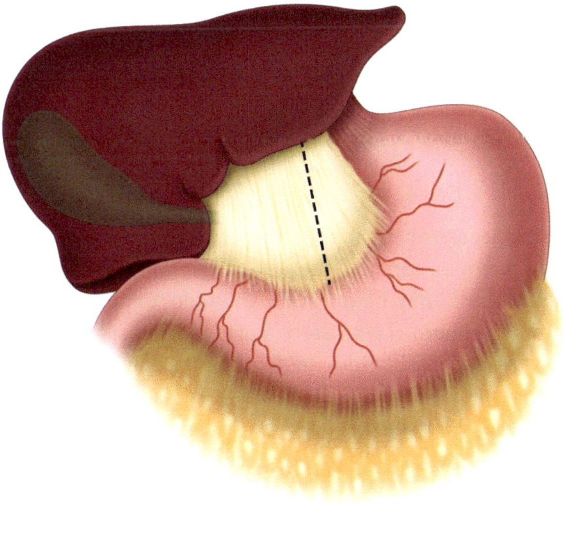

Fig. 7.2 Incision site in the gastrohepatic ligament initiating exposure of the supraceliac aorta

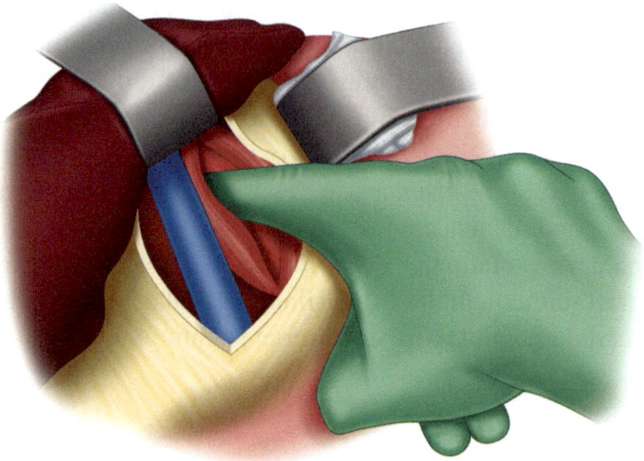

Fig. 7.3 Division and separation of the crural fibers of the diaphragmatic crus with exposure of the anterior surface of the aorta

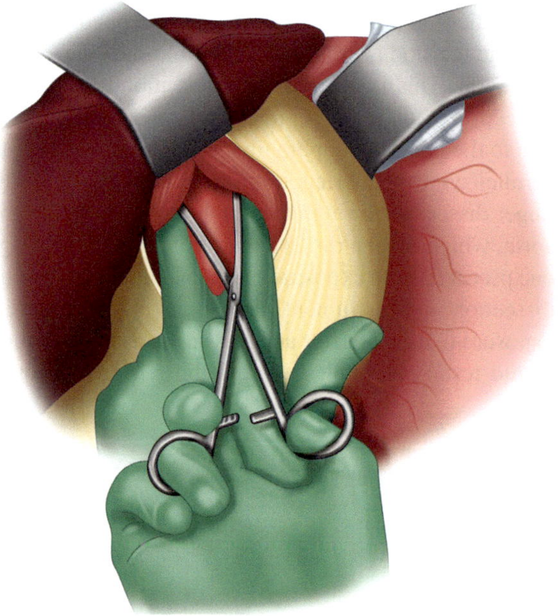

Fig. 7.4 Once lateral exposure is obtained on each side of the aorta, an atraumatic vascular clamp is applied; note there is no dissection of the posterior aorta

when necessary, of application of a vascular clamp (Fig. 7.4). Occasionally, because of a previous surgical operations and adhesions in the area, dissection of the supraceliac aorta may be difficult, and then, exposure is obtained via the standard infrarenal exposure. This can be particularly useful in situations where the initial graft was placed well below the level of the renal arteries in which a segment of normal infrarenal aortic neck is visible. It is also important during the entry into the abdomen that the omentum is carefully preserved as well as the vasculature to the omentum to allow for subsequent performance of the omental wrap.

At this point of the operation, the surgeon has the proximal control and proceeds with lysis of adhesions to allow for exposure of the distal vasculature. Distal control is usually accomplished at the iliac vessels with mobilization up to the area of the aortic bifurcation. The retroperitoneum is divided over the iliac vessels directly and distally to the prior graft placement. One needs to stay medial to the course of the ureters. Preoperative ureteral stents are beneficial in the identification of the ureters or immediate identification of a ureteral injury. Distal control may be required at the level of the femoral arteries with exposure in a standard fashion through longitudinal decisions. At this point, one begins the tedious aortic dissection around the aortoenteric fistula, recognizing that a portion of the duodenum will be stuck down to the graft (Fig. 7.5). This requires division and dissection of surrounding inflammatory tissue with some component of sharp dissection with eventual exposure of the aortic graft on its anterior surface. The dissection then proceeds superiorly. Again, it is important not to enter the aortoenteric fistula until one has completed as much of the dissection as possible. The conduit of choice should now be readily available. If bleeding is encountered, then supraceliac aortic control and digital control can be obtained with the dissection continuing expeditiously with the goal of exposing a segment of the infrarenal aorta. It is very common to need to continue the dissection into a segment of non-inflamed aorta, and this typically indicates exposure of the suprarenal aorta. Mobilization on each side of the aorta just superior to both the right and left renal artery is accomplished with gentle dissection. This area is usually free of previous scar tissue and some of the inflammatory process related to the infection. If the suprarenal aorta is freed of surrounding tissue, a suprarenal clamp in placed, the supraceliac clamp is removed, limiting visceral ischemia.

If possible, prior to proximal clamp placement, the patient is given an appropriate heparin dose, typically 70 mg/kg and intravenous mannitol 25 to 50 g. At this point, the patient will be experiencing either visceral or renal ischemia, and thus, it is important to proceed with the operation rather than spend excessive time with arterial wall and graft debridement. It is expected and anticipated that the third or fourth portion of the duodenum will be entered, and it is mandatory to limit the bowel enteric contamination; this is generally easily accomplished with the use of

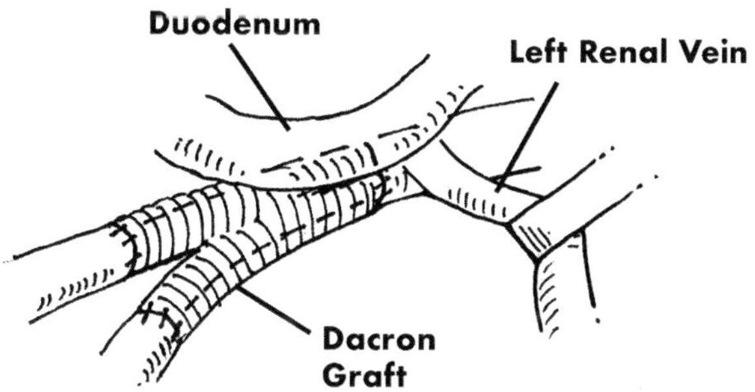

Fig. 7.5 The relationship of the left renal vein, the graft and the proximal anastomosis, and the duodenum

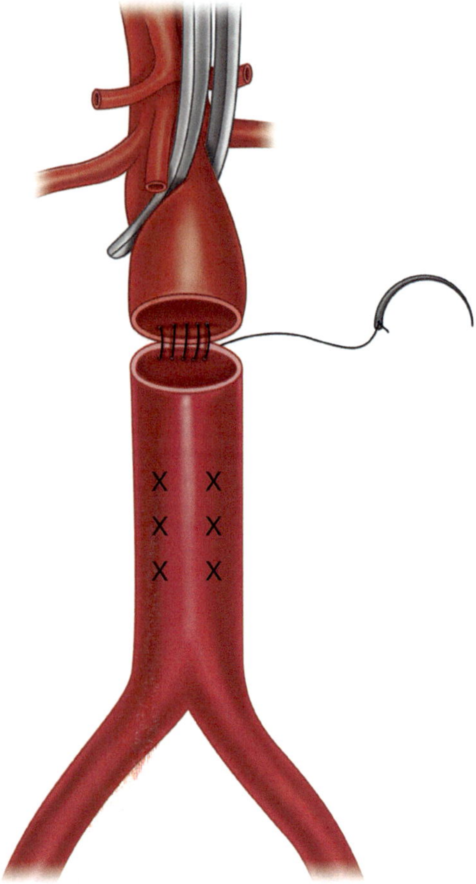

Fig. 7.6 The anastomosis is accomplished in a circumstantial fashion with 3-0 polypropylene suture with bites into the aortic wall near or at the level of the renal arteries. Adjusted suture bites and travel between bites accommodate any size discrepancy between the aorta and the conduit of choice (cryopreserved allograft or a Dacron graft)

bowel clamps and laparotomy pads. The duodenal repair is accomplished at a later point. The anastomosis is accomplished in a circumstantial fashion with 3-0 polypropylene suture with bites into the aortic wall near or at the level of the renal arteries accommodating any size discrepancy with adjusted bites into the conduit of choice, be it a cryopreserved allograft or a Dacron graft (Fig. 7.6). The anastomosis is checked, and if hemostatic, large Fogarty clamps with soft inserts are applied to the graft. With the release of the suprarenal clamp, renal perfusion is restored. Debridement of any inflammation or infection is completed including removal or excision of all the remaining graft material. Complete excision of the preexisting graft is mandatory. The time spent excising any grossly infected or inflammatory tissue is a critically important component of in-line replacement therapy and should not be accomplished in haste. This often requires a debridement of the aortic wall up to the level of the inferior vena cava. Following this, the anastomoses are performed to each uninvolved iliac artery, preferably beyond the prior graft anastomosis.

If the graft does extend down to the femoral arteries, the groin incisions are accomplished first with exposure of the femoral arteries and the graft. The native arteries are exposed proximal and distal to the site of the prior anastomosis. A two-team approach is beneficial to expedite the operation. Access to the retroperitoneal tunnels down to the level of the femoral arteries is maintained within umbilical tape; laparotomy pads can be passed through the tunnels accomplishing some additional debridement while maintaining access. Due to the significant retroperitoneal adhesions that are typically encountered, creation of a new tunnel is difficult with a significant risk of iliac vein injury. It is useful to divide the graft limb just above the anastomosis to allow for perfusion through the common femoral profunda–femoral-superficial femoral artery circuit, thereby limiting limb ischemia. The author has also placed a Sundt shunt through the end of the cryopreserved or Rifampin-soaked Dacron graft limb and the other end into the distal graft above the anastomosis; this maintains perfusion to one limb, while the other limb will be sewn to the distal artery. Once the distal anastomosis is ready to be performed, the arteries proximal and distal to the graft are clamped, any remaining graft material is completely excised, and the distal anastomosis is now performed. In most instances, when doing the groin reconstruction, the author attempts to preserve retrograde flow. However, in practice, many of the groin anastomoses are accomplished in an end-to-end fashion. Providing coverage of the groin anastomoses, the rotational sartorius muscle is useful and performed when possible. The skin of the groin wound is left open with the application of a VAC dressing.

Following both distal anastomoses, flow is completely restored, and attention turns toward the duodenal defect. The defect is typically closed in a transverse fashion (Fig. 7.7). If the duodenal defect is large, a segmental resection with end-to-end anastomosis is performed. Finally, a segment of the omentum is mobilized and wrapped around the recently placed cryopreserved arterial allograft or Rifampin-soaked Dacron graft (Fig. 7.8). The omental pedicles are created by dividing the omentum perpendicular to the omental arteries, typically using the right or left omental arteries as the inflow to the wrap.

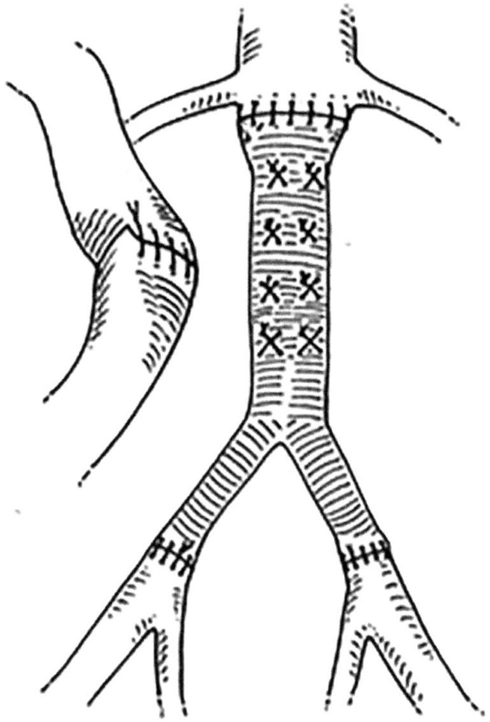

Fig. 7.7 The duodenal defect closed in a transverse fashion

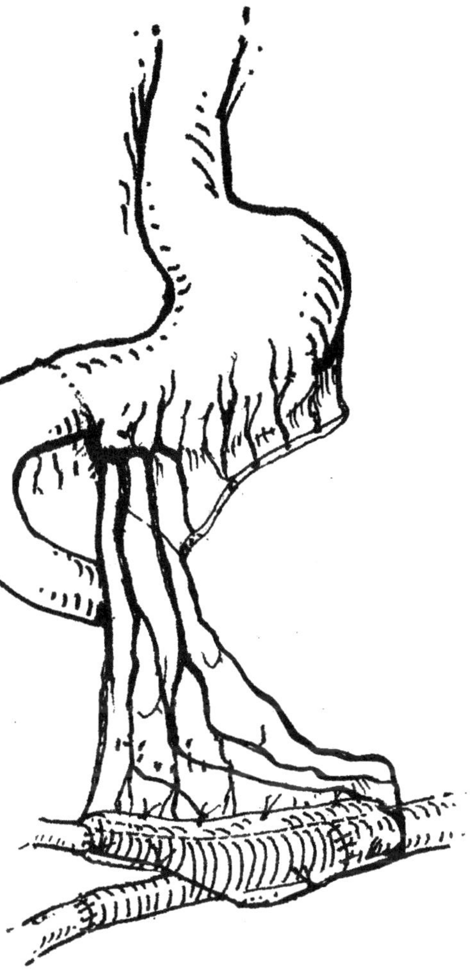

Fig. 7.8 Schematic representing the omental wrap based upon the right omental artery

Use of the Cryopreserved Arterial Allograft

When time allows, this is our preferred treatment method for in-line repair of AEF. The graft and appropriate sizes of the aortic allograft are determined to be available. The graft is prepared as the operation ensues as there is a defined manufactural de-thawing process in the preparation of the cryopreserved allograft. The thawing process averages approximately 30–40 min. Slits to enlarge the circumference of the proximal portion of the graft may have to be performed to accommodate the anastomosis due to the size discrepancy. Rather than using a single opening in the allograft, incisions are made into the allograft both 3 o'clock and 9 o'clock

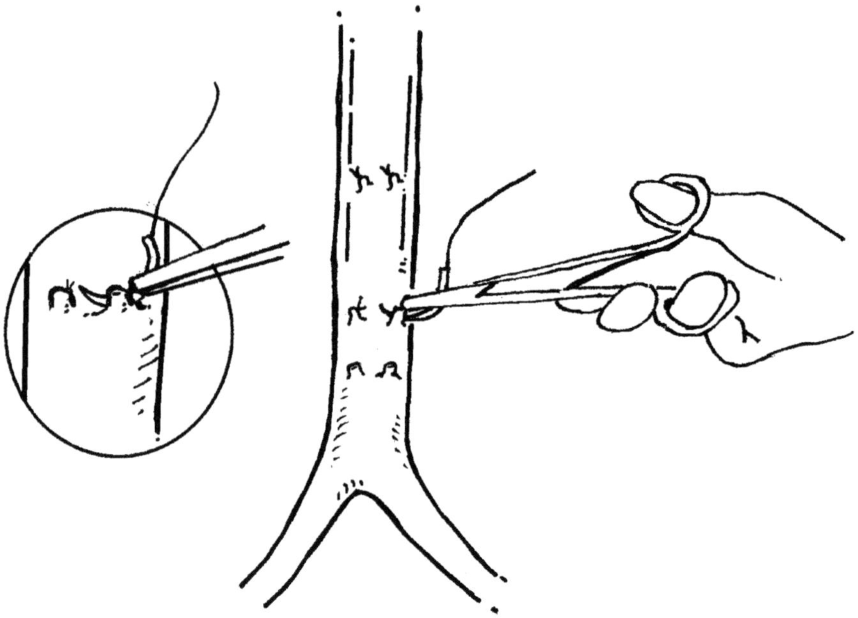

Fig. 7.9 Preparation of the cryopreserved graft with the graft rotated with the lumbar arteries oriented anteriorly. Insert: the lumbar branches are oversewn with 4-0 Prolene sutures, typically with a figure-of-eight suture

positions for appropriate sizing. The graft is rotated so that the lumbar orifices are positioned anteriorly—each lumbar artery is to be oversewn with interrupted sutures of 4-0 Prolene (rather than just tying off the branch). Any additional holes or leaks in the allograft are also suture ligated (Fig. 7.9).

Use of the Rifampin-Impregnated (Soaked) Dacron Graft

The most used agent for antimicrobial impregnation of prosthetic grafts is soaking the graft in the antibiotic solution of Rifampin. Prosthetic grafts form an ionic bond with the Rifampin primarily through the gelatin that is used in the sealant process. The antibiotic is released locally and gradually for a period of up to 5 days (Fig. 7.10).

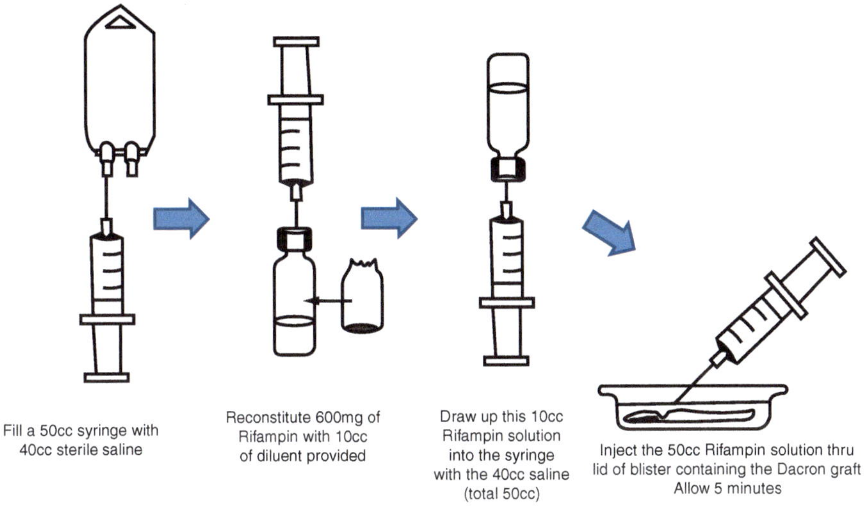

Fig. 7.10 Preparation sequence for the Rifampin-soaked Dacron graft

Complications

This is an extensive operation, one which has a significant physiologic insult to the patient. Complications are generally related to the systemic response (early) and the potential for additional infectious complications (late). Appropriate antibiotic coverage should be sustained for a minimum of 6 months and potentially lifetime.

Take-Home Points

1. This is a complex operation, technically difficult and challenging. Cryopreserved graft with in-line replacement is the procedure of choice in patients who are not prohibitive risk.
2. The cryopreserved graft will need to be prepared with suture ligation of lumbar vessels with the graft positioned so that the sutures ligatures (4-0 polypropylene) appear on the anterior surface (to easily allow repair if needed after restoration of flow).
3. Debridement of surrounding inflammatory aortic tissue is critically important to the long-term success of the operation; this is especially true when one is using Rifampin-soaked Dacron graft. This debridement can be accomplished after the proximal anastomosis is completed, thereby limiting visceral and renal ischemia.
4. One needs to ascertain that the cryopreserved graft is long enough to reach to the anticipated distal anastomotic site—this is critically important when going to the femoral levels. One also needs to make sure that the main body of the allograft is not too long as to be compressed in the retroperitoneal tunnels. Rather, the bifurcation needs to remain above where the retroperitoneal tunnels start.

Chapter 8
Open Repair of Ruptured Abdominal Aortic Aneurysm

Sachinder Singh Hans

Patients with a ruptured abdominal aortic aneurysm (AAA) typically presents in hypovolemic shock due to significant blood loss unless the rupture is contained. Hypovolemic shock is treated by volume replacement, but in patients with ruptured AAA, restricting fluid resuscitation and accepting lower systolic blood pressure (permissive hypotension) have been shown to be beneficial. Early transportation to the emergency room of the hospital, prompt diagnosis (ultrasound/CTA), and immediate proximal control have a positive impact in the outcome of patients with ruptured AAA. In most patients, there is time to obtain an emergency CTA of the abdomen and pelvis with 1 mm cuts to confirm the diagnosis and plan either endovascular or open repair depending on the anatomy of the AAA. In patients with a free rupture, CTA imaging may not be possible, and immediate transfer to the operating room is the best option.

Operative Technique

Patient is prepped from the nipple line to midthigh. To avoid cardiovascular collapse, anesthetic induction and intubation should be withheld until the surgeon is ready to make the incision, as induction of the anesthesia can lead to profound hypotension due to elimination of sympathetic tone. A rapid transfusion protocol is activated. Cell saver (autologous blood recovery system) and body warmer are both

S. S. Hans (✉)
Vascular and Endovascular Services, Henry Ford Macomb Hospital, Clinton Twp, MI, USA

S. S. Hans et al. (eds.), *Primary and Repeat Arterial Reconstructions*,
https://doi.org/10.1007/978-3-031-13897-3_8

necessary. In most patients, a midline transabdominal incision from xiphoid process to symphysis pubis is made. In few selected patients with ileostomy, urinary diversion, and contained rupture from leaking type IV thoracoabdominal aneurysm, a left flank approach through tenth intercostal space is preferable. The incision extends from the lateral border of the rectus abdominis muscle between symphysis pubis and umbilicus and extends upward and laterally into the tenth intercostal space with position of the table described in Chap. 3.

Proximal Control

In most hemodynamic stable patients, with associated small- to moderate-sized retroperitoneum hematoma, following mobilization of the ligament of Treitz with the help of finger dissection around the aortic neck, proximal control can be obtained with cephalad retraction of the left renal vein and proximal aortic clamp is applied (Figs. 8.1 and 8.2). In patients with extensive retroperitoneal hematoma and shock, supraceliac control is preferable. If severe hypotension develops during finger dissection, then proximal control can be obtained by inserting the index and middle finger of the operator's hand into the aorta and guiding a number 28 Foley catheter with a 30 cc balloon, which is inflated in the lower thoracic aorta.

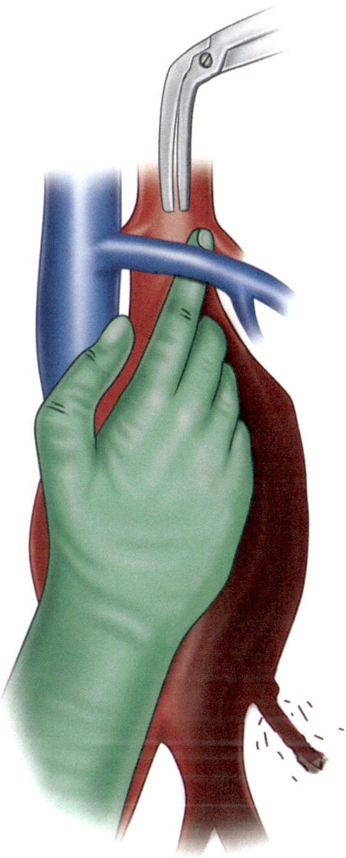

Fig. 8.1 Showing finger dissection of the ruptured AAA with the index finger of the right hand just behind the left renal vein making the plane between the aortic neck and the surrounding tissue. Proximal vascular clamp is shown

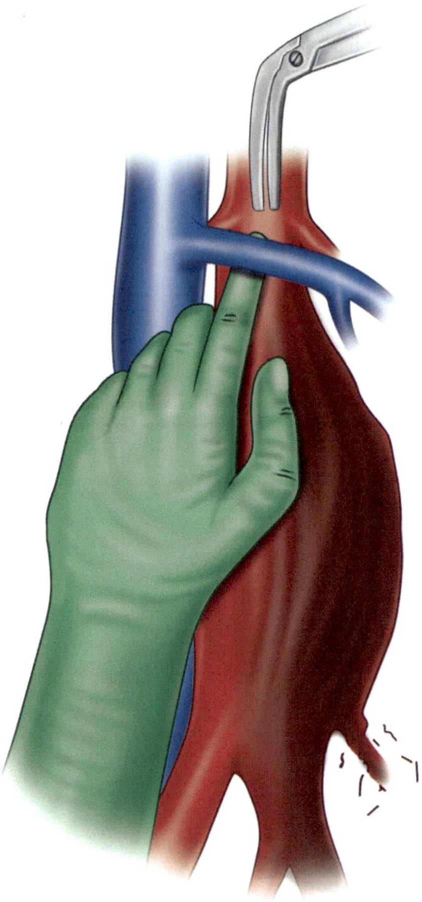

Fig. 8.2 Finger dissection with the index finger in the anterior wall so that the aortic neck and on both sides are separated from the surrounding tissues

Exposure of the Supraceliac Aorta

The left lobe of the liver is retracted toward the right following division of the left triangular ligament. The peritoneal reflection over the gastroesophageal junction is divided and retracted to the left by a Penrose drain. This is usually aided by an NG tube in the esophagus. Deep blades of the self-retraining retractor (Bookwalter III) should be applied and gastrohepatic omentum is opened through a longitudinal incision with ligation and division of the blood vessels in the omentum (Fig. 8.3). Fibers of the right crus are identified by using the right index finger, and one can feel an aortic pulse under the finger. About a 5 cm opening is made in the right crus using Metzenbaum scissors, and the fascia surrounding the aorta at this site is divided using the left hand and a long-angled vascular clamp is applied to the exposed supraceliac aorta (Figs. 8.4 and 8.5). Celiac artery is inferior to the clamp site. Circumferential dissection of the aorta and passage of silastic loop around the aorta are unnecessary and may be potentially risky.

In patients with aneurysmal dilatation of the suprarenal aorta, even if the site of rupture is infrarenal, the juxtarenal aorta may not be suitable for proximal anastomosis. Therefore, exposure of the proximal aorta by medial visceral rotation is necessary. This can be accomplished by incising the peritoneum along the lateral

Fig. 8.3 Showing suprarenal control of the aorta by opening gastrohepatic omentum

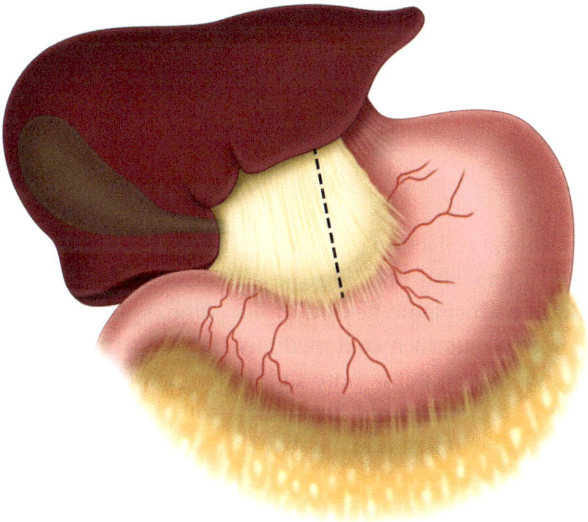

Fig. 8.4 The right crus of the diaphragm is separated using blunt finger dissection following application of Bookwalter retractor following division of the left triangular ligament and retracting the left lobe of the liver medially and esophagogastric junction laterally

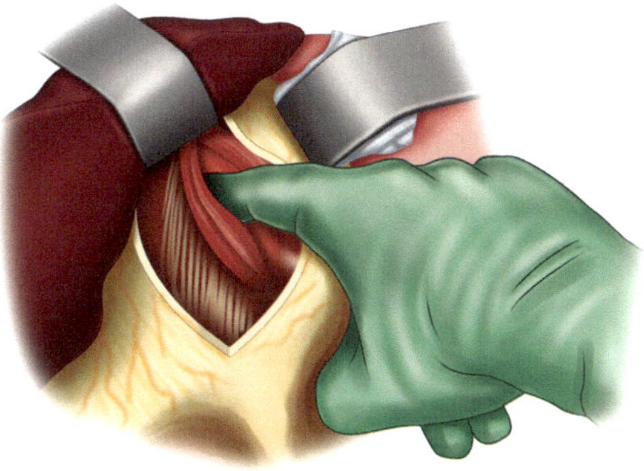

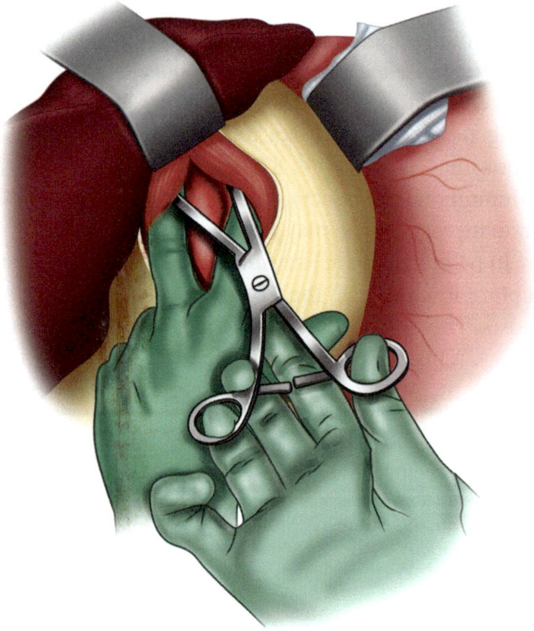

Fig. 8.5 With both fingers separating the supraceliac aorta from surrounding tissues anteriorly and on each side, a vascular clamp is applied to the supraceliac aorta

peritoneal reflection of the descending colon and sigmoid mesocolon (white line of Toldt) and also dividing the phrenicocolic ligament and the lienorenal ligament along with splenic flexure of the colon, spleen, and tail of the pancreas, which are reflected anteriorly and medially (Figs. 8.6 and 8.7). Though the left kidney can be left in its bed, but a more satisfactory exposure of the proximal abdominal aorta is obtained by reflecting the kidney from the psoas fascia medially and forward. Most of the attachments can be divided by electrocautery and bleeding is minimal if dissection is done in a proper tissue plane. One should look out for lumbar branch of the left renal vein, which needs to be clipped or sutured, as its tear can result in a significant blood loss. It is important to leave the shining fascia over the psoas muscle intact and not dissect underneath the fascia as it will result in excessive bleeding. The left renal artery is carefully exposed and preserved. The left crus of the diaphragm is divided with electrocautery, and this enables exposure of the superior mesenteric artery and the celiac artery so that a supraceliac clamp can be safely applied.

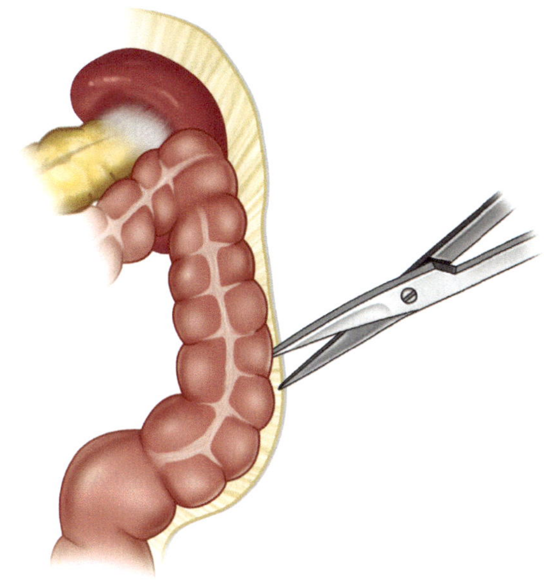

Fig. 8.6 Medial visceral rotation by division of the peritoneal reflection along the sigmoid mesocolon, descending mesocolon, and ligaments around the spleen

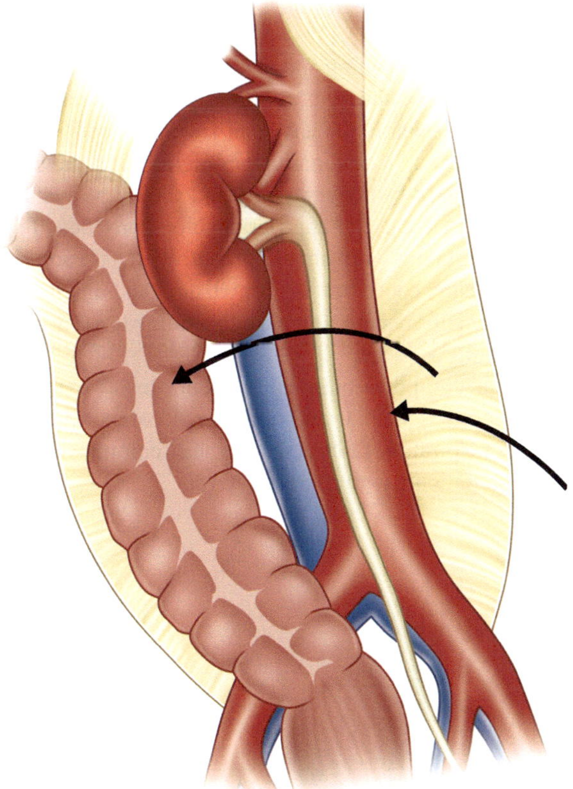

Fig. 8.7 Left colon including the Splenic flexure, kidney, and ureter with tail of the pancreas and spleen mobilized medially for exposure of the entire abdominal aorta from the celiac axis to its bifurcation and the left CIA and the left EIA

Balloon Occlusion Control

An alternative technique for proximal aortic control involves the insertion of a 12 F sheath in the femoral artery under local anesthesia to allow for a passage of a large-diameter occlusion balloon into the distal thoracic aorta. This sheath should be held by manual pressure as it tends to slip out. Arteriography can then be performed (if preoperative CTA was not obtained) to determine if endovascular open repair should be performed.

After obtaining proximal control, volume status (intravenous fluids and blood products for resuscitation) should be optimized. Intravenous heparin (smaller dose, 75 IU/kg) is administered by anesthesia in patients with small- to moderate-sized hematoma with a relatively stable hemodynamics. In patients with large hematoma and hypotension, proximal anastomosis is completed, and heparin is administered following the completion of proximal anastomosis if ACT is not prolonged due to dilutional coagulopathy. The remaining procedure proceeds as described in Chap. 3 on repair of intact juxtarenal and infrarenal AAA.

Complications

Bleeding

Intraoperative bleeding and postoperative bleeding can result in increased morbidity and mortality following ruptured AAA. Excessive intraoperative bleeding may result from a tear in the left renal vein or posterior collar renal vein (lumbar vein) or iliac veins and, occasionally, the inferior vena cava itself. Postoperative bleeding is usually caused by coagulopathy and should be evaluated by coagulation profile and managed by the use of appropriate blood products. In patients with a large retroperitoneal hematoma and shock, proactive transfusion consisting of two pooled buffy coat platelets concentrates immediately and again 30 min before aortic unclamping together with fresh frozen plasma administered in a 1:1 ratio with packed red blood cell should be given.

Other complications include acute lower extremity ischemia, colon ischemia, spinal cord ischemia, and abdominal compartment syndrome. Multiorgan failure (renal, respiratory failure, and cardiac complications) is associated with high mortality in patients with ruptured AAA.

Take-Home Points

1. Prompt diagnosis followed by expedient proximal aortic control is the key to success in this catastrophic condition. Patient should be immediately transferred to the operating room and definite treatment (either with EVAR or open repair) should be performed.
2. A well-qualified team consisting of anesthesia staff and operating room staff, availability of hybrid operating room with special radiology tech, and prompt support from blood bank are key to salvage patients who are otherwise going to succumb from ruptured AAA.

Chapter 9
Endovascular Aortic Stent Graft Explantation

Loay Kabbani, Khalil Masabni, and Timothy J. Nypaver

Introduction

With improvement in endovascular techniques and continued refinements/modifications of endovascular grafts, along with the technical experience accumulated over the past two decades, endovascular aneurysm repair (EVAR) has become the primary means of infrarenal abdominal aortic aneurysm (AAA) repair in approximately 80% of patients. In those patients with shorter aortic necks (aortic neck length < 15 mm) as well as those with challenging anatomic configurations (iliac tortuosity, aortic neck angulation, small diameter access vessels), EVAR is now often possible. Fenestrated EVAR has allowed endovascular means of repairing juxtarenal AAAs as well. While the initial morbidity and mortality of EVAR are lower compared to open AAA repair, EVAR patients will require lifelong radiographic surveillance to identify endoleaks, graft migration, limb thrombosis, and sac expansion. Thirty percent of EVAR patients develop endoleaks, with 30% of these patients requiring some type of endovascular intervention. Fortunately, the majority of

L. Kabbani (✉)
Department of Surgery, Henry Ford Hospital, Detroit, MI, USA

Wayne State University, Detroit, MI, USA

Michigan State University, Detroit, MI, USA

Henry Ford Hospital, Heart and Vascular Institute, Detroit, MI, USA
e-mail: LKABBAN1@hfhs.org

K. Masabni
Division of Vascular Surgery, University of Arizona, Tucson, AZ, USA

T. J. Nypaver
Division of Vascular Surgery, Wayne State School of Medicine, Henry Ford Hospital,
Detroit, MI, USA

S. S. Hans et al. (eds.), *Primary and Repeat Arterial Reconstructions*,
https://doi.org/10.1007/978-3-031-13897-3_9

post-EVAR endoleaks can be treated using endovascular techniques, whether through embolization of the feeding vessel (type II endoleak) or via proximal or distal extension (type I endoleak) of the stent graft. Additionally, type III endoleaks can often be treated with a bridging stent graft. However, these endovascular "rescue" techniques may also fail, leading to continued sac expansion or even rupture. Graft infections and recurrent graft limb thrombosis (in which endovascular techniques are no longer possible or indicated) are additional situations where endovascular aortic stent explantation and concomitant open aortic reconstruction will be required. Endovascular aortic stent graft explantations are complex procedures with unique and specialized techniques often required to ensure a successful outcome.

Indications for EVAR Explant

The incidence of late open conversion after EVAR should be less than 5% (range, 0–9%). In one recent series, the conversion rate was 1.5% [1]. The main indications for graft explantation include endoleak (with or without graft migration), graft infection, or refractory graft occlusion. Sac enlargement secondary to endoleaks can occur in up to 40% of EVARs. While the majority of these endoleaks can be repaired endovascularly, some persist despite several attempts at endovascular rescue, and thus, patients often require conversion to EVAR explant and open aortic reconstruction. Graft infection, while less frequent with EVAR compared to open repair, is a major life and limb-threatening complication which typically will require aortic stent graft explantation. This is further complicated by the infected field which, when performed with in-line aortic graft repair, will require a replacement conduit relatively resistant to infection. This mandates familiarity and experience with either use of cryopreserved allografts or Rifampin-soaked Dacron grafts. Many of the operative considerations and details will be similar to the management of infected aortic grafts that were placed via an open approach. Graft thrombosis is the least common indication for EVAR explant; graft thrombosis is usually confined to a graft limb and can be successfully managed with endovascular thrombolysis/thrombectomy or with an extra-anatomical bypass. Endovascular thrombolysis/thrombectomy will usually require relining of the graft limb with evaluation for and treatment of the underlying culprit lesion.

Type Ia endoleaks account for the majority of endoleaks that require explant [1–4]. Type Ia endoleaks and graft migration are noted to occur more commonly with EVARs placed outside indication for use (IFU) as detailed by the endograft manufacturer. EVARs performed on AAAs with short, heavily calcified necks, diseased distal iliac seal zones, or severe aortic neck angulation (> 60 degrees) are common underlying factors associated with EVAR failure. In one study, 56% of patients requiring graft explants had EVARs performed outside the recommended IFU criteria [1]. Additionally, it has been noted that pre-EVAR aortic neck diameters of 30 to 32 mm, despite meeting IFU criteria, can predispose to type Ia endoleaks [2].

Type II endoleaks occur in 14–30% of all EVARs. Most of the type II endoleaks do not cause sac expansion. Patients with persistent type II associated sac expansion, despite endovascular attempts to control or eliminate the endoleak, will often require an open repair, ranging from ligation of feeding vessels to open graft explantation and replacement. An additional option is direct opening of the aneurysm sac with internal ligation/oversewing of any back bleeding feeding vessels. One significant concern, in a patient with sac enlargement thought to be secondary to a type II endoleak, is the possibility of an unrecognized undiagnosed type I endoleak. Also, type II endoleaks that cause sac enlargement will often predispose for the development of a type I endoleak. One needs to take this into consideration when selecting the appropriate treatment of an enlarging aneurysm sac presumed to be secondary to a type II endoleak. Lastly, there is the real possibility, after direct ligation or internal suturing of feeding vessels (repair of type II endoleak), of developing new type II endoleaks, or even a type I endoleak.

Type V endoleaks are a unique concern with growth expansion despite the absence of an identified endoleak with imaging studies (computed tomographic angiography, catheter angiography, or ultrasound based duplex imaging). As no precise endoleak is identified and therefore cannot be targeted for treatment, aortic stent graft explantation will be necessary in the setting of continued sac expansion. It is presumed that many Type V endoleaks are really unrecognized Type I endoleaks.

Anatomy

The proximal seal zone for the majority of EVARs is infrarenal, with the exception for fenestrated EVARs that are performed for juxtarenal aneurysms. Most EVAR devices have suprarenal fixation, adding a further layer of complexity to EVAR explants. Exposure of the infrarenal aorta is mandatory to accomplish the repair and suture the replacement aortic graft to the native aortic neck. Exposure of either the supraceliac aorta or the suprarenal aorta will frequently be required for proximal aortic control. It is the authors' experience that one should be prepared to accomplish the proximal repair with a suprarenal clamp or supraceliac clamp in place as the infrarenal aortic neck following graft explantation may not have the integrity to allow infrarenal clamp placement.

Treatment

In endovascular aortic stent explantation, there exist several variables which greatly influence the conduct of the operation; this would include the indications for explant, the prior endograft utilized, the type of replacement graft being used, the operative exposure and approach (transabdominal vs. retroperitoneal), the cross-clamp position (suprarenal or supraceliac or infrarenal), and extent to which the endograft is explanted (partial vs. complete).

Proximal

We prefer the transperitoneal transabdominal approach when an infrarenal clamp is possible. This is often in the case when proximal graft migration has occurred, and a suitable infrarenal neck is still available for clamp placement. When suprarenal or supraceliac control is required (as is the case in most patients) or when patients have had extensive prior abdominal operations, the retroperitoneal approach is utilized preferably.

Transperitoneal Transabdominal Approach

Clamp position will be dictated by the anatomic findings as noted on preoperative imaging. Factors which influence clamp position are the relationship of the renal and visceral vessels to the endograft and the superior extent of the suprarenal fixation component. In one series, supraceliac clamping was used in only 25% of patients [3]. However, exposure of the supraceliac aorta is time well spent as paravisceral aortic dissection is often difficult. Inflammation in the proximal neck, potentially secondary to metal penetration by endo-hooks, can make the pararenal dissection difficult, rendering placement of a suprarenal clamp problematic.

The steps for supraceliac aortic exposure (transperitoneal) are as follows: the left lobe of the liver is retracted toward the right following division of the left triangular ligament; the peritoneal reflection over the gastroesophageal junction is divided; the gastrohepatic ligament is opened through a longitudinal incision; deep blades of self-retaining retractor are applied; and finally, an opening is made through the overlying crus. With careful blunt finger dissection, the anterior surface of the aorta is exposed and the fascia surrounding the aorta entered. The aorta with then dissected on each side downward, enough to allow aortic clamp placement. Circumferential dissection of the aorta is unnecessary and may be potentially risky.

Suprarenal clamping remains technically feasible in patients without an inflammatory response and in whom an adequate distance between the renal ostia and the superior mesenteric artery exists.

The aortic neck and the proximal extent of the endograft are exposed via an inframesocolic approach, with the fourth portion of duodenum and ligaments of Treitz mobilized. The transverse colon, stomach, and greater omentum are packed and retracted with the small bowel retracted to the right and sigmoid colon retracted downwards. The left renal vein is encountered and carefully exposed to allow cephalad retraction. It may be necessary to ligate the lumbar, gonadal, and adrenal veins, keeping in mind that if the renal vein is to be divided, these vessels should be preserved. Mobilization is facilitated by the placement of a Penrose drain positioned around the renal vein allowing further superior retraction and exposure.

The extent of endograft excision often depends on the pre-existing device seal, presence (or absence) of suprarenal fixation struts, and whether underlying graft infection is suspected. Suprarenal stents and barb fixation can make complete excision challenging. There are several technical aids to facilitate this maneuver that are detailed below.

Retroperitoneal Approach

The retroperitoneal approach is favored by the authors when suprarenal or supraceliac exposure will be required to gain proximal control. The advantages include complete single plane exposure of the paravisceral aorta to allow for selection of the proximal clamp site. This approach may be problematic if distal right iliac artery exposure is anticipated. Exposure is accomplished through a left flank incision in the ninth intercostal space extending from the intercostal space to the lateral rectus sheath with division of the musculature of the abdominal wall and entry into the retroperitoneal space. Mobilization of the peritoneum and intraperitoneal contents to the midline ensues, maintaining the psoas muscle on the posterior aspect of the exposure and then developing a plane posterior to the left kidney. The dissection continues superiorly to the level of the diaphragmatic crus which is then divided allowing exposure of the supraceliac aorta. The crus can be divided slowly with Bovie cauterization with a right-angle clamp protecting the underlying aorta. Suprarenal or supraceliac exposure can then ensue with the intention of clamping the aorta above the most superior hooks of suprarenal attachment.

Intraoperative Challenges

In the absence of infection, we commonly suture proximally to the fabric of a well-incorporated endograft, while incorporating native aortic tissue in the anastomosis (Fig. 9.1a and b). When complete excision of the EVAR graft and suprarenal stent is required, we use several strategies to facilitate complete excision of these suprarenal struts. One method is to circumferentially release barbs from the main body with a wire cutter. Also, a 20-mL syringe can be used as a sheath to encircle and collapse the suprarenal component (described with the Zenith Cook Endograft). Iced saline can be placed on nitinol elements to help collapse the metal to the

a b

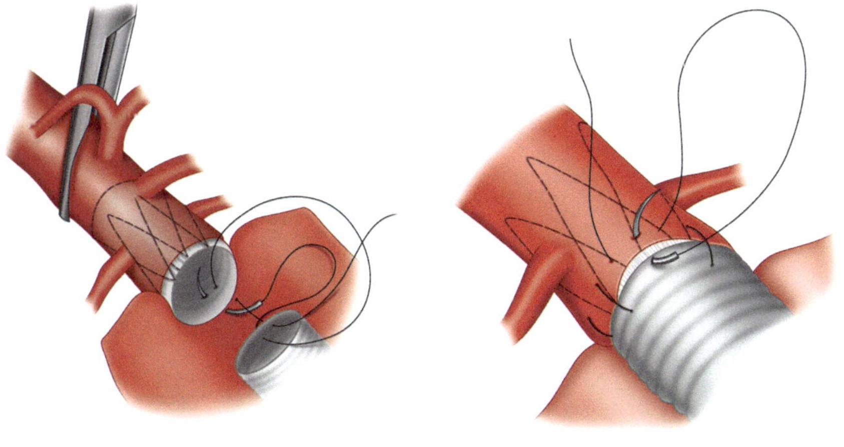

Fig. 9.1 (**a** and **b**) Supraceliac control of aorta with suturing of the prosthetic graft proximally with incorporation of the divided endograft into the suture line

pre-deployment state and facilitate removal from the arterial wall. If these techniques are unsuccessful, we do not hesitate to leave the bare stent segments in situ even in an infected setting (assuming all graft material has been excised).

It is important to note that complete removal of an endograft with suprarenal fixation can tear the aorta, injure the adjacent renal or visceral artery origins, and prolong suprarenal cross-clamp time, all contributing to adverse outcomes. Complete excision of the endograft can necessitate extension of the aortotomy above the level of the renal orifices. When this is required, we perform a beveled anastomosis to incorporate SMA and right renal arteries and then perform left renal artery reimplantation or bypass (Fig. 9.2). A retroperitoneal approach simplifies this maneuver with greater direct exposure to allow the construction of a proximal beveled anastomosis.

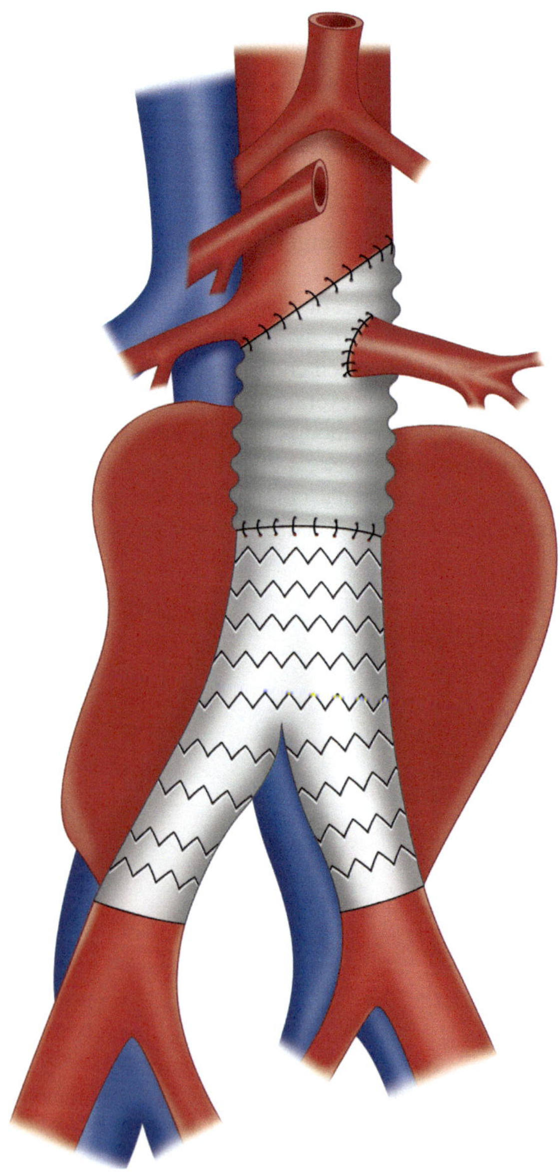

Fig. 9.2 Proximal prosthetic graft (beveled) with reimplantation of the left renal artery with distal endograft remaining in situ

Distal

Given the extensive inflammation in the pelvis, obtaining distal control can be challenging. As such, several techniques are available to obtain distal control. One method is utilizing Pruitt occlusion balloons, placed and positioned directly into each of the limbs of the aortoiliac endograft. This is especially useful when infection is not suspected and the distal segment of the endograft, already noted preoperatively to be adequately sealed, can be left in situ. Also, transfemoral balloon occlusion of both iliac limbs is an alternative option. Occasionally, we transect the iliac limbs of an endograft if there is extensive inflammation in the pelvis. The transected iliac limbs of the stent graft are then incorporated (Fig. 9.3) into the distal

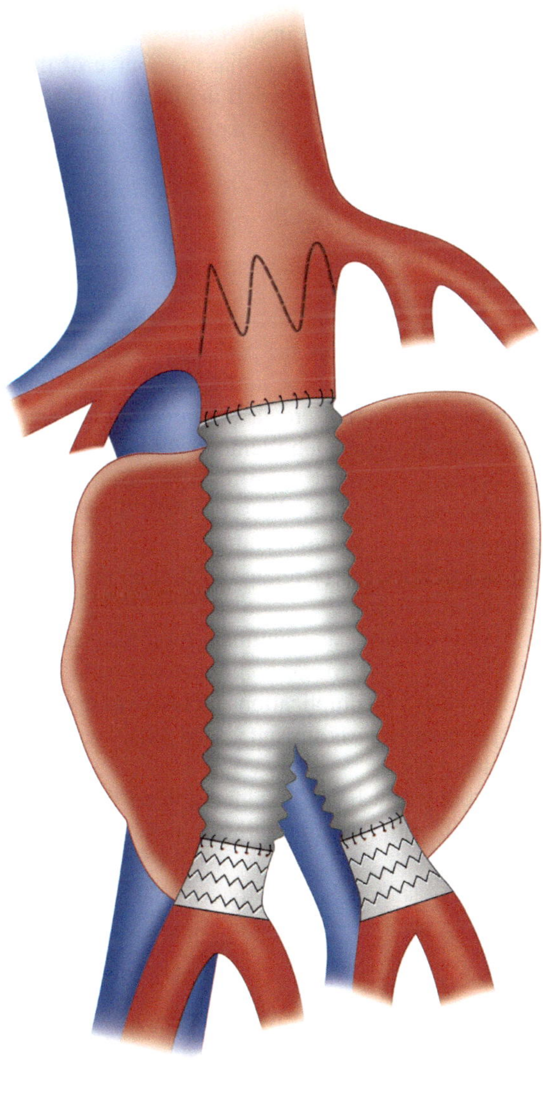

Fig. 9.3 Proximal prosthetic graft anastomosed to distal limbs of endograft (left in situ) with incorporation of iliac vessel wall

anastomosis. This technique is particularly useful in patients with ruptured aneurysms where time and blood loss are of the essence. It is preferred that with distal suturing, the graft limb is also incorporated into the native iliac vessels. Alternately, suturing the medial margins of iliac limbs together to create a new aortic bifurcation or "new carrefour" can be performed. This allows a tube graft to be used for the distal anastomosis. It is advantageous to ensure that the stitches are passed through the graft fabric and the aortic wall to obtain better hemostasis and attachment. The intent of this technique is to reduce the extent of dissection and decrease operative time with the potential secondary effect of decreasing morbidity.

A less common situation occurs with a type Ib endoleak in which it is determined that the proximal attachment site is intact and the problem leading to the sac expansion is related to distal seal, either unilaterally or bilaterally. Most type Ib endoleaks can be managed via extension of the iliac limbs into the distal common iliac or further down into the external iliac. The hypogastric artery in this situation can be embolized or if preservation is desired, an iliac branch device can be deployed. Rarely, in the emergent open repair setting of a rupture AAA with a prior endograft (and once it is determined that the source of the rupture is a distal Type Ib), the proximal endograft can be left in place with the new graft sutured to the prior endograft and extended into the native iliac vessel beyond the prior seals zones of the endograft (Fig. 9.4).

Complications

This is an extensive operation, one which has significant physiologic insult to the patient. Bleeding from the proximal anastomosis can result from inadequate incorporation of healthy native aortic tissue into the anastomosis. If graft infection is the indication for explant, recurrent infection remains a risk, but should be minimized by performing wide debridement and by utilizing an omental wrap.

Similarly, bleeding from distal anastomosis can occur secondary to failure to incorporate healthy iliac vessel into the distal anastomosis. Iliac artery degeneration progressing to iliac rupture after complete endograft removal from the iliac arteries can occur. This may be related to disruption of iliac artery wall integrity while excising the iliac limbs.

EVAR explant has significant morbidity and mortality with a complication rate of 27–60% [4, 5]. Major complications include renal dysfunction, respiratory failure, and cardiac complications inclusive of myocardial infarction. Due to concern of the potential for significant blood loss, we recommend using cell saver in non-infected cases.

Outcomes for EVAR explantation are dependent upon the indication for excision and repair with mortality rates of 40% reported in the setting of post—EVAR ruptured AAAs [4, 5]. However, when EVAR explants are performed electively, mortality rates should be less than 5%. Therefore, patients with EVAR failures not

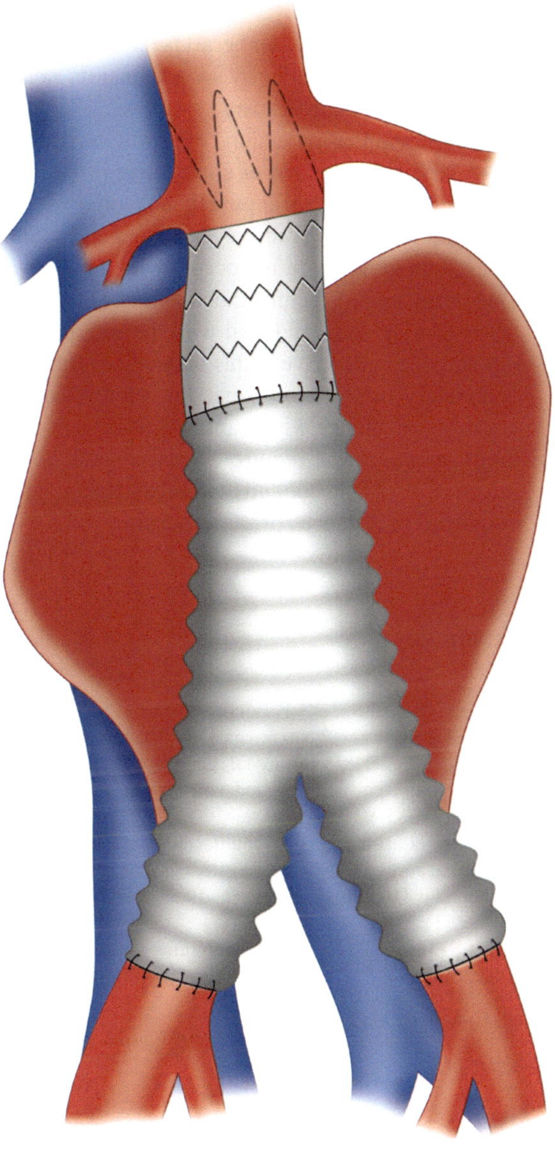

Fig. 9.4 Incorporated proximal endograft anastomosed into the distal main body of the new aorto-bi-iliac prosthetic graft

amenable to endovascular salvage need expeditious evaluation for EVAR explantation so that an emergent operation can be avoided. Referral to tertiary care centers that perform high volumes of aortic repair is recommended. Postoperative imaging surveillance is of paramount importance particularly for those patients who have had partial graft explantation.

Take-Home Points

1. Explantation of aortic stent graft is required in the setting of prior EVAR complicated by endoleak-induced sac expansion, aortic rupture, graft infection, and recalcitrant graft thrombosis.
2. This is a complex procedure with worse outcomes compared to standard open AAA repair. Suprarenal or supraceliac proximal control is frequently required, and the retroperitoneal approach is favored when infrarenal clamping is not possible or anticipated. Transperitoneal exposure and infrarenal clamping is suitable when stent graft migration occurs with a preserved infrarenal neck.
3. One of the unique technical challenges of explantation of the aortic endograft is the need to manage and deal with the suprarenal fixation apparatus. The operating surgeon must have in his arsenal several different and tailored methods to completely or partially excise the suprarenal fixation and to allow the secure construction of a proximal anastomosis.
4. Graft infection will require complete graft excision (and replacement with an infection resistant conduit), whereas partial graft excision can be judiciously employed in instances of sac expansion and rupture secondary to endoleak.

References

1. Kansal V, Nagpal S, Jetty P. Editor's choice - late open surgical conversion after endovascular abdominal aortic aneurysm repair. Eur J Vasc Endovasc Surg. 2018;55(2):163–9.
2. McFarland G, et al. Infrarenal endovascular aneurysm repair with large device (34-to 36-mm) diameters is associated with higher risk of proximal fixation failure. J Vasc Surg. 2019;69(2):385–93.
3. Dubois L, et al. A Canadian multicenter experience describing outcomes after endovascular abdominal aortic aneurysm repair stent graft explantation. J Vasc Surg. 2021;74(3):720–728.e1.
4. Arnaoutakis DJ, et al. Strategies and outcomes for aortic endograft explantation. J Vasc Surg. 2019;69(1):80–5.
5. Lyden SP, et al. Technical considerations for late removal of aortic endografts. J Vasc Surg. 2002;36(4):674–8.

Chapter 10
Open Repair of Splanchnic Artery Aneurysms

Sachinder Singh Hans

Surgical Anatomy

The abdominal aorta has three anterior branches: celiac trunk, superior mesenteric artery (SMA), and inferior mesenteric artery (IMA) which supplies the GI tract.

Celiac Trunk

The celiac trunk is the first major branch of the abdominal aorta and arises just below the aortic hiatus and 1–3 cm long and runs horizontally and forward slightly to the right above the pancreas and splenic vein. It divides into left gastric, common hepatic, and splenic arteries.

Superior Mesenteric Artery

The superior mesenteric artery (SMA) arises from the aorta 1–2 cm below the celiac trunk at the level of L1 vertebral body. It lies posterior to the body of the pancreas and splenic vein. It passes forward and inferiorly anterior to the uncinate process of the pancreas and the third portion of the duodenum to enter the root of the mesentery of the small intestine and supplies the midgut. The superior mesenteric vein (SMV) lies to the right side of the SMA. In about 15% of individuals, hepatic artery may arise from the SMA.

S. S. Hans (✉)
Vascular and Endovascular Services, Henry Ford Macomb Hospital,
Clinton Twp, MI, USA

S. S. Hans et al. (eds.), *Primary and Repeat Arterial Reconstructions*,
https://doi.org/10.1007/978-3-031-13897-3_10

Inferior Mesenteric Artery

The inferior mesenteric artery (IMA) is smaller in size than the SMA and arises from the anterolateral aspect of the aorta at the level of L3 vertebral body 3–4 cm above the aortic bifurcation.

Splanchnic Artery Aneurysms

Splanchnic artery aneurysms are uncommon. In contemporary vascular practice, splanchnic artery aneurysms are diagnosed with increasing frequency due to widespread utilization of imaging modalities. Splanchnic artery aneurysms may be associated with aneurysms in the thoracic aorta, abdominal aorta, renal arteries, and popliteal and femoral arteries.

Splanchnic artery aneurysms may be true aneurysms or false aneurysms (pseudoaneurysms). True aneurysms are usually caused by atherosclerosis (degenerative), fibromuscular dysplasia, collagen vascular disease, and Ehlers–Danlos syndrome. Pseudoaneurysms are often related to trauma, iatrogenic injury, local inflammatory process, or infection. Because of the rare occurrence of splanchnic artery aneurysms, their natural history and risk of rupture are not well defined. The widespread adoption of endovascular therapy has significantly impacted the therapeutic management of splanchnic artery aneurysms and is now often the preferred treatment modality. However, open repair of splanchnic artery aneurysms remains an option when endovascular therapy is not appropriate. Aneurysms of the celiac trunk and its branches are the most common among all splanchnic artery aneurysms.

Splenic Artery Aneurysms

Asymptomatic splenic artery aneurysms larger than 3.0 cm should be considered for repair. In women of childbearing age, even smaller aneurysms should be repaired. All false aneurysms should be repaired. Smaller calcified aneurysms (less than 2 cm) can be observed. Splenic artery aneurysms have a female preponderance of four to one. Aneurysms in mid and distal portion of the splenic artery are often saccular. Most splenic artery aneurysms are asymptomatic. Hemodynamic instability with hemorrhage shock may occur due to free rupture and is often associated with pregnancy. Initial bleeding from rupture may be contained in the lesser sac. Endovascular repair with coil embolization or stent graft is successful in vast majority of cases. If catheter-based approach is not feasible due to excessive tortuosity of splenic artery, open treatment may either involve exclusion of the aneurysm with proximal and distal ligation or ligation with interval reconstruction. Splenectomy is reserved for distal and hilar lesions not suitable for ligation or reconstruction.

Incision

1. Either a midline laparotomy or a bilateral subcostal incision is preferred. In patients with suspected rupture, a midline incision is preferable.
2. Proximal splenic artery aneurysms are exposed by incising the gastrohepatic ligament and entering the lesser sac (Fig. 10.1). An aneurysm from the mid to distal splenic artery is exposed through the gastrocolic omentum.
3. Posterior wall of the stomach is separated from the anterior surface of the pancreas.
4. The entire length of the pancreas is exposed from its head to the body and tail toward the hilum of the spleen.
5. An incision is made in the posterior peritoneum. The splenic artery aneurysm can be exposed from the origin to the middle portion of the splenic artery (Fig. 10.2).
6. For aneurysms located in the distal splenic artery, gastrosplenic ligament is divided and the posterior peritoneum over the distal splenic artery is divided after its careful palpation. Proximal control of splenic artery is obtained by using a right-angle clamp and passing a silastic vessel loop. Care is taken not to injure the splenic vein, which courses next to the splenic artery. If the splenic artery aneurysm extends to the hilum of the spleen, splenectomy with aneurysm resection is performed en bloc. Arterial reconstruction following proximal and distal ligation of the splenic artery is not necessary because of the abundant collaterals.
7. In patients with giant splenic artery aneurysms, the normal proximal and distal splenic artery may be difficult to visualize because of the size of the aneurysm.

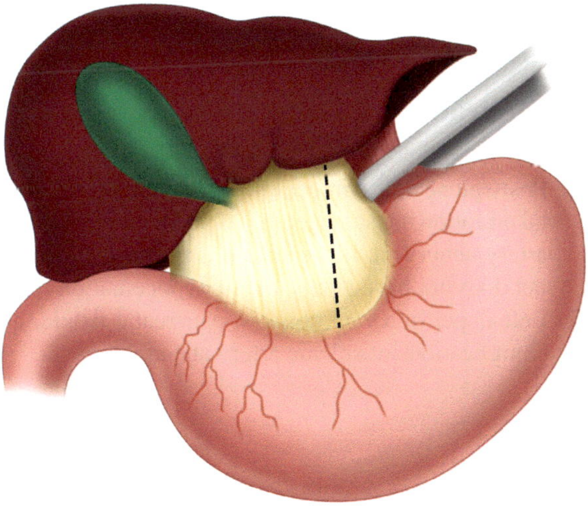

Fig. 10.1 Opening in the gastrohepatic omentum for exposure of proximal splenic artery aneurysm, celiac artery aneurysm, and hepatic artery aneurysm

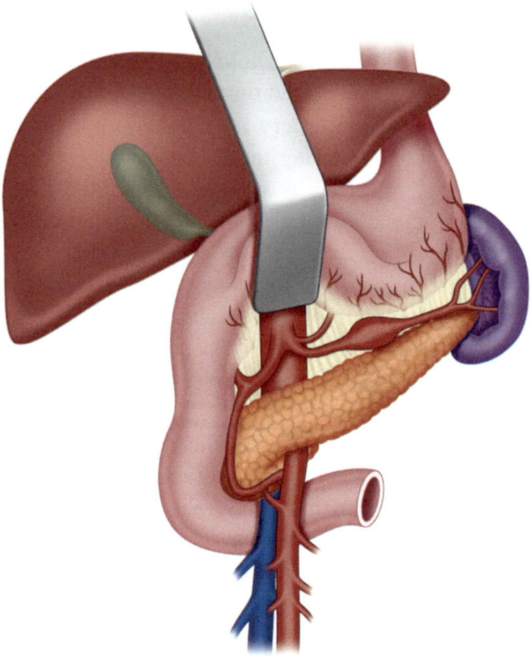

Fig. 10.2 Stomach retracted superiorly. Exposed proximal and mid splenic artery aneurysm at the superior border of the pancreas

Once the proximal control is obtained, aneurysm sac is opened, and pancreatic branches of splenic artery are ligated from within. In such patients with ligation of the distal splenic artery, the spleen remains viable via its arterial supply from the left gastric artery branches.

Complications

1. Post-splenectomy infection: Appropriate vaccination regimen should be undertaken following splenectomy if performed in association with removal of splenic artery aneurysm. If the spleen is viable following ligation of the splenic artery but does not have a pulsatile flow, vaccination regimen should be considered.
2. Left upper quadrant abscess, pancreatic fistula, and pancreatitis are other rare complications of splenic artery aneurysm repair.

Hepatic Artery Aneurysms

Hepatic artery aneurysms are the second most common splanchnic artery aneurysms. Most are extrahepatic and are more common in the common hepatic artery. Most hepatic artery aneurysms are asymptomatic. Hepatic artery aneurysm has the highest incidence of rupture among all splanchnic artery aneurysms. Hepatic artery aneurysm may present as right upper quadrant or epigastric pain followed by upper GI hemorrhage and jaundice. Repair of hepatic artery aneurysms should be considered for all symptomatic patients and for aneurysms greater than 2 cm in diameter. All intrahepatic pseudoaneurysms should be considered for repair.

The anatomical relationship of the hepatic artery aneurysm to the gastroduodenal artery and associated liver disease is a major determinant for treatment options. When anatomically feasible, catheter-based therapeutic approach should be considered as the first line of management. As the gastroduodenal artery provides an excellent collateral flow to the liver, common hepatic artery aneurysm can be treated with ligation. If the gastroduodenal artery is small, arterial reconstruction will be necessary. Hepatic artery ligation should not be considered in the presence of cirrhosis of the liver. For intrahepatic pseudoaneurysm, a catheter-based approach is preferred. Hepatic resection (segment) may be necessary in select group of patients.

Incision

Both midline laparotomy and bilateral subcostal incisions are appropriate for repair of nonemergent hepatic artery aneurysm.

Exposure of the Hepatic Artery

The lesser sac is entered through an opening in the gastrohepatic omentum. Proximal portion of the hepatic artery arising from the celiac artery trunk is exposed by elevating the stomach with further exposure of the lesser sac as the dissection is continued. The junction of the common hepatic artery and the proper hepatic artery is marked by the origin of the gastroduodenal artery. Interposition grafting following aneurysmorrhaphy should be performed in cases where gastroduodenal artery needs to be sacrificed.

Interposition Graft

Proximal and distal control is obtained, and patient is given systemic bolus of heparin 100 units/kg. The aneurysm is opened, and small feeding arteries are ligated and "normal" hepatic artery proximal and distal to the aneurysm is identified. In patients with more proximal common hepatic artery aneurysms near the origin of the celiac axis, proximal anastomosis of the interposition graft may need to be performed to the supraceliac aorta. Interposition graft using PTFE graft or reversed greater saphenous vein (GSV) is selected depending upon the clinical situation as vein graft is preferred in the presence of associated inflammation or infection such as pancreatitis (Fig. 10.3).

Proximal anastomosis to the common hepatic artery is preferred as an end-to-end anastomosis and to the supraceliac aorta as an end-to-side anastomosis (Fig. 10.4). The exposure of the supraceliac aorta is described in the chapter on ruptured abdominal aortic aneurysms (AAA). In patients with urgent or emergent symptoms, proximal anastomosis may be performed to the right common iliac artery and tunneled through the right transverse mesocolon.

Distal hepatic anastomosis is performed in an end-to-end fashion using continuous 5-0 or 6-0 cardiovascular polypropylene sutures.

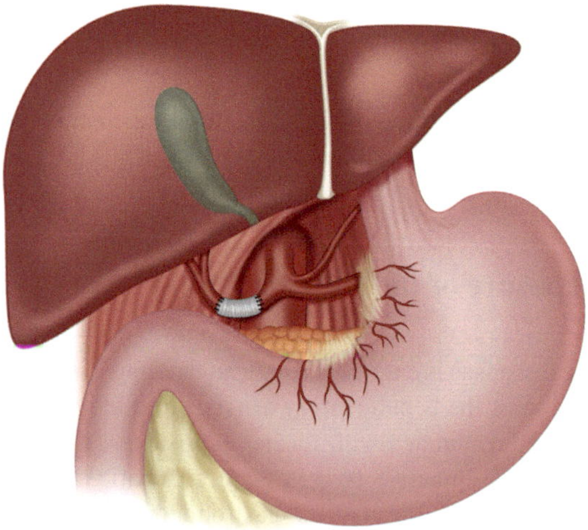

Fig. 10.3 Hepatic interposition graft following resection of hepatic artery aneurysm with proximal anastomosis to the origin of the hepatic artery

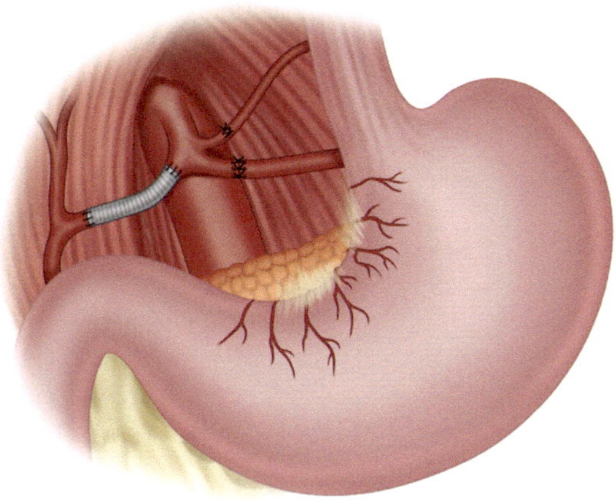

Fig. 10.4 Repair of hepatic aneurysm with proximal anastomosis to the supraceliac artery and distal anastomosis to the hepatic artery proximal to the gastroduodenal artery. The left gastric and splenic artery are lighted

Celiac Axis Aneurysm Repair

Aneurysm arising from the proper celiac axis is uncommon and is usually present in association with other splanchnic or aortic aneurysms. Most celiac aneurysms are diagnosed incidentally on imaging for diagnosis of other intra-abdominal pathology. Rupture is associated with significant mortality and aneurysm greater than 2.0 cm should be considered for repair.

Options for open repair include ligation alone and aneurysm resection with bypass, and in selected cases of isolated saccular aneurysms, aneurysmorrhaphy may be considered. When ligation alone is considered, adequate collateral circulation must be present, and this treatment modality should be avoided in the presence of liver disease or in patients with prior splenectomy. In case of aneurysm resection with a bypass grafting, an aortoceliac bypass is performed with a prosthetic conduit.

Exposure is either a midline abdominal or bilateral subcostal incision. The lesser sac is entered through an opening in the gastrohepatic omentum. The celiac artery trunk and its branches are exposed by elevating the stomach with further exposure of the lesser sac as the dissection is continued. Careful dissection around the origin of the celiac axis is performed. The main three branches of the celiac axis are exposed, and when an aneurysm involves trifurcation of the celiac trunk, splenic, and left gastric arteries, these can be sacrificed and aortohepatic bypass should be performed (Fig. 10.5a, b).

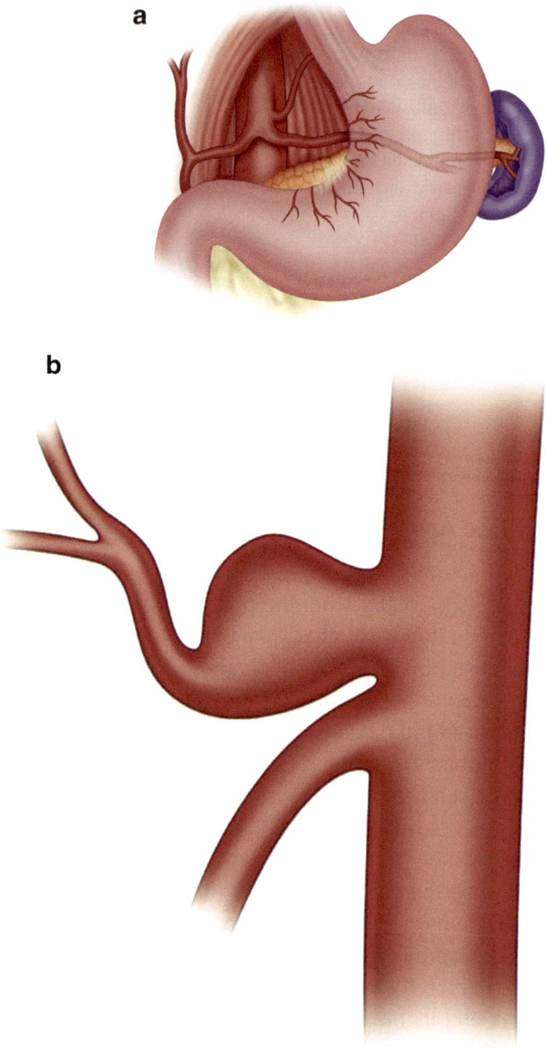

Fig. 10.5 (**a**) Celiac artery aneurysm, AP view. (**b**) Celiac artery aneurysm, lateral view

For proximal celiac axis aneurysms, bypass requires proximal anastomosis to the supraceliac aorta, which is exposed by separating the fibers of the right crus after making an opening in the gastrohepatic omentum and retracting the esophagus with a Penrose drain to the left and retraction of the left lobe of the liver, following division of the left triangular ligament. The supraceliac aorta is relatively free of atherosclerotic disease in most patients and is a satisfactory site of proximal inflow in most instances. Median arcuate ligament and the fascia over the supraceliac aorta are divided. Gentle blunt finger dissection should be performed medially and laterally to expose the supraceliac aorta.

Arterial reconstruction is then performed. Aortic control is obtained via application of an occlusion clamp to the supraceliac aorta after adequate heparinization is performed. Though Satinsky clamp (partially occluding clamp) can be used, we prefer complete clamping of the supraceliac aorta almost perpendicular to the aorta by an angled DeBakey clamp proximally and distally by an angled vascular clamp so that any bleeding from the lumbar branches will not interfere with a clean dry field after aortotomy incision is made. The blood pressure should be kept slightly low (mean pressure, 70–80 mmHg) before application of the clamp as the blood pressure tends to increase following clamping of the aorta. This enables proximal anastomosis to be completed safely in a "dry" field.

Proximal anastomosis to the supraceliac aorta is performed using 3-0 or 4-0 cardiovascular polypropylene suture, and distal anastomosis is performed end to end with 5-0 or 6-0 CV polypropylene suture to the celiac trunk above its division into its three branches (Fig. 10.6), and if adequate distal anastomotic site, splenic and left gastric artery are ligated and divided and distal anastomosis is performed to the hepatic artery. Care should be taken to avoid kinking of the conduit in patients in whom interposition vein graft is used.

Open treatment of proximal celiac artery aneurysms may consist of ligation in the presence of adequate collateral circulation. Ligation without arterial bypass should be avoided in the presence of liver disease or in patients with prior splenectomy. Aneurysmectomy with aortoceliac bypass grafting using prosthetic graft is performed when arterial reconstruction is required.

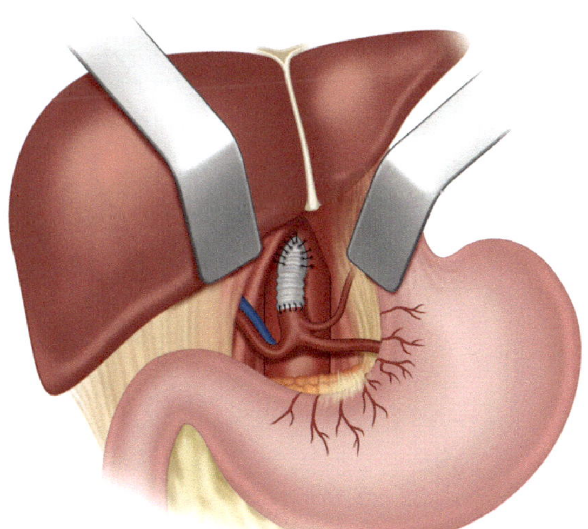

Fig. 10.6 Repair of celiac artery aneurysm with graft from the supraceliac aorta to the celiac artery proximal to its branches

Superior Mesenteric Artery

The superior mesenteric artery tends to occur in the proximal 4–5 cm of the artery (Fig. 10.7a, b). Superior mesenteric aneurysms are more common among males. Most SMA aneurysms are due to mycotic etiology (60–70%) with *Staphylococcus* and *Streptococcus* species being the dominant microorganisms. Mycotic SMA aneurysms occur more frequently in patients with a history of intravenous drug abuse or bacterial endocarditis. They are more frequently symptomatic as compared to other splanchnic artery aneurysms. Rupture rate of SMA aneurysm ranges from 35% to 50%. Repair in symptomatic/mycotic aneurysms or in aneurysms should be undertaken regardless of their size.

Fig. 10.7 (**a**) Superior mesenteric aneurysm exposed at the root of the mesentery. The superior mesenteric vein to the right of the artery. (**b**) Superior mesenteric artery aneurysm 3–4 cm from its origin, lateral view

a

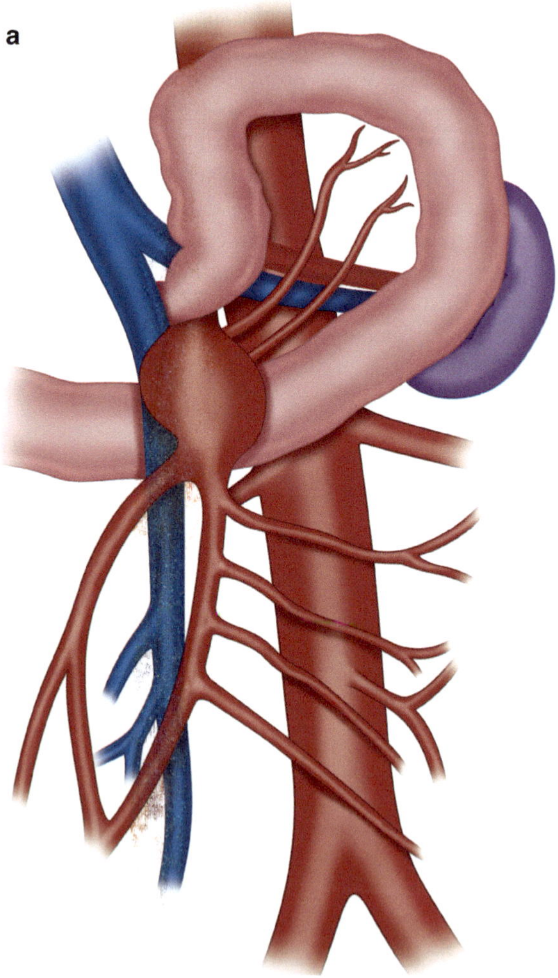

Fig. 10.7 (continued)

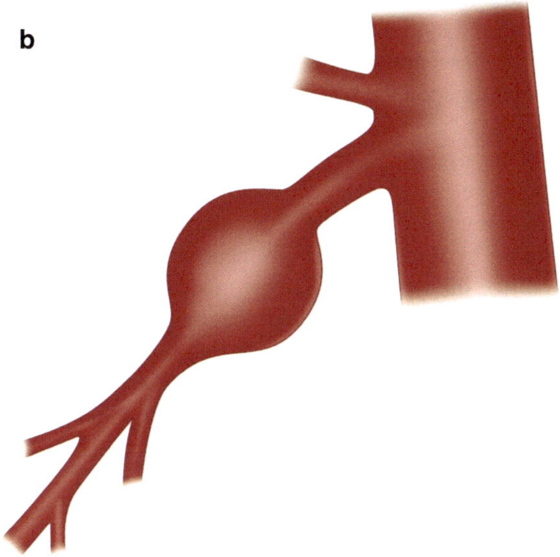

Operative Management

Branch SMA aneurysms can be ligated. Superior mesenteric artery aneurysm should be repaired via a midline laparotomy with direct exposure of the SMA by retracting the transverse colon with its mesocolon upward and small bowel mesentery to the right following mobilization of the ligament of Treitz. Dissection is done in the root of the mesentery and branches of SMA are controlled. In most patients, interposition graft is from the proximal SMA with distal anastomosis to the SMA, followed by resection of the SMA aneurysm performed in an end-to-end to fashion. Distal SMA aneurysms are suited for aneurysmorrhaphy and with plication or patch angioplasty. In the presence of infection, autogenous vein bypass is required.

Large saccular aneurysms can be treated with aneurysmorrhaphy. The injury to the superior mesenteric vein should be avoided as it lies to the right of the SMA.

If the SMA aneurysm involves its ostia (uncommon), antegrade superior mesenteric bypass from the supraceliac aorta to mid SMA is performed following resection of the aneurysm. In that situation, the proximal anastomosis is end to side and the distal anastomosis can be performed end to end.

Exposure of the supraceliac aorta has been previously described. Exposure of the SMA in the root of the mesentery is performed by lifting the transverse colon and mesocolon superiorly and palpating the artery in the root of the mesentery. The superior mesenteric artery is exposed by making a longitudinal incision in the root of the mesentery, and a retro pancreatic tunnel (preferred) or prepancreatic tunnel is made by blunt finger dissection for allowing the passage of a graft from the supraceliac aorta to the exposed portion of the SMA for distal anastomosis.

If a retrograde bypass is planned, the infrarenal aorta or left common iliac artery is explored by retracting the duodenum to the right and incising or medially reflecting the descending and sigmoid colon. Proximal site of anastomosis is selected depending upon the plaque burden and the graft is directed in a gradual curved path like a lazy "C." Potential kinking of the graft and the presence of significant atherosclerotic disease in the aortoiliac segment make this a poor second choice for inflow site.

A more useful alternative for transcural approach to the SMA is medial visceral rotation by incising the peritoneal reflection from the diaphragm to the pelvis to mobilize the descending colon medially. Next, the splenorenal and phrenicocolic ligaments are divided. The descending colon, stomach, body and tail of pancreas, and spleen are rotated anteriorly and medially by replacing the hand underneath the visceral bundle. This plane can be either anterior or behind the left kidney. The operating table should be tilted toward the right to aid in mobilization of the viscera medially.

Other Splanchnic Artery Aneurysms

Gastric artery and gastroepiploic artery aneurysms are rare. Most patients present with intraperitoneal rupture with a high mortality rate. Therefore, repair should be recommended in patients with gastroepiploic artery aneurysm and gastric artery aneurysms. The operation consists of operative ligation with or without arterial reconstruction.

Aneurysms involving jejunal, ilial, and colic arteries comprise a very small portion of all splanchnic artery aneurysms. Rupture of jejunal and ilial aneurysms is less common than colic aneurysms. Rupture usually occurs into the peritoneal cavity. All mesenteric branch artery aneurysms should be repaired by ligation or resection with intraoperative assessment of the bowel viability. Occasionally, simultaneous small bowel resection or colon resection may need to be performed.

Gastroduodenal artery and pancreaticoduodenal artery aneurysms are uncommon and account for a small portion of all splanchnic artery aneurysms. These aneurysms are more often pseudoaneurysms secondary to pancreatitis. When true pancreaticoduodenal artery aneurysms are associated with occlusive disease of the celiac axis, both aneurysm and lesion of the celiac axis need treatment. In that situation, the celiac axis should be revascularized to minimize the risk that the embolization of the pancreaticoduodenal artery aneurysm will interrupt the major collateral arterial circulation to the celiac axis.

Chapter 11
Renal Aneurysm Repair

Abdul Kader Natour and Alexander D. Shepard

Renal artery aneurysms (RAAs) are rare entities that the average vascular surgeon will encounter very infrequently. The overwhelming majority are asymptomatic and discovered incidentally on imaging performed for other reasons. Ruptured RAAs carry significant morbidity and mortality, and patients at risk for rupture should be repaired electively. The major risk factors for rupture are size and pregnancy. There has been considerable debate recently over the size threshold for aneurysm repair. Traditionally a 2 cm diameter was considered the threshold for repair, but many now advise watching until >3 cm. Symptoms of hypertension can sometimes result from aneurysms arising from fibromuscular dysplasia (FMD) associated with a stenosis or from micro-embolization of mural thrombus (less common).

Preoperative imaging is performed with a thin-cut, high-quality computed tomographic angiogram (CTA) of the abdomen. Careful review of this study with three-dimensional (3-D) reconstruction is imperative to define RAA and branch anatomy preoperatively (Fig. 11.1). Most of these aneurysms are saccular and arise at bifurcation/branch points and 15% are bilateral. Creation of a 3-D printed model can be very helpful in planning repair.

A. K. Natour
Division of Vascular Surgery, Henry Ford Hospital, Detroit, MI, USA
e-mail: anatour1@hfhs.org

A. D. Shepard (✉)
Division of Vascular Surgery, Henry Ford Hospital, Detroit, MI, USA

Wayne State University School of Medicine, Detroit, MI, USA
e-mail: ASHEPAR2@hfhs.org

S. S. Hans et al. (eds.), *Primary and Repeat Arterial Reconstructions*,
https://doi.org/10.1007/978-3-031-13897-3_11

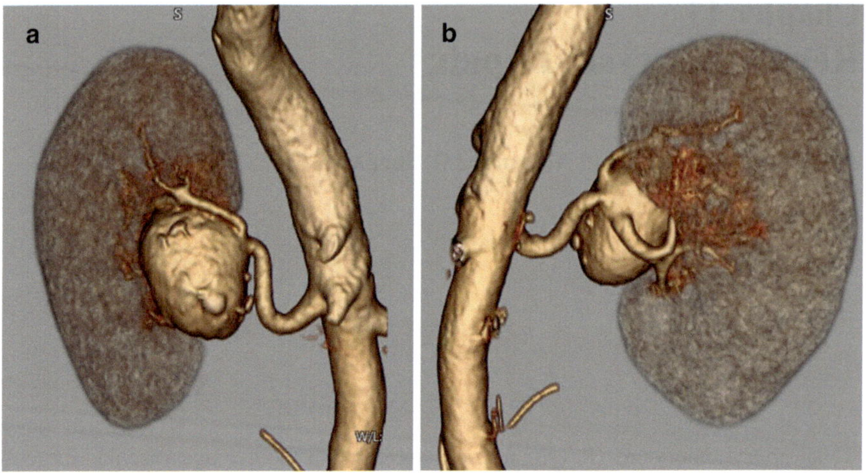

Fig. 11.1 Three-dimensional reconstruction of a large right RA aneurysm. (**a**) Anterior view; distal main RA to the lower pole of the kidney is obscured on this view. (**b**) Posterior view clearly defines distal main RA arising from posterior surface of aneurysm and its relationship to a large upper pole segmental artery

Operative Steps

These procedures are usually best performed through a modified transverse supraumbilical ("frown") incision, though some surgeons prefer a standard midline celiotomy with a transperitoneal (TP) approach to the kidney. The patient is placed on the table supine with the contralateral arm tucked at the side to create a space for anchoring a mechanical retraction system (e.g., Thompson or Omni-Tract) to the table. A firm foam pad is placed under the ipsilateral flank to slightly elevate the involved kidney. An upper abdominal transverse incision from the contralateral anterior axillary line to the ipsilateral posterior axillary line is made if treating unilateral disease or extending to both flanks if treating bilateral disease (unusual). The rectus abdominis muscles are transected and the oblique muscles divided in the direction of their fibers.

Right renal artery (RA) exposure: An incision is made in the lateral peritoneal reflection from the hepatic flexure to the cecum, and with blunt dissection, the hepatic flexure mobilized toward the midline. The duodenum and pancreas overlying the right kidney are displaced medially to the left (Kocher maneuver) exposing the aorta, inferior vena cava (IVC), and renal vessels (Fig. 11.2). Dissection of the right renal vein (RV) from the surrounding tissue is performed from its junction with the IVC to the renal pelvis. Ligation and division of any small tributaries are performed to allow complete mobilization and subsequent retraction of the right RV to expose the underlying right renal artery (RA).

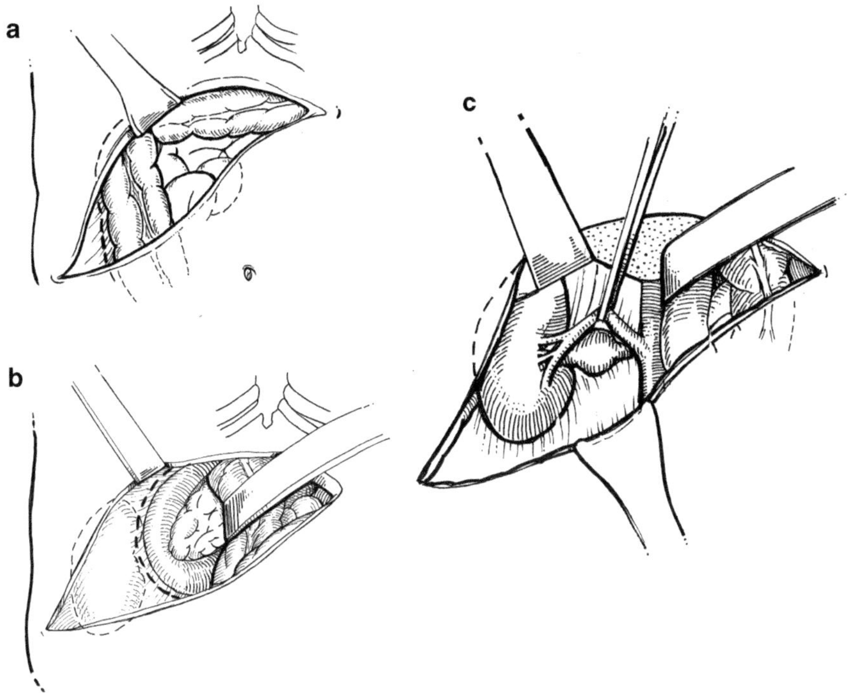

Fig. 11.2 Exposure of the right RA using limited right medial visceral rotation. (**a**) Dotted line is incision in peritoneal reflection used to mobilize hepatic flexure and part of the ascending colon. (**b**) Dotted line is incision to mobilize the duodenum off the right kidney (Kocher maneuver). (**c**) Right RA aneurysm exposed by mobilizing and retracting right RV cephalad

Dissection of the renal artery is carried out in a proximal-to-distal fashion relative to the aneurysm. When exposing the proximal-most right RA under the IVC, it is usually necessary to divide small branches of the IVC including lumbar veins. Larger branches should be suture ligated to avoid inadvertent dislodgement with problematic bleeding during subsequent medial IVC retraction. After gaining control of the proximal RA, branches distal to the aneurysm are identified and controlled with small-caliber elastic loops. Careful review of preoperative imaging will ensure that no branches are inadvertently missed. This usually requires some dissection of the aneurysm itself, which should be minimized as large aneurysms are thin walled and can be easily torn if care is not taken. Once both inflow and outflow vessels have been controlled, the aneurysm itself is mobilized. Control of posterior branches may have to await resection of the aneurysm itself.

Left renal artery (LRA) exposure: Exposure of the left RA follows a similar retroperitoneal dissection as performed on the right but with a partial left medial visceral rotation. The peritoneal reflection lateral to the left colon and spleen is incised from the proximal sigmoid colon cephalad toward the aortic hiatus (Fig. 11.3). A retroperitoneal plane is developed anterior to the left kidney with the spleen, tail of the pancreas, and splenic flexure of the colon retracted medially. A plane anterior to the kidney is developed using a combination of blunt and sharp dissection taking care not to injure the mesocolon medially; this plane is more difficult to develop than a retrorenal plane. This approach provides a much better exposure of the RA than from the midline through the mesocolon. Exposure of proximal and mid left

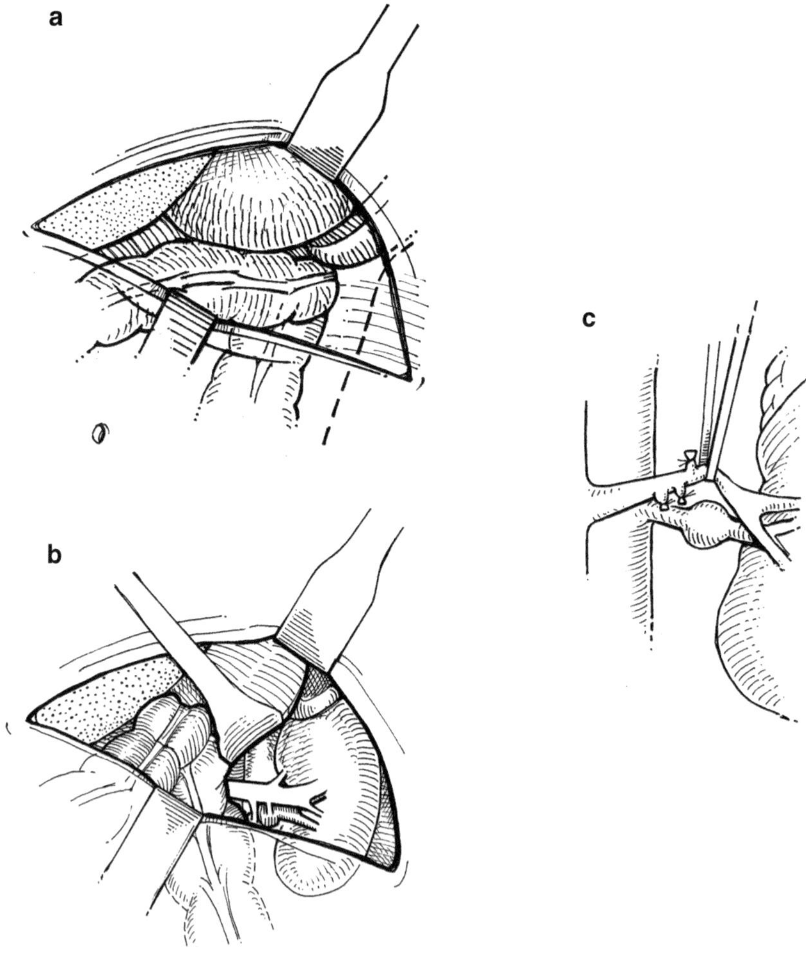

Fig. 11.3 Exposure of the left RA using limited left medial visceral rotation. (**a**) Dotted line is incision in peritoneal reflection used to mobilize the splenic flexure and descending colon along with the spleen, which are retracted medially. (**b**) The spleen and left colon are retracted medially to expose the left kidney and left renal vasculature; left RV is anterior to left RA. (**c**) Left RA aneurysm exposed by mobilizing and retracting RV cephalad after ligating and dividing its lumbar, gonadal, and adrenal branches

RA aneurysms requires mobilization of the overlying left RV with ligation and division of its lumbar and gonadal branches. A retrorenal approach with elevation of the left kidney can be helpful for aneurysms arising posteriorly off the RA. This approach avoids the need for RV mobilization but often places the RA on significant stretch, which can complicate subsequent repair. A left flank oblique incision in the tenth intercostal space is helpful if such an approach is chosen. Dissection of the left RA follows the same steps as the ones described for the right RA.

Following proximal and distal control and aneurysm mobilization, the patient is systemically heparinized to an activated clotting time of 250 s. Until recently, we also routinely administered 25 g of mannitol 20 min prior to clamping to induce an osmotic diuresis. Recent studies, however, have shown that mannitol may not have a specific renal protective effect, so we now just ensure that the patient is volume loaded with a good urine output prior to clamping. We believe strongly in the utility of cooling to reduce renal metabolic demands and minimize ischemic injury when RA clamp times more than 30 min are anticipated *or* in the presence of significant preoperative renal dysfunction. Some authors have favored mobilizing the entire kidney and surrounding it with ice, a technique we find quite cumbersome. We prefer cold renal perfusion with an iced Ringer's lactate solution (4 °C containing heparin, mannitol, and methylprednisolone). Following proximal RA clamping, the distal RA is infused with 250–300 cc of this solution over 5–6 min. With large aneurysms, a 16G angiocath or balloon-tipped irrigation catheter can be placed directly in the aneurysm. Alternatively, individual branches can be perfused with a pediatric feeding tube after opening the aneurysm, taking great care not to injure them. Following completion of perfusion, the distal arteries are occluded with microvascular clamps. For these small-caliber vessels, we prefer the use of Yasargil (cerebral aneurysm) microclips. These low-profile clips reduce the clutter associated with larger clamps and provide a less-obstructed surgical field. Conventional clamps are suitable for the main renal artery. The aneurysm sac is next resected leaving a small rim of aneurysmal tissue attached to the involved arteries. Care must be taken to preserve all sizeable branches including those originating from the posterior surface of the aneurysm. Cutting across their origins may make subsequent reconstruction difficult if not impossible.

Reconstruction Techniques

There are a variety of in situ reconstruction techniques available for RAA repair including aneurysmorrhaphy (defined as excising only the aneurysmal portion of a saccular RA aneurysm) and more commonly aneurysm resection with either bypass or interposition vein grafting. Studies have chosen that there is little to no difference in short- or long-term outcomes between these two types of reconstruction when chosen appropriately. The technique chosen is thus dependent on the anatomy of the patient's RA and aneurysm.

For aneurysms of the main RA, aortorenal bypass or interposition grafting is most commonly performed, but for saccular aneurysms, resection and primary closure or patch angioplasty, to avoid narrowing, are also suitable. When using primary closure, it is important to leave a small (1–2 mm) rim of aneurysmal wall attached to the artery. This minimizes the risk of narrowing the lumen with vessel closure. Closure with interrupted stitches as opposed to a running suture may also be helpful (Fig. 11.4). For RAA associated with FMD, aortorenal bypass reduces the risk of future problems; it is also appropriate for main RAA associated with FMD or atherosclerosis. Extra-anatomic bypasses based on the hepatic or splenic arteries may also be suitable. A description of these procedures is covered in the chapter on RA bypass.

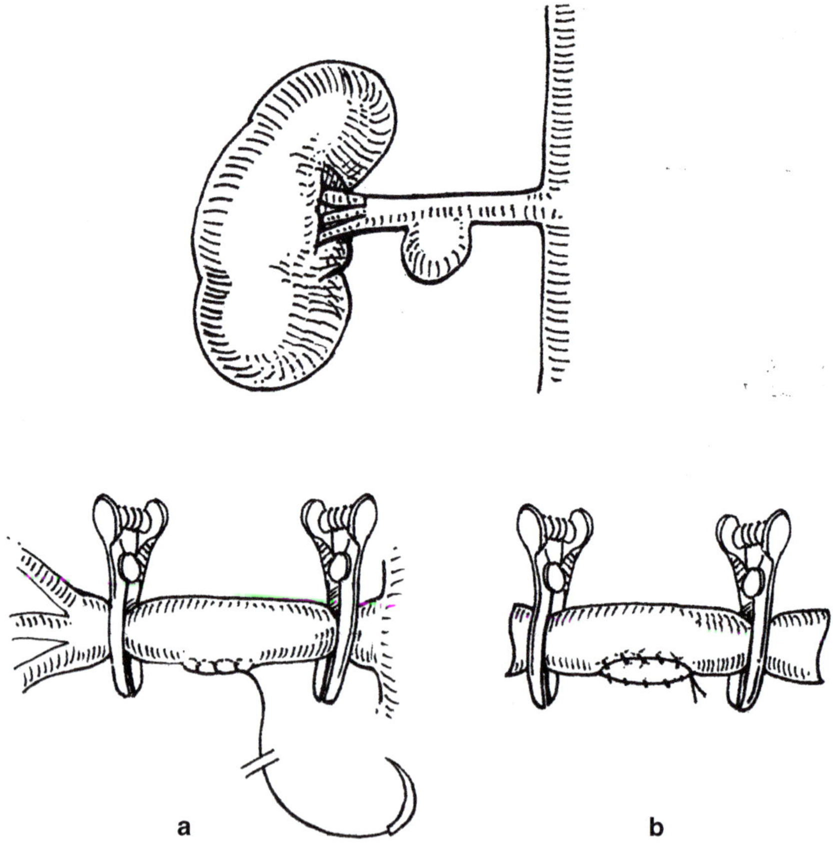

Fig. 11.4 Techniques for reconstructing aneurysms of the main RA. (**a**) Saccular aneurysms can be treated with lateral aneurysmorraphy using either primary repair, or. (**b**) Longitudinal patch closure. (**c**) For aneurysms involving the full circumference, interposition grafting, or. (**d**) Formal aortorenal bypass is suitable

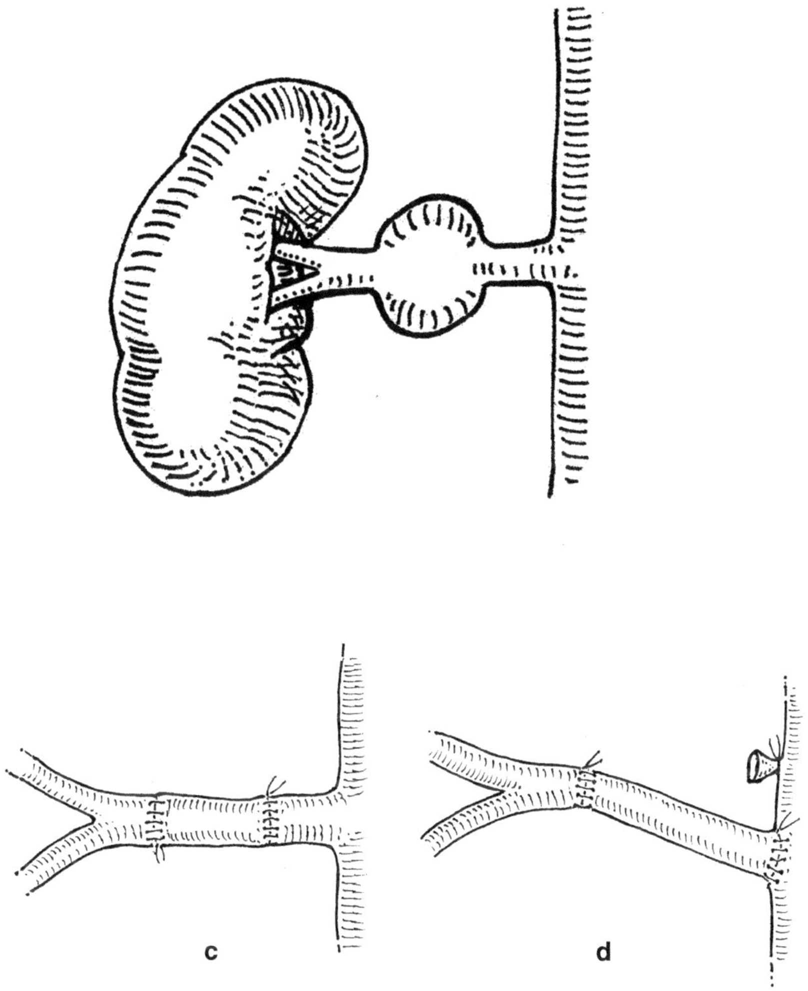

Fig. 11.4 (continued)

Aneurysms at branch points, most commonly the main RA bifurcation, are more frequent than main RA lesions and require more complex repairs. For saccular aneurysms, aneurysmorrhaphy with or without patching can be performed, but salvage of all branches frequently requires resection and grafting +/− branch reimplantation (Fig. 11.5). Reimplantation of a segmental artery into the main RA is preferred over bypass when possible. After aneurysm excision, separate branches near each other can be conjoined to create a common orifice for reimplantation or bypass (Fig. 11.5c). Saphenous vein grafts are preferred to prosthetic grafts; though in the reconstruction of large-caliber main RAAs, prosthetic grafts are probably adequate, and in young adults avoid the very-long-term risks of vein graft aneurysmal degeneration. Regardless of repair method, meticulous technique with loupe magnification and fine (6-0 or 7-0) polypropylene suture is mandatory. For very small branches, interrupted sutures as opposed to running may be more appropriate to avoid "purse-stringing" the anastomosis. At the completion of the reconstruction, technical adequacy is confirmed with intraoperative duplex scanning and any significant defects fixed immediately.

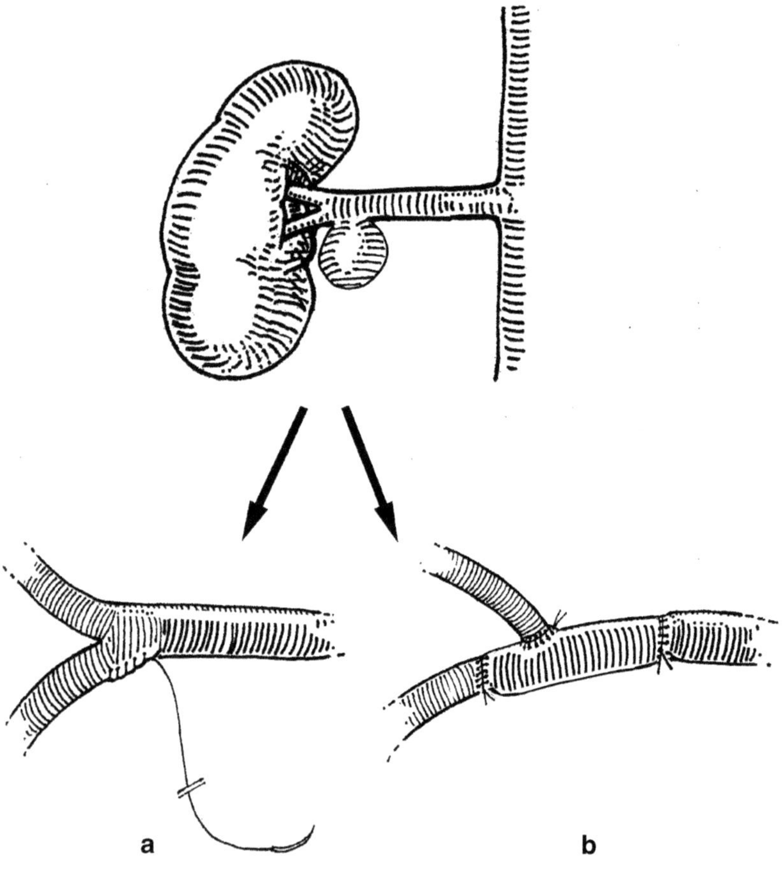

Fig. 11.5 Techniques for reconstructing aneurysms involving the RA bifurcation or segmental arteries. (**a**) Primary closure or vein patch closure (not shown). (**b**) Interposition vein grafting to larger RA branch with reimplantation (end to side) of smaller branch(es) into the vein graft. (**c**) Sewing two large branches together to create a common channel for distal anastomosis for either a redundant main RA or more commonly an interposition vein graft. RA, renal artery; RV, renal vein

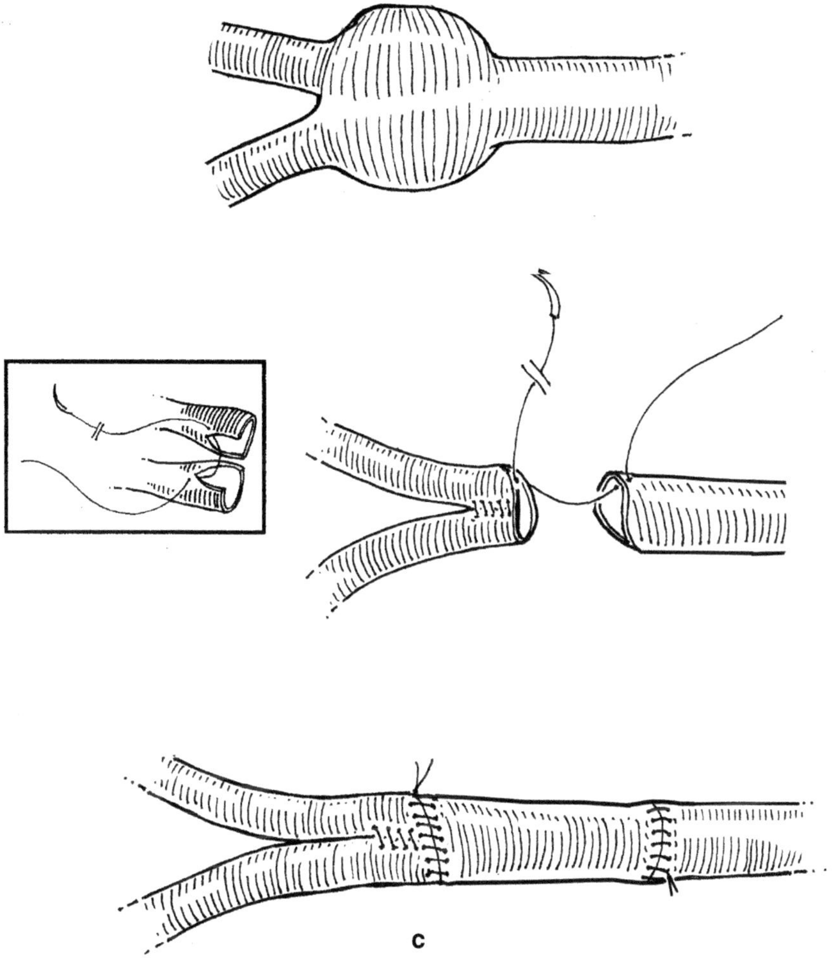

Fig. 11.5 (continued)

Other Less Frequently Used Described Techniques

Aneurysm plication: Plication of small (<1 cm in diameter) branch aneurysms has been suggested when such are encountered during operations for larger, clinically significant aneurysms. The redundant arterial wall is oversewn with a running 6-0 or 7-0 polypropylene suture. Aneurysms of very distal branches supplying limited parenchyma can be ligated in similar circumstances.

Ex vivo *repair and auto-transplantation*: This approach is helpful for some complex distal branch aneurysms that were previously treated with nephrectomy. A full description of this approach is beyond the scope of this chapter.

Nephrectomy: Nephrectomy is still required for non-reconstructible aneurysms, in the presence of a nonfunctioning, atrophic kidney or with uncontrollable RAA rupture.

Endovascular Repair

Endovascular techniques can be used to treat anatomically appropriate RAAs particularly in patients with poor operative risk. Localized aneurysms of the main RA can be repaired with a covered stent though there is no good data regarding long-term patency of such reconstructions. Inferring from contemporary experience with small-caliber stent grafts in the performance of branched endograft repair of thoracoabdominal aneurysms, however, patency of these grafts is probably reasonable. Embolization therapy is also appropriate for distal intraparenchymal aneurysms where there is low risk for significant loss of renal mass. The possibility of inducing renovascular hypertension from a resulting small segment of ischemic parenchyma must be weighed against the risk of the aneurysm. Small-necked saccular aneurysms, regardless of location, can also occasionally be treated with intra-sac coiling using techniques like those used for cerebral artery aneurysms.

Post-operative Care

Patients with a prolonged renal ischemia time may experience a significant diuresis during the immediate post-op period that will require attention to intravenous fluids and close monitoring of potassium and magnesium levels. Acute thrombosis of the reconstructed renal artery is a potential complication and may be heralded by a sudden drop in urine output. Small branch occlusions are usually well tolerated though renovascular hypertension may result from ischemic renal parenchyma. A thin-cut CTA is usually performed on post-operative day 4 or 5 in patients with normal renal function to ensure a technically adequate repair. Patients are maintained on aspirin (or other antiplatelet medications) plus a statin for at least 6 months. Follow-up in the outpatient clinic includes regular measurement of blood pressure and renal function and surveillance renal duplex ultrasound every 6 months for the first 2 years. Any detected abnormality should be further studied with a CTA or a catheter-directed arteriogram.

Outcomes

Renal artery aneurysm repair is an uncommonly performed operation, which can be quite challenging. Open repairs should only be undertaken in reasonable risk patients by experienced surgeons. In centers of excellence, renal artery reconstructions have durable outcomes with good long-term patency (95%) and freedom from recurrence.

Further Reading

Henke PK, Cardneau JD, Welling TH, et al. Renal artery aneurysms: a 35-year experience with 252 aneurysms in 168 patients. Ann Surg. 2001;234:454–62.

English WP, Pearce JD, Craven TE, et al. Surgical management of renal artery aneurysms. J Vasc Surg. 2004;40:53–60. https://doi.org/10.1016/j.jvs.2004.03.024.

Klausner JQ, Lawrence PF, Harlander-Locke M, et al. The contemporary management of renal artery aneurysms. J Vasc Surg. 2015;61:978–84. https://doi.org/10.1016/j.jvs.2014.10.107.

Coleman DM, Stanley JC. Renal artery aneurysms. J Vasc Surg. 2015;62(3):779–85. https://doi.org/10.1016/j.jvs.2015.05.034.

Chaer RA, Abularrage CJ, Coleman DM, et al. The Society for Vascular Surgery clinical practice guidelines on the management of visceral aneurysms. J Vasc Surg. 2020;72(1S):3S–39S. https://doi.org/10.1016/j.jvs.2020.01.039.

Chapter 12
Femoral and Femoral Anastomotic Aneurysms

Sachinder Singh Hans

Anatomy

Arterial aneurysms in the lower extremity have the potential to cause limb-threatening ischemia from thrombosis or embolization from the mural thrombus. Rupture of the femoral and popliteal aneurysms is extremely rare. Most femoral and popliteal aneurysms are degenerative in nature. Pseudoaneurysms are often related to anastomotic, traumatic, and mycotic etiology.

True femoral artery aneurysms are more common in the common femoral artery (CFA) than they are in the superficial femoral artery (SFA) or deep femoral artery (DFA). Aneurysms confined to the CFA are classified as type 1, while those involving the origin of the DFA are type 2. Femoral aneurysms are asymptomatic in 40% of patients and in another 40% present with signs of lower extremity ischemia, and in the remaining 20%, patients may present with a groin mass, which may become painful as the aneurysm enlarges and causes symptoms secondary to the pressure on surrounding structures.

Indications

The common femoral artery measures 10.5 mm in men and 8.5 mm in women (AP/Tr diameter). The guidelines for surgical repair of CFA aneurysms have recently been increased from 2.5 to 3.5 cm for asymptomatic patients. All symptomatic patients should undergo repair to prevent complications regardless of their size.

S. S. Hans (✉)
Vascular and Endovascular Services, Henry Ford Macomb Hospital,
Clinton Twp, MI, USA

S. S. Hans et al. (eds.), *Primary and Repeat Arterial Reconstructions*,
https://doi.org/10.1007/978-3-031-13897-3_12

Preoperative planning by imaging of the aorta, iliac, SFA, and popliteal arteries with CT angiography should be performed to evaluate the presence of concurrent aneurysms. Patient should undergo lower extremity arterial Doppler study including segmental pressures in patients with suspected associated arterial occlusive disease. The surgical treatment involves open repair as the aneurysmal segment is replaced with Dacron or polytetrafluoroethylene (PTFE) graft.

Operative Procedure

A hockey stick incision is made in the groin extending from the apex of the femoral triangle (upper thigh) curving slightly laterally and upward toward the anterior superior iliac spine (Fig. 12.1). Dissection is continued into the subcutaneous tissue, which is incised longitudinally by electrocautery or by a 15-blade scalpel.

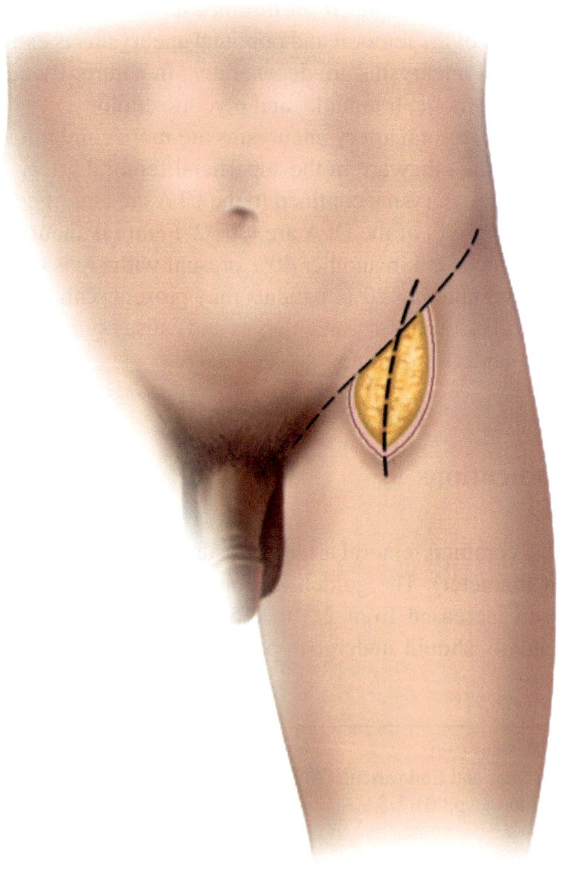

Fig. 12.1 Hockey stick incision in the left groin for exposure of the femoral and femoral anastomotic aneurysm

The inguinal lymph nodes are mobilized medially, and the lymphatics are tied with 3-0 silk free tie or silver clips (Fig. 12.2). The medial border of the sartorius is exposed and further medial dissection exposes the femoral sheath, which is opened longitudinally. Superficial veins crossing the femoral vessels are tied and divided. The common femoral artery is exposed. Shelving of the inguinal ligament is exposed, and dissection is done by lifting the inguinal ligament with peritoneal sac and fascia superiorly by a "baby" Deaver retractor. This enables one to expose the distal external iliac artery and its two branches: medially deep epigastric artery and laterally deep circumflex iliac artery. The deep circumflex iliac vein is visualized crossing the distal external iliac artery and should be ligated with 3-0 silk free tie and divided.

The shelving edge of the inguinal ligament may have to be partially divided if the aneurysm is large with inadequateexposure. A silastic loop doubled on itself is passed around the distal external iliac artery. Deep epigastric artery and deep circumflex iliac artery are exposed and preserved. Attention is then paid to the proximal SFA and a silastic loop doubled on itself is passed as well. Dissection of the DFA may be technically difficult. Dissection is kept close to the lateral wall of the aneurysm. A branch of the profunda femoral vein is seen crossing the origin of the

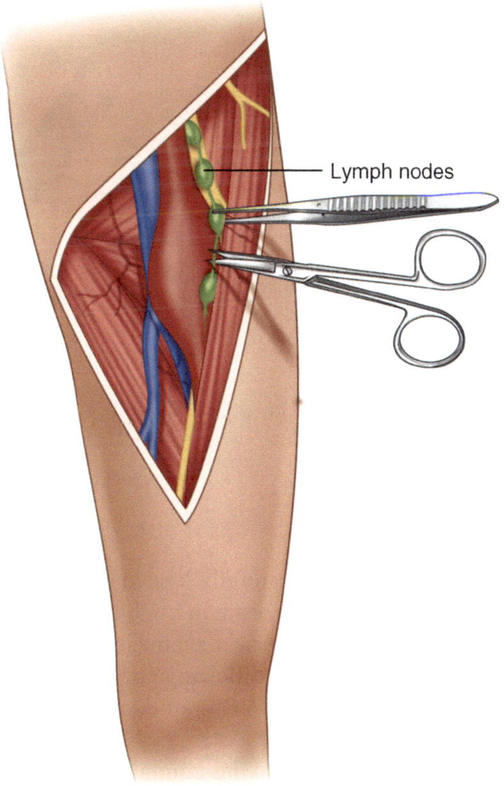

Fig. 12.2 Left inguinal lymph nodes mobilized medially

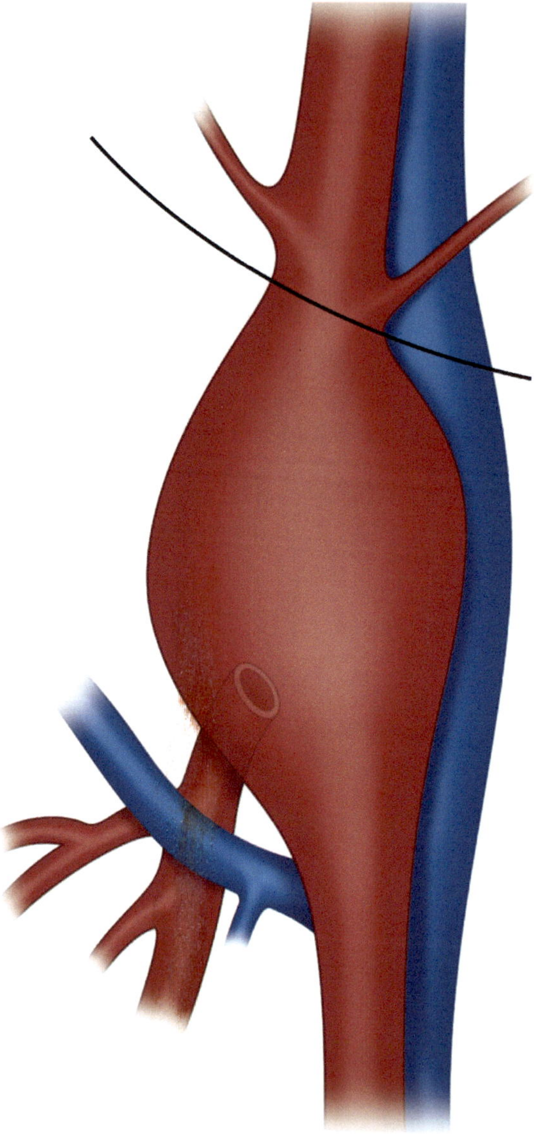

Fig. 12.3 Exposed right common femoral artery aneurysm. Vein crossing the origin of deep (profunda) femoral artery

DFA and should be carefully ligated and divided (Fig. 12.3). Failure to expose this vein and ligate it may result in troublesome bleeding in this area. If the origin of the DFA is difficult to expose, then the intraluminal control can be obtained after opening of the aneurysm following the application of proximal and distal vascular clamps and passage of a Garrett dilator (no. 5 or 6 Teleflex Inc.) into the mouth of the DFA.

In patients with leaking common femoral artery aneurysms, a retroperitoneal approach through a short transverse suprainguinal incision to obtain proximal control of the external iliac artery is performed. Intravenous heparin is administered (100 units/kg) by the anesthesia team.

In most aneurysms, the anterior wall is excised leaving the posterior wall intact. An 8 mm interposition Dacron graft is anastomosed to the distal external iliac artery end to end and the distal anastomosis to the proximal SFA. A small opening (5–6 mm) is made in the posterolateral aspect of the Dacron/PTFE graft, and the DFA is sutured to the opening in the prosthetic graft from inside the opened aneurysm using a continuous 5-0 cardiovascular polypropylene suture (Figs. 12.4 and 12.5). In patients with difficulty in implantation of the DFA into the interposition graft from the CFA to the SFA, an interposition 6 mm PTFE graft is sutured from the DFA to an opening into the interposition graft (Fig. 12.6)

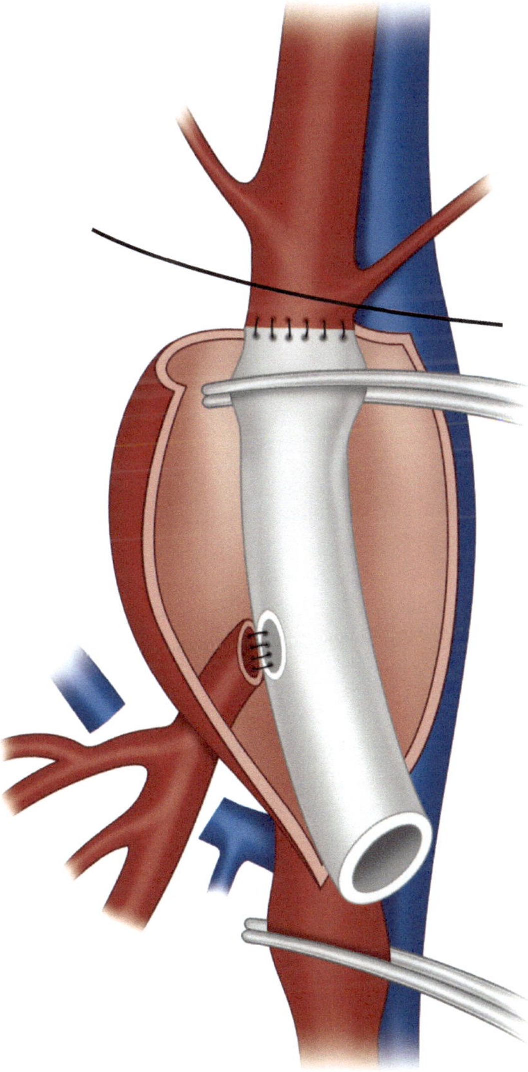

Fig. 12.4 Partial resection of the anterior wall of aneurysm. Vascular clamp applied to the prosthetic graft following completion of proximal end-to-end anastomosis. Vein crossing the deep femoral artery is ligated and divided. The deep femoral artery is being implanted into an opening in the posterolateral wall of the prosthetic graft. Vascular clamp applied to the proximal superficial femoral artery

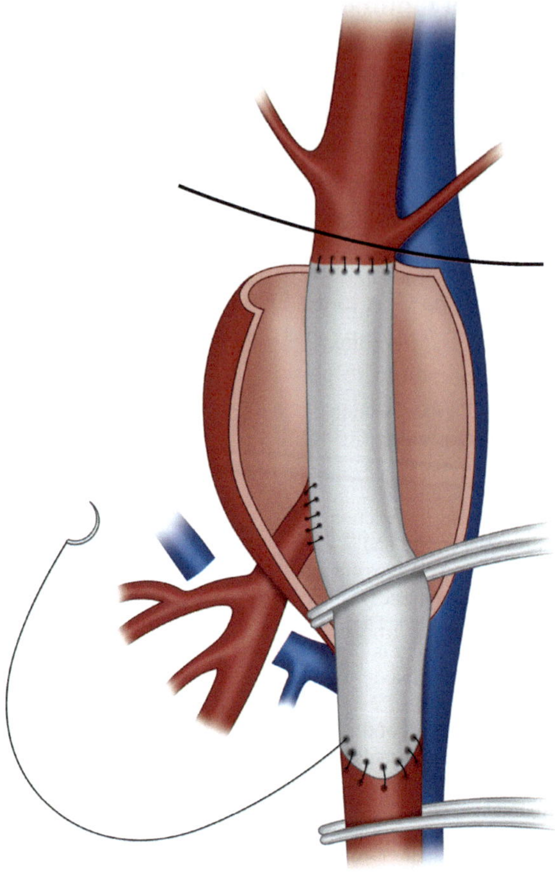

Fig. 12.5 Completed suture line for the deep femoral artery implantation. Completion of distal end-to-end anastomosis of the prosthetic graft to the proximal superficial femoral artery

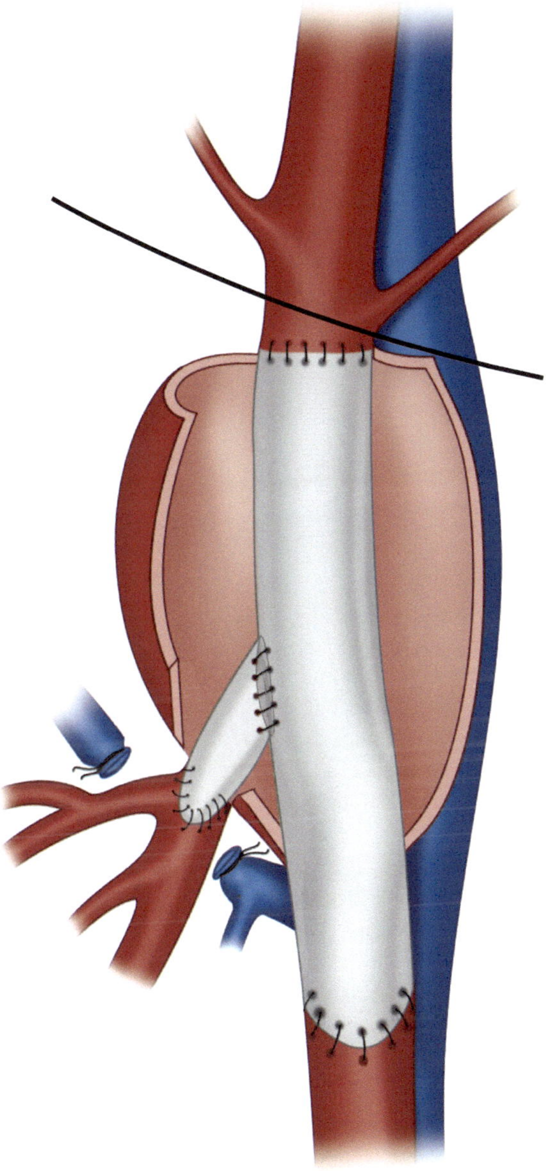

Fig. 12.6 Repair of right femoral aneurysm with interposition graft. A separate interposition graft from the common femoral artery to superficial femoral artery graft with end-to-end anastomosis and a separate graft to the deep femoral artery

In patients with chronic occlusion of the SFA, interposition graft to the DFA should be performed.

Femoral Anastomotic Aneurysm

Femoral anastomotic aneurysms most commonly occur at the site of femoral anastomosis of aortofemoral bypass graft. Femoral anastomotic aneurysm is most often caused by degeneration in the wall of the femoral artery. Anastomotic aneurysms typically present 5 years or later following aortofemoral bypass graft. Aneurysms greater than 2.5 cm in diameter should be repaired. Symptomatic aneurysm with local compression symptoms also should undergo operative repair. Leaking femoral anastomotic aneurysm should be repaired on an emergent basis. Patients with suspected anastomotic aneurysms should undergo femoral duplex imaging followed by CT angiography of the entire graft to evaluate the remote possibility of infection (gas bubbles or fluid) around the graft.

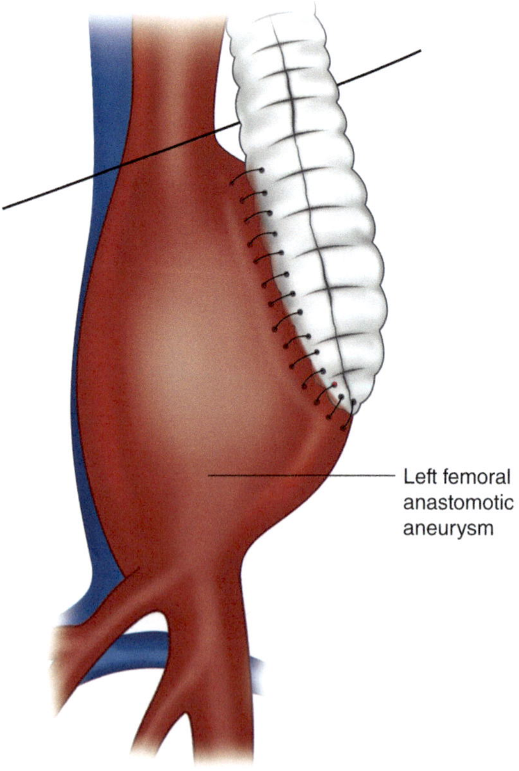

Fig. 12.7 Femoral anastomotic aneurysm

Operative Repair

The previously placed groin incision for aortofemoral grafting is extended proximally and distally depending upon the relationship of the aneurysm to the SFA and DFA. The dense scar tissue around the aneurysm necessitates a sharp dissection with a 15-blade scalpel cutting at an angle. It is important to stay on the outer wall of the aneurysm. The graft is exposed under the inguinal ligament in a similar manner as described in the femoral aneurysm repair. The graft is usually well incorporated and is surrounded by sheath (Fig. 12.7). The common femoral artery posterior to the prosthetic graft is most often occluded. In most patients, the CFA proximal to artery anastomosis is usually sacrificed as the anastomosis at this site following removal of the femoral anastomotic aneurysm is not recommended. Mobilization of the DFA in the proximal SFA is like as described in femoral artery repair chapter. Systemic heparin (100 units/kg) is administered by the anesthesia team. Aneurysm is opened following proximal clamping and placing vascular clamps on the SFA and DFA. As the aneurysm is opened, the sutured line of the anastomotic aneurysm from the previously placed femoral anastomosis of the aortofemoral graft is exposed and the graft is then circumferentially removed from the host artery (CFA and proximal SFA).

After removal of the aneurysm, a proximal anastomosis is performed end to end to the femoral limb of the aortofemoral graft and distal anastomosis is performed end to end within an oblique orientation incorporating the proximal SFA and DFA. In some patients, distal anastomosis is performed end to end to the proximal SFA and DFA, which will need to be reimplanted into the interposed Dacron graft with a continuous suture of 4-0 or 5-0 cardiovascular polypropylene (Fig. 12.8).

In patients with critical limb ischemia and the presence of anastomotic aneurysm, repair of aneurysm and simultaneous infrainguinal bypass may need to be of the aneurysm followed by an interposition of an 8 mm or 10 mm knitted Dacron graft to the remotely placed femoral limb of the graft in an end-to-end fashion, which is performed using 4-0 cardiovascular polypropylene suture representing proximal anastomosis. Distal anastomosis of this new Dacron graft is performed in an end-to-end fashion just above the common femoral artery bifurcation with a continuous 5-0 cardiovascular polypropylene suture carefully maintaining flow to the deep femoral artery. In its distal portion, anastomosis is not completed and Dacron graft at its apex is divided transversely. A 2–3 cm long incision is made in the proximal superficial femoral artery. Endarterectomy of the proximal superficial femoral artery is performed if necessary. The terminal portion of the greater saphenous vein is disconnected from the common femoral vein. The terminal portion is

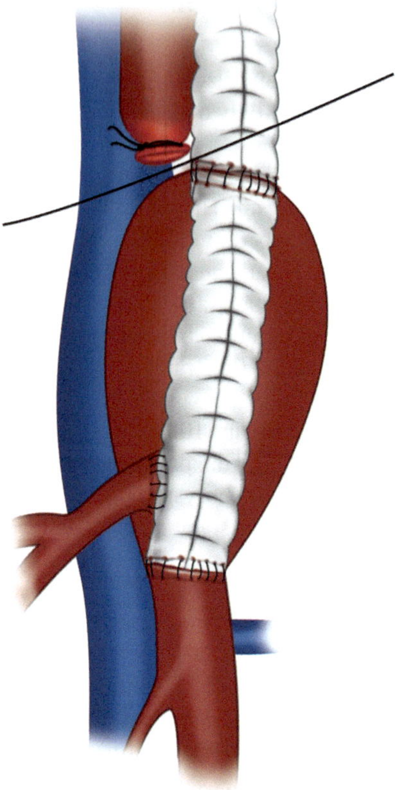

Fig. 12.8 Repair of femoral anastomotic aneurysm with interposition graft and reimplantation of the deep femoral artery into newly interposed prosthetic graft

Fig. 12.9 Repair of femoral anastomotic aneurysm with interposition of a Dacron graft. A simultaneous in situ bypass to proximal superficial femoral artery is shown. The distal anastomosis of the "new" Dacron graft with its anastomosis to the distal common femoral artery in an end-to-end fashion is shown. The apex of Dacron graft cut transversely is sutured to the saphenous vein also cut transversely and are sutured to each other in a continuous fashion

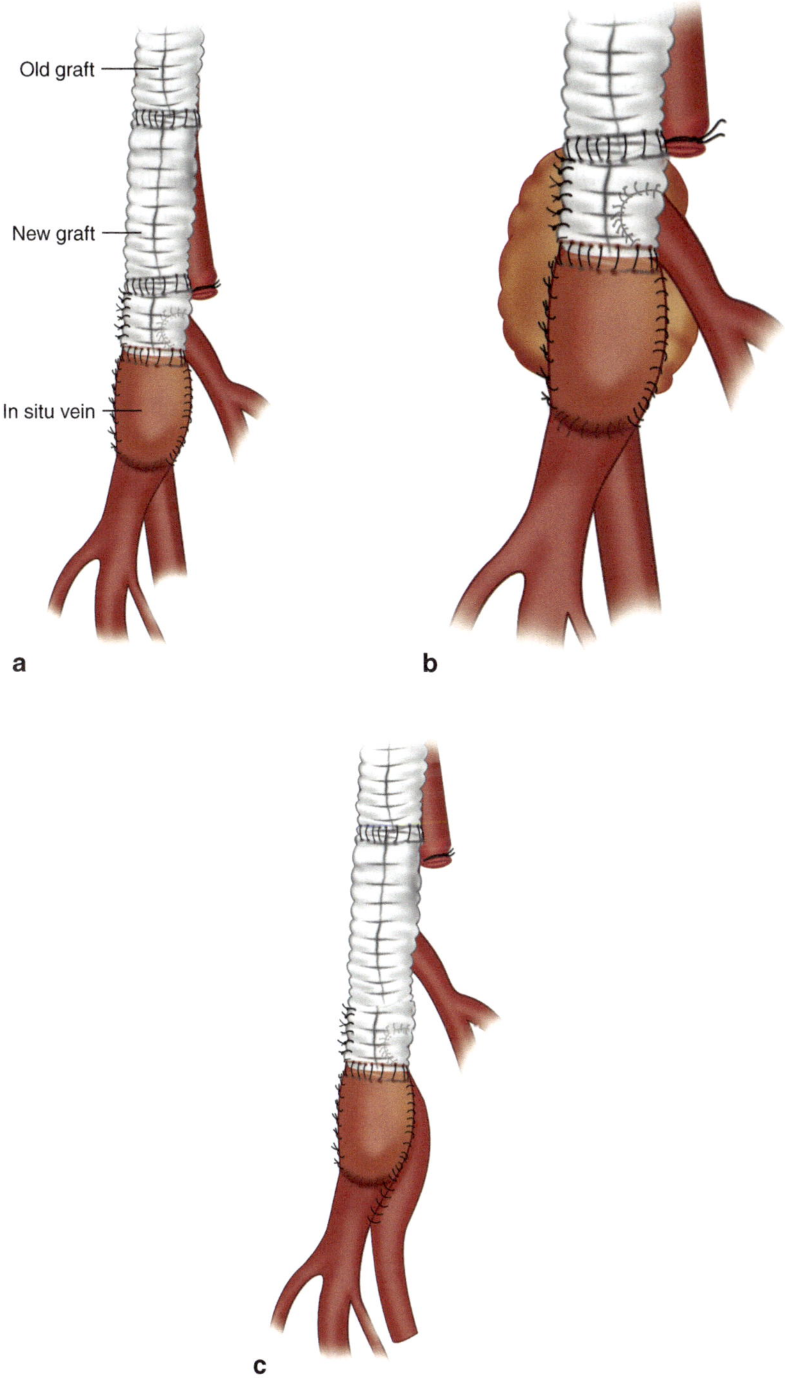

Completed repair of left Femoral anastomotic aneurysm

slit longitudinally for about 3 cm (in-situ vein) and is anastomosed to the proximal superficial femoral artery in an end-to-side fashion using 5-0 or 6-0 cardiovascular polypropylene suture in a continuous fashion using parachute technique. The apex of the terminal greater saphenous vein is divided transversely and is sutured to transversely shape apex of the Dacron graft with a continuous 5-0 cardiovascular polypropylene suture (Fig. 12.9). Bringing the terminal portion of the vein conduit and its anastomosis to the Dacron limb in an end-to-side fashion as a piggyback technique should preferably be avoided.

Postoperative Complications

Postoperative complications include hemorrhage, lymphatic leak, surgical site infection, and recurrent femoral anastomotic aneurysm. Graft occlusion and major limb amputation should be extremely uncommon.

Take-Home Points

1. The dissection during the repair of femoral and femoral anastomotic aneurysm should be kept very close to the aneurysmal wall, and proximal and distal control should be obtained before the aneurysm is opened.
2. In some patients where mobilization of the DFA is difficult to the large size of the aneurysm, intraluminal control of the DFA may be a better option.
3. In patients with leaking femoral and femoral anastomotic aneurysms, proximal control should be obtained via a short transverse incision in the lower quadrant of the abdomen 3–4 cm above the inguinal ligament.

Chapter 13
Popliteal Artery Aneurysm Repair Primary and Recurrent

Mitchell R. Weaver

Clinical Presentation and Indications for Repair

Popliteal artery aneurysms (PAA) are the most frequently encountered true peripheral artery aneurysm that a vascular surgeon repairs. PAA are most commonly seen in older men and are associated with aneurysms at other locations, specifically the contra lateral popliteal artery and the abdominal aorta. While less frequently encountered in clinical practice, iatrogenic and traumatic popliteal artery pseudoaneurysms do occur.

PAA may have an asymptomatic presentation such as a pulsatile mass behind the knee, noted on physical exam, or as an incidental finding on an imaging study. Symptomatic presentations include acute limb-threatening ischemia secondary to sudden thrombosis of the aneurysm or distal embolization of PAA mural thrombus, or more rarely as rupture. Chronic symptoms of ischemia may also occur leading to claudication or tissue loss, which may have an insidious onset due to chronic silent embolization. Local compression of the nerve or vein may lead to pain, paresthesia, or limb swelling.

In general, a PAA that is causing symptoms has indication for repair. For asymptomatic PAA, a size of 2 cm has been a traditionally accepted size to consider elective repair in good risk patients. Other considerations beyond size include degree of thrombus within aneurysm, status of tibial vessel runoff, and ambulatory status, along with consideration of comorbidities and overall health status of the patient.

M. R. Weaver (✉)
Henry Ford Hospital, Detroit, MI, USA

Wayne State University School of Medicine, Detroit, MI, USA
e-mail: mweaver1@hfhs.org

S. S. Hans et al. (eds.), *Primary and Repeat Arterial Reconstructions*,
https://doi.org/10.1007/978-3-031-13897-3_13

Significant PPA mural thrombus in a good risk patient would make the argument for earlier repair, whereas lack of thrombus in a poorer surgical risk patient would advocate for a watchful waiting approach.

Preoperative Evaluation

Several imaging modalities including duplex ultrasound, computed tomography angiography (CTA), magnetic resonance angiogram (MRA), and catheter-based digital subtraction angiography, are available and may be of use in the diagnosis and management of PAA. Duplex ultrasound is a good screening tool for identifying PAA and is also useful for surveillance of asymptomatic PAA that have not reached criteria for repair. Duplex ultrasound is also valuable in identifying the vein preoperatively that will be used as conduit for bypass during repair of PAA. In planning PAA repair, imaging studies must define the extent of the aneurysm and identify any arterial disease proximal or distal to the PAA. CTA is the author's preferred imaging modality for this. Catheter-based digital subtraction angiography is typically reserved for cases of acute PAA occlusion, where catheter-directed thrombolysis is initiated to recover outflow vessels. Catheter-based digital subtraction angiography is also employed when other imaging studies are unable to define the tibial vessel runoff well enough to plan the arterial reconstruction. Ankle brachial index (ABI) along with digital photoplethysmography (PPG) is obtained to objectively document the preoperative physiologic limb perfusion status.

Anatomy

The popliteal artery runs deep within the popliteal fossa and is a continuation of the superficial femoral artery beginning at the level of the adductor hiatus in the adductor magnus muscle of the thigh. The popliteal artery gives off several geniculate branches, and ends at the inferior border of the popliteus muscle where it branches into the anterior tibial artery and the timiperone trunk, which shortly branches into the peroneal and posterior tibial arteries.

Operative Approach

The standard approaches for repair of PAA include posterior approach and medial approach. Advantages of the medial approach include its familiarity to most surgeons and the versatility it allows for proximal and distal exposure such as in cases of superficial femoral artery involvement or a tibial artery being the distal arterial target for bypass. The medial approach also allows ready access to the great saphenous vein. Advantages of the posterior approach include the option for complete excision of the aneurysm in cases of nerve or vein compression. However, this approach is only useful for focal aneurysms as exposure is limited proximally to the adductor canal and to the anterior tibial artery takeoff distally. This approach also limits ready access to an appropriately sized vein to be used as bypass conduit.

Posterior Approach

The posterior approach is performed through and S or step incision (Fig. 13.1). This incision avoids a perpendicular incision across the knee crease, staying medial to the major nerves and veins in approaching the artery. The incision for posterior exposure starts on the posterior medial aspect of the thigh within 1 to 2 cm posterior to the course of the great saphenous vein and is carried down to just below the

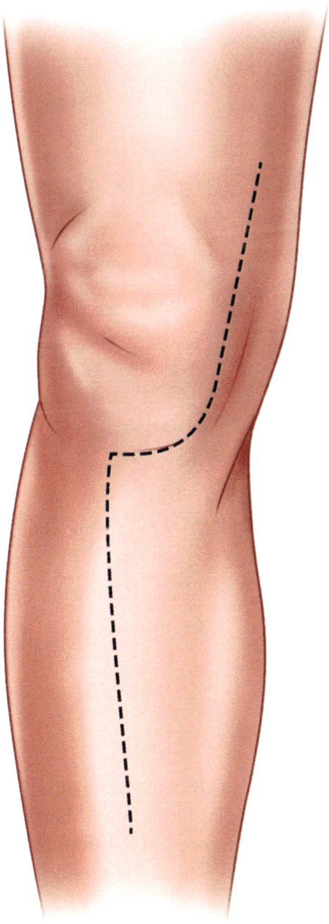

Fig. 13.1 Image demonstrating S or step incision for posterior to popliteal artery, which avoids a perpendicular incision across the knee crease

popliteal crease at which point the incision is sharply curved laterally to the middle of the leg at which point the incision is sharply curved downward. Below the knee, the incision and dissection remain just medial to the small saphenous vein and sural nerve. This incision theoretically provides access to harvest the great or small saphenous vein to be used as autogenous bypass graft. The author's preference is to use the saphenous vein as conduit for arterial reconstruction and typically uses the most proximal great saphenous vein, which tends to offer the best size match. This is performed with the patient in the supine position after which the patient is placed in a prone position for the posterior exposure.

The route to the neurovascular structure in the popliteal fossa is direct, with the popliteal artery the deepest of these structures (Fig. 13.2a, b). Dissection proceeds between the heads of the gastrocnemius muscle, staying medial and avoiding injury to the small saphenous vein and sural nerve. As the gastrocnemius muscle heads are retracted apart, a nerve to the medial head of the gastrocnemius muscle will be encountered and may be difficult to preserve in more distal exposures. In these

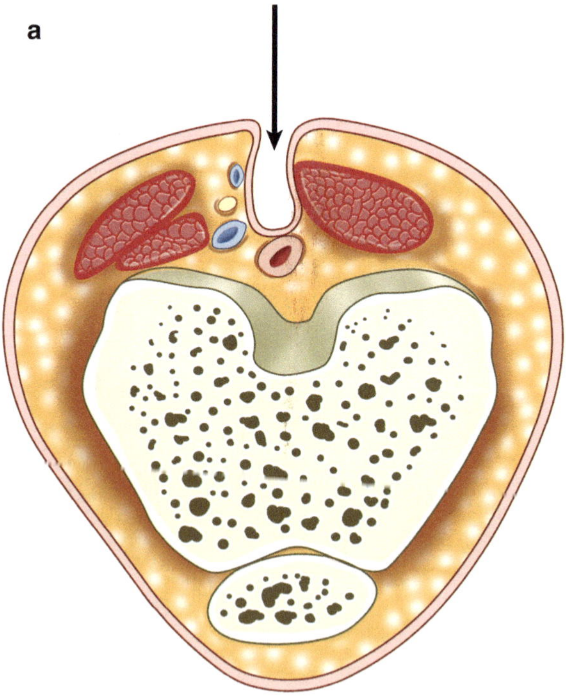

Fig. 13.2 (**a**) Image demonstrating course of dissection for posterior approach to popliteal artery, staying medial to the major nerves and veins in approaching the artery. (**b**) Image demonstrating posterior exposure of the popliteal artery

b

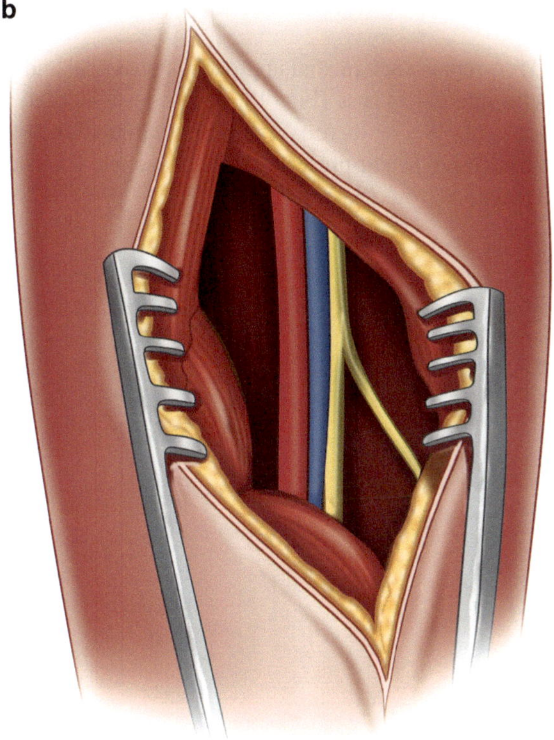

Fig. 13.2 (continued)

typically elderly patients, if a nerve is divided, it does not result in discernable disability. Dissection continues medial to the popliteal vein and usually requires ligation of a few small branches to the vein. Venae comitantes around the artery will require division as well. This exposure usually allows access of the popliteal artery proximally at the level of the adductor hiatus and distally to the origin of the anterior tibial artery.

At this point, the aneurysm is isolated as well as normal artery proximally and distally to the aneurysm. Geniculate branches are ligated. Arterial control is accomplished with application of vascular clamps to the arteries proximal and distal to the aneurysm or alternatively with inflation of a tourniquet in the thigh proximal to the incision after exsanguination of the distal limb with an Esmarch wrap. Then, the aneurysm may be excised or open longitudinally similar to open infrarenal aortic aneurysm repair, and then, the chosen bypass conduit is sewn in place with end-to-end anastomosis proximally and distally in the standard fashion with running polypropylene suture.

Medial Approach

The concept of PAA repair via a medial approach is proximal and distal ligation of the aneurysm with interval bypass (Fig. 13.3). During which attempt is made to ligate side branches of PAA as there is a risk of continued aneurysm growth if it remains pressurized from patent-preserved side branches. Exposure is via above and below knee incisions (Fig. 13.4).

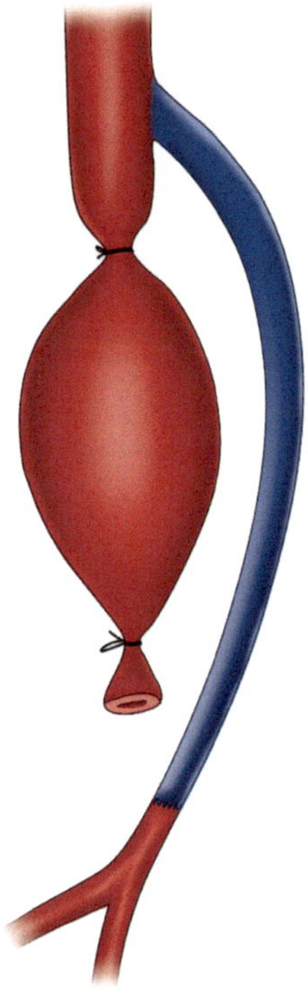

Fig. 13.3 Image demonstrating proximal and distal ligation of popliteal artery aneurysm with interval bypass

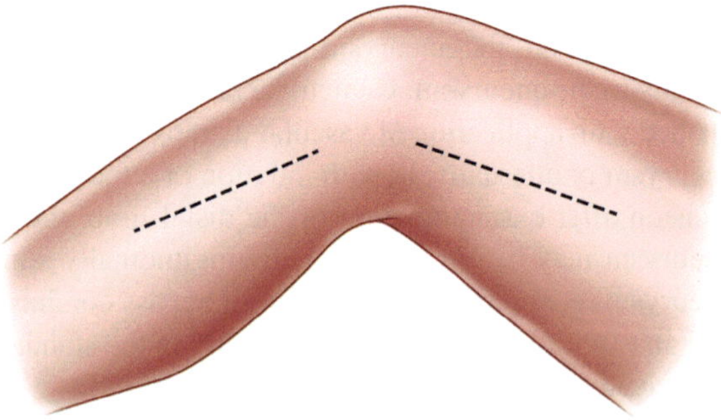

Fig. 13.4 Image demonstrating medial aspect of the lower limb with the knee slightly bent with the site of incisions for medial exposure of the above and below knee popliteal artery

The medial incision to expose the popliteal artery above the knee is made longitudinally over the palpable depression between the vastus medialis above and the sartorius muscle below. If the greater saphenous vein will be needed, the incision can be made closer to it. Once the skin and superficial fascia are opened, the deep fascia will be seen as well as the more opaque outline of its junction with the medial intermuscular septum and the fascia is incised below/posterior to this junction. After incising the fascia just below the intermuscular septum and above the sartorius muscle, the popliteal space is entered (Fig. 13.5a, b). The proximal popliteal artery is surrounded by venae comitantes with the popliteal vein behind it. Exposure of the popliteal artery requires dividing and dissection away these venae comitantes. It should be noted during this dissection that the saphenous nerve exits the adductor hiatus and travels superficially and distally, usually joining the great saphenous vein at or just below the knee. It should be identified and protected. If the nerve is injured, dividing the nerve and leaving the patient with an area of numbness is often better tolerated than ongoing causalgic pain of a partially injured or entrapped nerve.

The medial exposure of the below knee popliteal artery is performed via an incision placed just posterior to the edge of the tibia and in front of the great saphenous vein. Again, if the great saphenous vein is being harvested to use as conduit, the incision may be made closer to the vein. The course to the below knee neurovascular structures is direct (Fig. 13.6a, b), by first incising the fascia into the deep posterior compartment and then taking down fibers of the soleus muscle with electric cautery. Having divided the fibers of the soleus muscle and providing retraction the popliteal vein will come into view. The tibial nerve will be found adjacent to it superiorly and slightly deeper in the incision. The artery will be found deeper between these two structures. For exposure of the more proximal below knee popliteal artery to the anterior tibial artery, the popliteal vein is retracted posteriorly. Exposure including the anterior tibial artery and tibioperoneal trunk requires a greater mobilization of the vein including ligation and division of the anterior tibial vein and possibly other small tributaries.

Once exposure and control of normal artery proximal and distal to the popliteal artery aneurysm have been obtained, working through both incisions, further dissection of the aneurysm is performed to identify and ligate branches. The artery just proximal and distal to the aneurysm is ligated. Arterial reconstruction is then performed, typically with greater saphenous vein graft. Considerations for tunneling of the graft include anatomically or subcutaneously. If the decision is made to tunnel the graft anatomically, one must make certain that it will not be compressed by the residual aneurysm. If the graft is tunneled subcutaneously, it is often advantageous to divide the distal below knee popliteal artery and perform the distal anastomosis end to end. This is done to provide a better course for the graft to follow, as end-to-side anastomoses often result with the graft coming to meet the artery at a right angle and leads to kinking and graft failure.

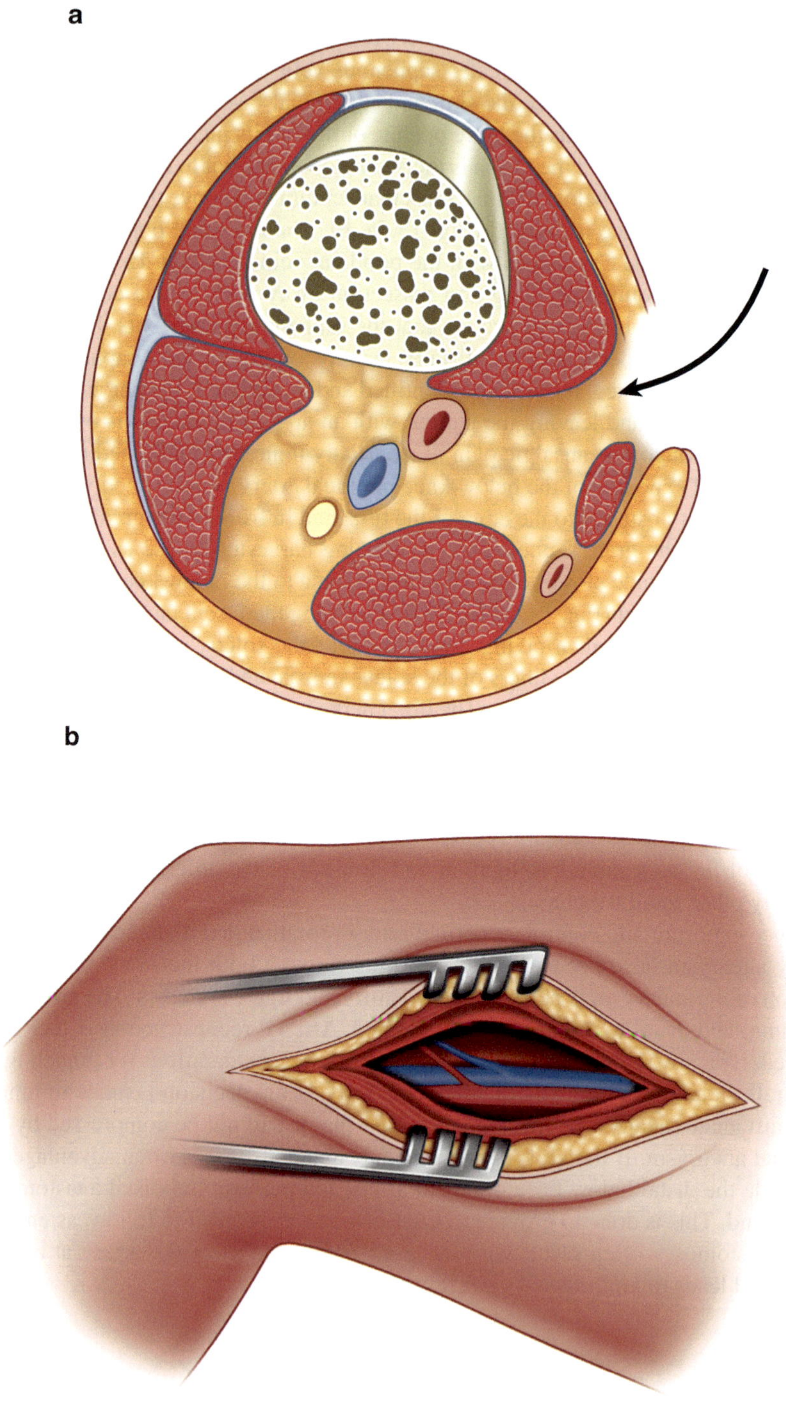

Fig. 13.5 (**a**) Cross-sectional image demonstrating course to the above knee popliteal artery via medial approach. (**b**) Image demonstrating exposure of the above knee popliteal artery via a medial approach

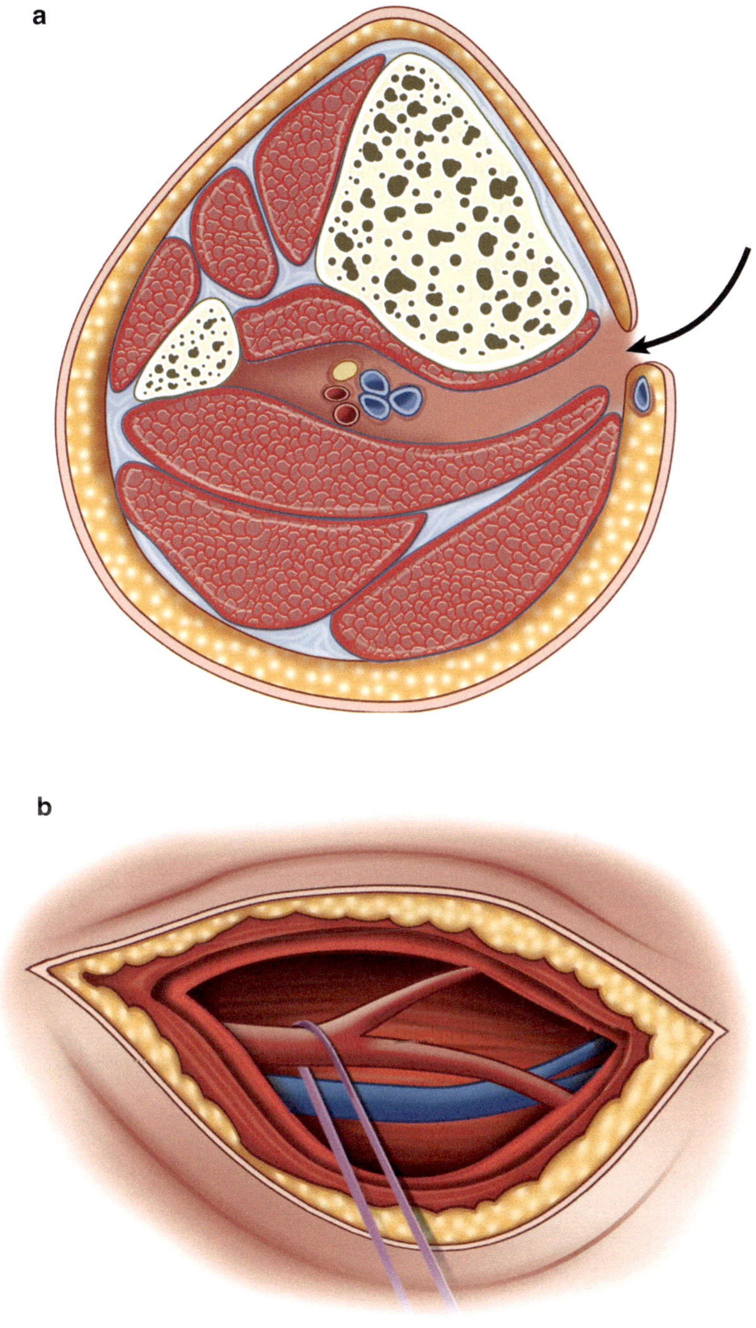

Fig. 13.6 (**a**) Cross-sectional image demonstrating course to the below knee popliteal artery via medial approach. (**b**) Image demonstrating exposure of the below knee popliteal artery via a medial approach

Recurrence and Remedial Interventions

While popliteal artery aneurysm repairs tend to be very durable, recurrent aneurysm may occur from progression of disease of the artery proximally or distally to the repair and, in such cases, require either bypass from a more proximal site or to a more distal site and exclusion of the aneurysmal artery. Also, aneurysms treated with ligation and interval bypass may also continue to grow if pressurized from non-ligated side branches, akin to type 2 endoleaks in endovascular aortic aneurysm repair. In such cases, if aneurysm is symptomatic, treatment requires occlusion of these branches via either open or endovascular techniques.

Chapter 14
Extracranial Carotid Artery Aneurysms

Sachinder Singh Hans

Aneurysms of the extracranial carotid artery are rare and account for less than 1% (0.3–0.6%) of all arterial aneurysms. The aneurysm is most often located in the common carotid artery (CCA) and the internal carotid artery (ICA) junction. The mid to distal ICA is the second most common location of such aneurysms. Atherosclerosis is by far the most common cause, but fibromuscular dysplasia (dysplastic) trauma and prior surgical intervention, congenital anomaly and infection can result in the formation of true carotid aneurysm as well as pseudoaneurysm.

Extracranial carotid aneurysm can be fusiform or saccular. Fusiform carotid artery aneurysms are often bilateral and degenerative in etiology and are located near the carotid bifurcation. Saccular aneurysms are more often unilateral and occur in the midsegment in the ICA in the neck. Pseudoaneurysm results from the disruption of the vessel wall, usually occurring at the site of patch grafting secondary to infection of the prosthetic patch, arterial dissection, and/or blunt/penetrating carotid artery trauma.

Patient may present with asymptomatic neck mass or symptoms of TIA or stroke secondary to embolization. Large aneurysms may cause compression of the surrounding nerves and upper aerodigestive tract. Dysphagia, headache, occipital pain, and retro-orbital pain may occur. Patient may present with Horner syndrome or voice hoarseness. Tracheal compression from ruptured carotid aneurysm can result in airway compromise.

On physical examination, a pulsatile mass in the neck may be palpable. Patient should undergo carotid duplex study followed by CT angiography of the neck. Catheter-based carotid/cerebral arteriography is often helpful in evaluating cross-over intracranial circulation in the event: ICA ligation may become necessary in patients with inaccessible location of the aneurysm.

S. S. Hans (✉)
Vascular and Endovascular Services, Henry Ford Macomb Hospital, Clinton Twp, MI, USA

S. S. Hans et al. (eds.), *Primary and Repeat Arterial Reconstructions*, https://doi.org/10.1007/978-3-031-13897-3_14

Operative Repair

The primary aim of the treatment is resection of the aneurysm and maintaining the flow through the ICA. The incision in the neck is like the one used for carotid endarterectomy (see Chap. 17). The internal jugular vein is mobilized after ligating and dividing of its branches. The hypoglossal vagus nerve and, in patiens with aneurysms extending cephalad, glossopharyngeal nerve are preserved if the dissection extends close to the stylohyoid muscle and the stylohyoid process.

During preoperative planning, if there is any concern for the necessity of exposure of the distal ICA, a mandibular subluxation should be considered, and patient should have nasotracheal intubation and have an ENT surgeon or a maxillofacial surgeon available for performing the subluxation (Figs. 14.1 and 14.2). Mandibular subluxation helps in obtaining distal exposure, which otherwise, may not have been be possible in patients with large aneurysms extending towards the base of the skull.

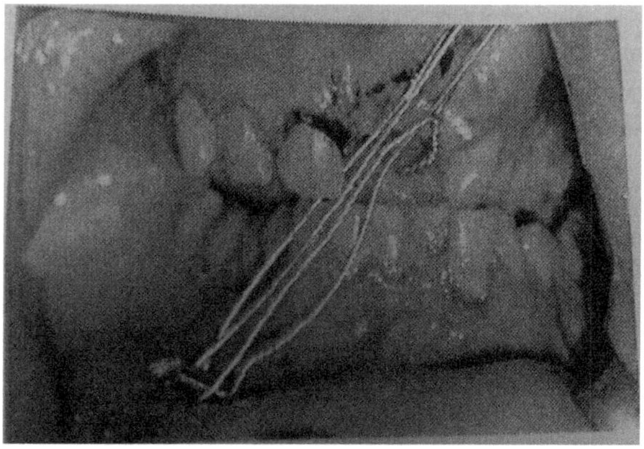

Fig. 14.1 Intraoral wiring for mandibular subluxation

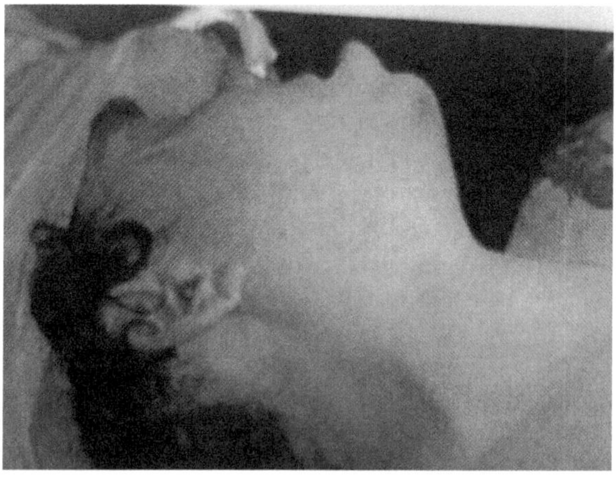

Fig. 14.2 Nasotracheal intubation with mandibular subluxation

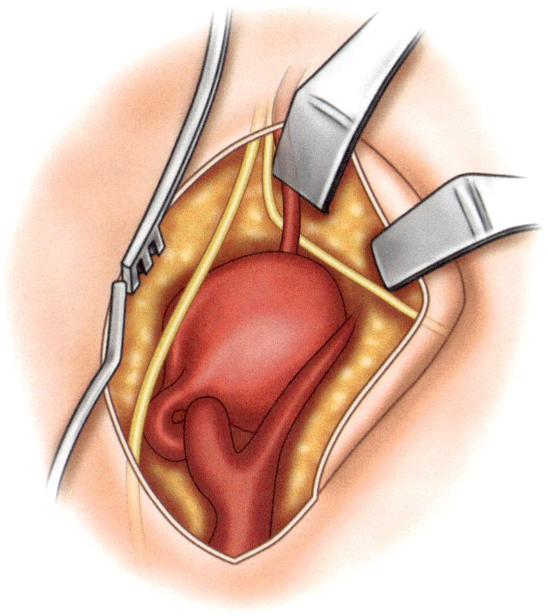

Fig. 14.3 Internal carotid artery aneurysm and its relationship to the vagus nerve with Hypoglossal nerve seen cephaled near the two retractors

Intraoperative shunting is rarely necessary. EEG monitoring, median nerve evoked potentials, and back pressure of the ICA are necessary if shunt placement is required. Heparin is administered intravenously by the anesthesia to keep the ACT 250–300 s. After mobilization of the carotid bifurcation in patients with mid-ICA aneurysms, the external carotid artery (ECA) is looped with a silastic loop and is pulled with the tape caudally. The internal carotid artery with the aneurysm is very carefully mobilized, and this mobilization helps in obtaining distal exposure of the ICA (Fig. 14.3).

Small aneurysms with redundant ICA can be resected in an end-to-end anastomosis performed using 6-0 or 7-0 cardiovascular polypropylene suture (Ethicon, Somerville, NJ). The internal carotid artery should be spatulated so that an end-to-end (functional side-to-side) anastomosis is performed (Figs. 14.4 and 14.5).

Partial resection of the aneurysmal wall with patch angioplasty using prosthetic patch is another option available in patients with anatomically high lesions. All the thrombotic material in the aneurysm should be carefully removed in such instances. In most patients, the anterior wall of the aneurysm should be resected to prevent injury to the nerves lying posterior to the aneurysm.

In some patients, interposition grafting may be necessary A synthetic graft (ringed PTFE WL Gore, Newark, DE) should be considered. A greater saphenous vein or superficial femoral artery harvested from the groin and upper thigh can also be used as a conduit following resection of the aneurysm. In mycotic aneurysms involving CCA/ICA, autologous conduit is preferred. In patients with large extracranial ICA aneurysm extending to the base of the skull, ICA ligation may be the

Fig. 14.4 Resected ICA aneurysm

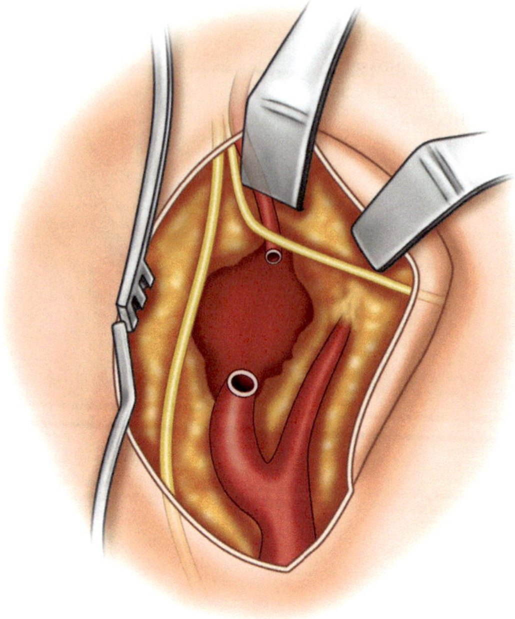

Fig. 14.5 Spatulated end to end ICA anastomosis following resection of ICA aneurysm. Hypoglossal nerve is placed behind the ICA

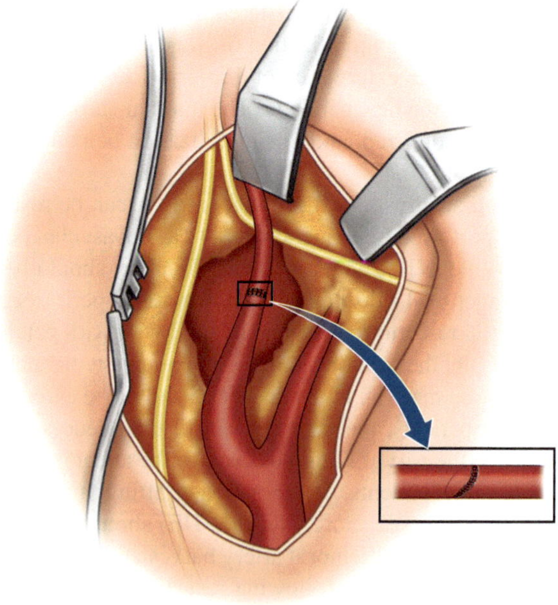

only option available for repair. Preoperative arteriography and intermittent balloon occlusion of ICA at its origin should be performed to evaluate the cross circulation in the circle of Willis. This treatment option is rarely necessary, as in most patients, arterial reconstruction following resection of the carotid aneurysm is feasible.

Complications

The most common complication of carotid artery aneurysms repair is cranial nerve injury. Perioperative stroke is the second common complication.

Chapter 15
Subclavian Artery Aneurysm

Mitchell R. Weaver

Presentation

Asymptomatic subclavian artery aneurysm may be found on physical exam as a pulsatile mass or incidentally on an imaging study. Symptoms of subclavian aneurysms include upper extremity ischemia from distal thromboembolization, hemorrhage from rupture, or compressive symptoms. Compressive symptoms may include brachial plexopathy, ipsilateral Horner's syndrome, or dysphagia lusoria, which may be seen with subclavian artery aneurysms developing at the origin of aberrant right subclavian arteries (Fig. 15.1a, b).

Several imaging modalities including computed tomography angiography (CTA), magnetic resonance angiogram (MRA), and catheter-based digital subtraction angiography, which are available and may be of use in the diagnosis and management of subclavian artery aneurysms. In planning subclavian artery aneurysm repair, imaging studies must define the extent of the aneurysm and identify any arterial disease proximal or distal to the aneurysm. CTA is the author's preferred imaging modality for this. Upper extremity segmental pressures and Doppler waveform analysis, along with digital photoplethysmography (PPG) are obtained to objectively document physiologic limb perfusion in case of ischemia.

M. R. Weaver (✉)
Henry Ford Hospital, Detroit, MI, USA

Wayne State University School of Medicine, Detroit, MI, USA
e-mail: mweaver1@hfhs.org

S. S. Hans et al. (eds.), *Primary and Repeat Arterial Reconstructions*,
https://doi.org/10.1007/978-3-031-13897-3_15

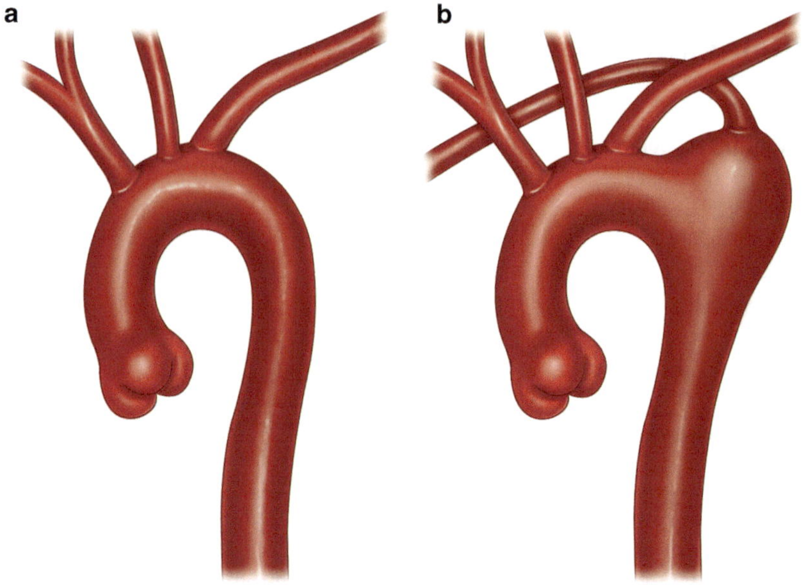

Fig. 15.1 (**a**) Image demonstrating typical aortic arch anatomy. (**b**) Image demonstrating aortic arch anatomy with aberrant right subclavian artery with aneurysm at origin

Management

Given the rarity of subclavian artery aneurysms, the exact size at which asymptomatic aneurysm should be repaired is not clearly defined; however, the presence of symptoms is an indication for repair. Aneurysms of the proximal subclavian artery, which are intrathoracic such as those associated with an aberrant right subclavian artery, prior to the development of endovascular therapies, required direct repair via a left thoracotomy and aortic replacement. This operation would typically be preceded by a right carotid subclavian artery bypass or transposition (see Chap. 22). In current practice, a hybrid approach is often used with performance of right carotid subclavian artery transposition followed by deployment of a thoracic stent graft (Fig. 15.2). Given difficulty in exposure of the subclavian artery secondary to the bony structures around it, endovascular repairs with stent grafting have been increasingly utilized especially in emergent settings with hemorrhage (Fig. 15.3a, b).

However, cases of aneurysms involving the more distal subclavian artery, especially those secondary to external compression as in arterial thoracic outlet, require open repair. Open repair is required not only to the repair of the artery but also for resection or repair of the compressive elements that led to the arterial injury, which are typically cervical rib, anomalous first rib, or clavicle. Most of these aneurysms extend beyond the lateral border of the first rib and thus are subclavian–axillary aneurysms. Open repair of subclavian–axillary aneurysms associated with cervical rib requires supra- and infraclavicular exposure (Fig. 15.4).

Fig. 15.2 Image demonstrating hybrid repair of aberrant right subclavian artery aneurysm with right carotid subclavian transposition and thoracic endograft

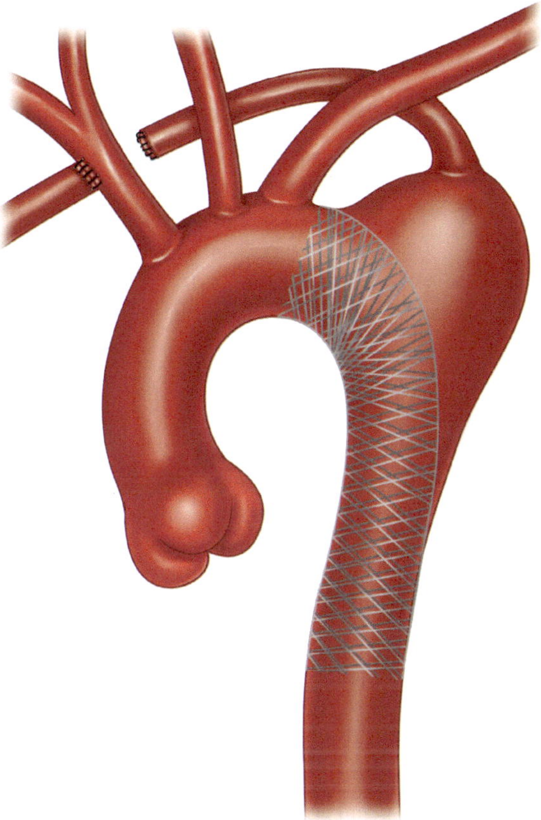

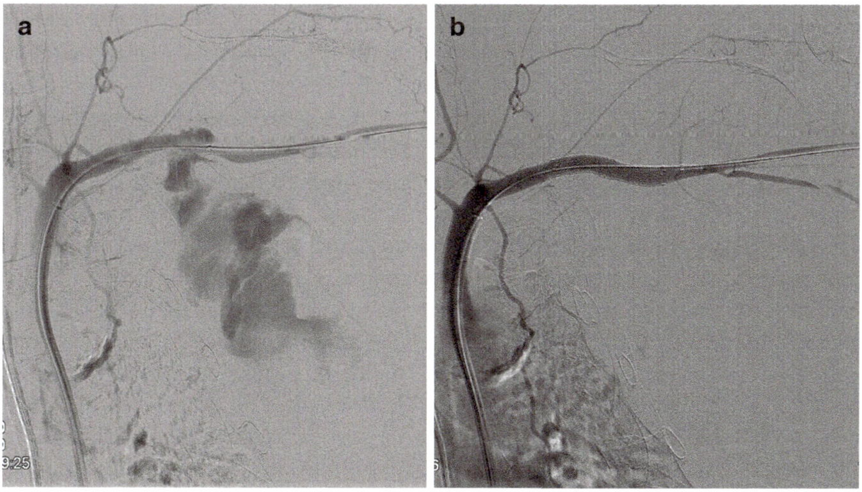

Fig. 15.3 (**a**) Digital subtraction angiogram demonstrating ruptured traumatic left subclavian pseudoaneurysm. (**b**) Digital subtraction angiogram following repair of pseudoaneurysm with stent graft

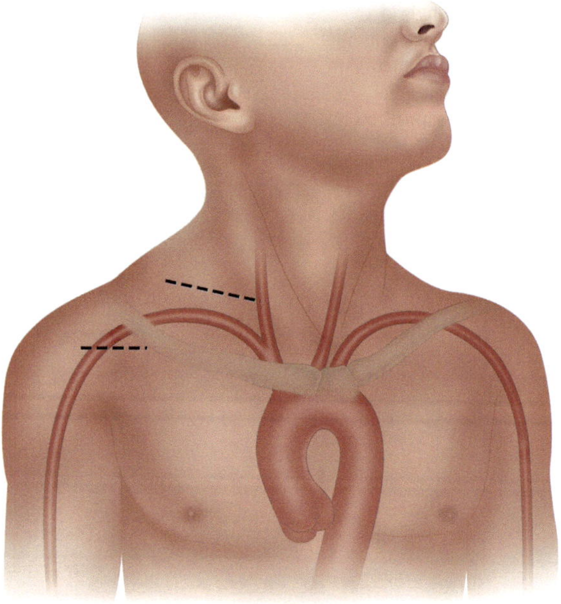

Fig. 15.4 Image demonstrating sites of supra- and infraclavicular incisions for exposure of subclavian and axillary arteries

Anatomy

The right subclavian artery arises from the innominate artery posterior to the sternoclavicular joint. Near the subclavian artery's origin, the right recurrent laryngeal nerve branches off of the vagus nerve, which is coursing anteriorly and wraps around the subclavian artery to ascend in the neck. The subclavian artery from its origin passes upward and then laterally behind the anterior scalene muscle, with the subclavian vein coursing anterior to the anterior scalene muscle. The subclavian artery then exits through the thoracic outlet between the clavicle and the first rib with the subclavian vein anterior and the brachial plexus posterior to the artery. Once past the outer boarder to the first rib, it becomes the axillary artery. Branches of the subclavian artery include the vertebral artery, internal thoracic artery, thyrocervical trunk, costocervical trunk, and dorsal scapular artery. An exception to the anatomy is cases of aberrant right subclavian arteries, which usually arise distally and posteriorly on the aortic arch coursing posterior to the esophagus, which may lead to compressive symptoms. The left subclavian artery typically is the last great vessel to arise from the aortic arch, which fist travels cephalad and then laterally posterior to the anterior scalene muscle. The thoracic duct ascends in the chest behind the aortic arch and left subclavian artery as it eventually courses anterior to the anterior scalene muscle and drains in the venous system near the junction of the left internal jugular and subclavian veins.

Open Repair

After general anesthesia is induced with the patient in a supine position, a rolled-up sheet is placed underneath the patient's shoulder and the table positioned with the head and torso raised approximately 30°. The neck is extended and rotated slightly to the contralateral side. The supraclavicular incision is made starting approximately 1 cm lateral to the midline and continued laterally approximately 6–8 cm, approximately 1–2 cm above the clavicle. The platysma muscle is divided with cautery and flaps are developed superiorly approximately 5 cm and inferiorly to the clavicle. The sternocleidomastoid muscle is mobilized along its lateral border, and if necessary, the clavicular head of the sternocleidomastoid muscle is freed off at the clavicle to allow for extended medial exposure. The omohyoid muscle is encountered and divided, furthering exposure of the anterior scalene fat pad. Starting on the medial edge of the anterior scalene fat pad is separated from the internal jugular vein and then its inferior border mobilized while carefully ligating all lymphatics as they are divided. On the left side, care is taken not to injure the thoracic duct; however, if injured or divided, it is meticulously oversewn with fine monofilament polypropylene suture. Once mobilized, the anterior scalene fat pad is retracted laterally and superiorly.

The anterior scalene muscle is then exposed along with the phrenic nerve, which runs lateral to medial, anterior to, and within the investing fascia of the muscle (Fig. 15.5). The nerve is carefully mobilized off the muscle, incising the fascia a few millimeters on either side of it. The edges of the anterior scalene muscle are then freed, and the muscle is divided exposing the subclavian artery (Fig. 15.6). Further dissections of the subclavian artery proximally can be performed, if necessary, by continuing medially and identifying and mobilizing the internal mammary and vertebral arteries. The vertebral vein is often encountered superficial to the subclavian artery and is divided to facilitate exposure. On the right side, additional exposure can be obtained with resection of the clavicular head, which will allow exposure to the distal innominate artery. Laterally abnormal fibrous band and the cervical rib if present are freed from around the artery and resected.

Infraclavicular exposure is obtain through incision starting just lateral to the sternal head of the clavicle overlying the deltopectoral groove, beginning about 1 cm below the clavicle and ending laterally about 2 cm below the clavicle (Fig. 15.4). The pectoralis major muscle fibers are split exposing the clavipectoral fascia with the pectoralis minor muscle in the lateral half of the incision. Care is taken to preserve nerve branches to the pectoralis major muscle. The cephalic vein may also be encountered as it passed between the heads of the pectoralis major muscle to join the axillary vein. Dividing the clavipectoral fascia will expose branches of the thoracoacromial trunk, which can be followed down to the first portion of the axillary artery (Fig. 15.7). The axillary vein that runs inferior and superficial to the artery is usually encountered first. Laterally, the pectoralis minor muscle is divided near its insertion to the coracoid process where the muscle is more tendinous to further expose the axillary artery as necessary.

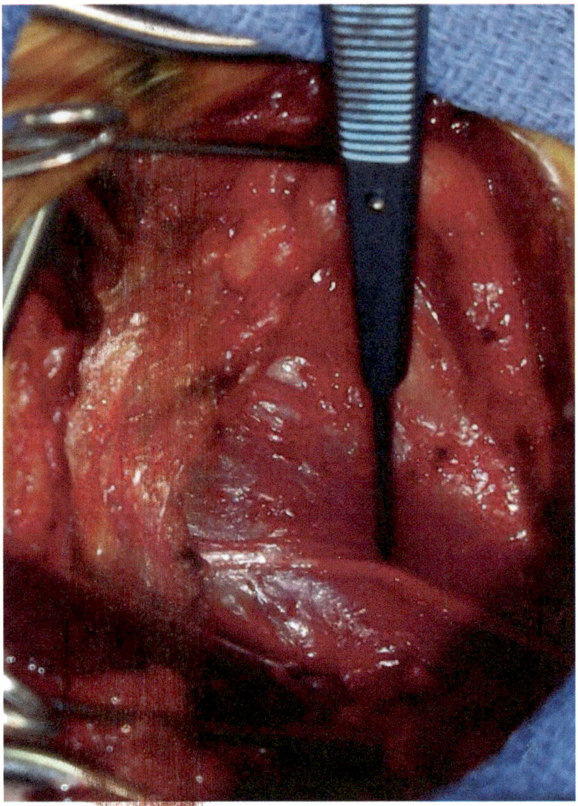

Fig. 15.5 Image demonstrating exposure of the anterior scalene muscle with phrenic nerve running over it

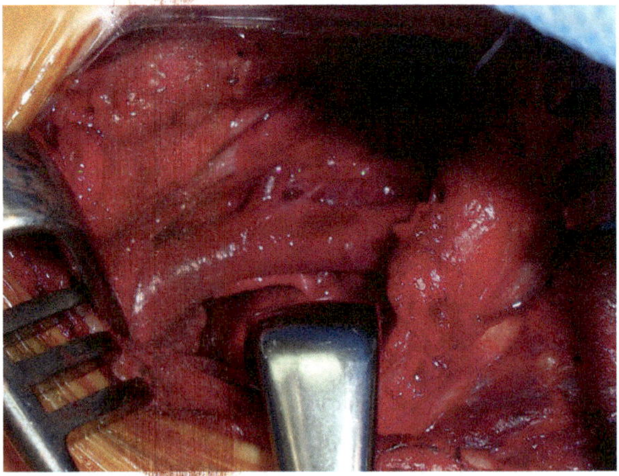

Fig. 15.6 Image demonstrating the subclavian artery after division of the anterior scalene muscle

Having obtained arterial control proximal and distal to the aneurysm working from both incisions, the aneurysm is freed from the neighboring neurovascular structures and any arterial branches are ligated and divided. Having the aneurysm

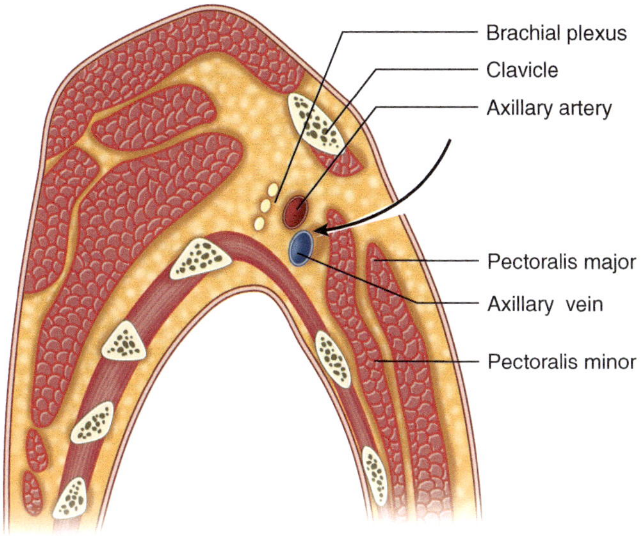

Fig. 15.7 Sagittal image demonstrating course to the axillary artery with splitting of the fibers of the pectoralis major muscle and division of the pectoralis minor muscle near its insertion to the coracoid process

Fig. 15.8 Image demonstrating interposition graft from the subclavian artery to the axillary artery passing anatomically between the clavicle and first rib for repair of aneurysm

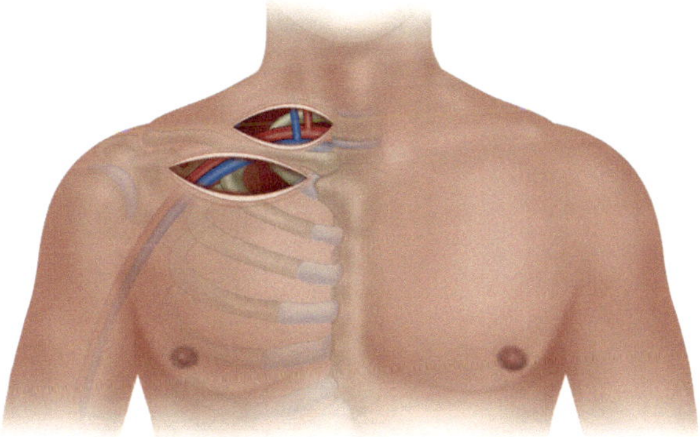

completely free, the patient can be systemically heparinized with the arteries clamped, the aneurysm resected, and arterial reconstruction performed with interposition vein graft (Fig. 15.8). With one's finger placed within the thoracic outlet the arm can be moved in multiple stress positions to make sure that no residual compression remains. If compression remains resection of the first rib may need to be performed in addition to the cervical rib.

Potential complications include nerve injury to the brachial plexus or phrenic nerve and lymphatic injuries, specifically on the left side, an injury to the thoracic duct. There is a low threshold for reexploration of any significant or persistent lymph leak.

Chapter 16
Axillary and Brachial Aneurysms

Farah Hanif Ali Mohammad

Surgical Anatomy

Axillary Artery

The axillary artery has three parts based on pectoralis minor. The first part is superior and medial to the pectoralis minor and begins as continuation of the subclavian artery at the lateral edge of the first rib. Here it gives off its first branch named the superior thoracic artery. The second portion lies underneath the pectoralis minor and gives off thoracoacromial and lateral thoracic artery. Third portion lies lateral to the pectoralis minor and gives off subscapular, anterior, and posterior humeral circumflex artery. It continues on to become brachial artery at the lower margin of teres major. The axillary vein runs along its entire course medially. The brachial plexus runs posterior to the first and then interlaces the second and third part.

Brachial Artery

The axillary artery continues on to become the brachial artery past the inferior border of teres major. The brachial artery passes between the biceps and triceps muscles. In the antecubital fossa, it divides into the radial, interosseous, and ulnar arteries to supply the soft tissues of the forearm. The median nerve runs along the artery crossing from relatively lateral to medial position as it goes distally. Its first

F. H. A. Mohammad (✉)
Henry Ford Hospital, Detroit, MI, USA

S. S. Hans et al. (eds.), *Primary and Repeat Arterial Reconstructions*,
https://doi.org/10.1007/978-3-031-13897-3_16

major branch called the deep brachial artery runs posteriorly and serves as a major collateral in the setting of brachial injury. Two brachial veins closely run along the artery in the brachial sheath.

Axillary and Brachial Artery Aneurysms

Axillary and brachial artery aneurysms are uncommon and account for less than 1% of peripheral artery aneurysms. True aneurysms may be congenital, degenerative, or inflammatory in nature. Chronic repetitive trauma of the axillary artery can also cause aneurysmal degeneration. This phenomenon is seen in patients who are chronically dependent on crutches. Axillary aneurysms have also been reported in baseball pitchers. They can also arise from first rib compression in thoracic outlet syndrome. Pseudoaneurysms can occur after penetrating and blunt trauma. They can also be iatrogenic in nature. Brachial artery is frequently used as an access during cardiac catheterizations and arterial lines. Mycotic brachial artery pseudoaneurysms have also been reported in patients with history of IV drug abuse.

All symptomatic true or pseudoaneurysms should be repaired. Most common presentation is distal embolization leading to digital ischemia. They may also present with neurologic symptoms associated with brachial plexus (axillary) or median nerve (brachial artery) compression. Pseudoaneurysms may also present in the setting of infection, in which case ligation may be well tolerable due to significant collaterals. Asymptomatic true aneurysms should be repaired if >2 cm. Pseudoaneurysms from iatrogenic injury may be amenable to ultrasound-guided thrombin injection. If the neck is wide or there are pressure-induced skin changes from the aneurysm, it will need an open repair. Most commonly management includes simple primary repair, resection with end-to-end anastomosis, patch angioplasty, and interposition bypass.

Operative Steps for Axillary Artery Aneurysms

The patient is positioned supine with the ipsilateral arm abducted to 90 degrees. The first and second portions of the axillary artery are best exposed with an infraclavicular incision approximately 2 cm below the clavicle. The incision is made from mid-clavicle to anterior surface of deltoid, approximately 7–8 cm in length. Subcutaneous soft tissue and clavipectoral fascia are divided. The pectoralis major muscle fibers are either retracted or split (Fig. 16.1). The axillary sheath lies in the fatty areolar tissue underneath the fascia. The artery lies just deep and slightly cephalad to the vein. The vein should be carefully dissected and retracted caudally. The nerves lie behind the first portion of the axillary artery at this level; thus, clamps should be placed carefully. Pectoralis minor muscle may need to be divided for exposure for

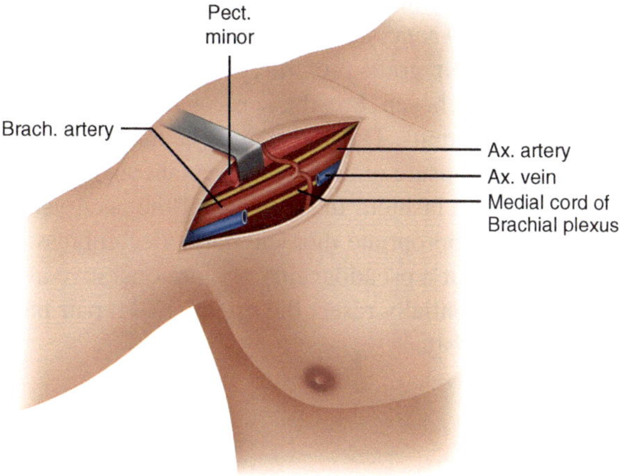

Fig. 16.1 Infraclavicular exposure of axillary artery. Division of Pectoralis minor tendon at its insertion

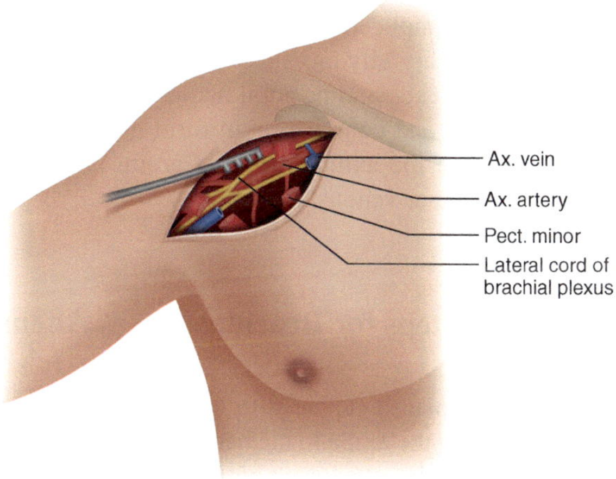

Fig. 16.2 Distal axillary and proximal brachial artery exposure

the second portion of the axillary artery. The pectoral nerves should be identified and protected if the pectoralis minor is resected near the coracoid process. Ligation and division of the thoracoacromial artery help in exposure. The cords of the brachial plexus run anterior and around the artery in this region; thus, careful dissection is required. If more lateral or if the third portion needs exposure, the incision would have to be extended on to the deltopectoral groove (Fig. 16.2). The pectoralis major may be resected near its insertion if necessary. The cephalic vein is dissected along its medial border and retracted laterally along with deltoid muscle. Here the clavipectoral fascia is divided along the inferior border of the coracobrachialis muscle up to the coracoid process. The neurovascular bundle lies in the areolar tissue underneath the fascia. The median nerve is the most superficial portion in the sheath. The nerve can be carefully retracted cephalad. The vein and ulnar nerve lie medial the artery in this segment. Once the artery is exposed and encircled, decision is made for the repair. Aneurysm repair usually involves resection and interposition bypass. Autogenous vein grafts preferably lower extremity veins (great saphenous veins are better) can be chosen. Prosthetic reconstruction may be utilized if there are no adequate vein conduits. The conduit can be tunneled anatomically if aneurysm is focal and within exposure or tunneled subcutaneously if proximal and distal incisions are made in a skip fashion. In rare cases if the aneurysm is due to thoracic outlet syndrome, then appropriate thoracic outlet decompression will need to be performed. In the setting of a pseudoaneurysm, intraoperative assessment of the vessel may be needed to potentially resect the pseudo and repair the artery primarily or with vein patch angioplasty.

Pearls

Understanding the relation to the artery to the surrounding structures is key to avoiding technical complications. The vein lies medial to the artery and may be adherent and should be carefully mobilized especially due to the surrounding inflammation. The brachial plexus and pectoral nerves lie behind the first part but then wrap the second portion and continue on to form the median nerve lying superficial to the third portion of the axillary artery. Careful meticulous dissection is necessary to avoid any nerve or venous injuries.

Operative Steps for Brachial Artery Aneurysm

The patient is placed supine with the arm abducted to 90° over an arm board. The entire arm from the axilla to the hand is prepped and draped. This helps with checking perfusion at the conclusion of the procedure. To expose the brachial artery in the arm, an axial incision is made on the medial aspect of the arm between the biceps and triceps muscles (Fig. 16.3). Care should be taken to avoid the superficial basilic vein running medially in the lower portion of the arm. The biceps muscle is retracted anteriorly, and the deep fascia over its medial border is incised. This exposes the neurovascular bundle. The most superficial structure is the median nerve and should be carefully mobilized and retracted. The artery lies underneath the nerve surrounded

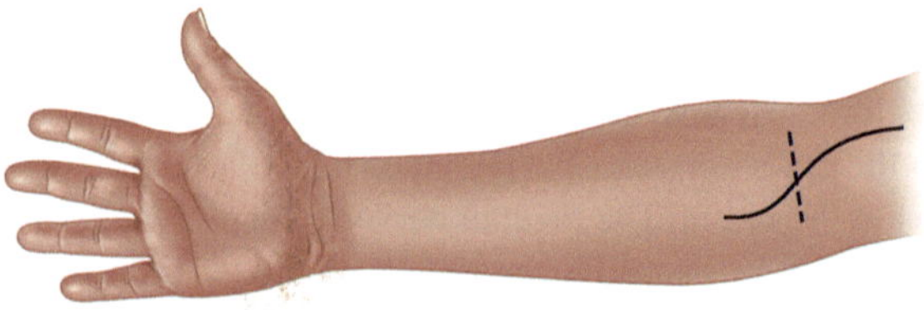

Fig. 16.3 Type of incisions (transverse and S-shaped) for exposure of the brachial artery at the elbow

by two brachial veins. The deep brachial artery should be identified and protected while exposing the proximal brachial artery. Other branches including the superior and inferior ulnar collateral arteries may need to be controlled in the mid or distal exposure. Interconnecting veins over the artery can be carefully ligated. Surgeon should be aware of the possibility of high bifurcation if two large branches are seen.

At the antecubital fossa, usually a transverse incision just inferior to the antecubital crease may be sufficient (Fig. 16.4). However, if the aneurysm is large or more extensive exposure is needed, then an S-shaped incision is more suitable. The superior longitudinal portion is made along the medial border of the biceps muscle, and horizontal portion runs along the crease, and inferior portion extends laterally onto the forearm. As the incision is deepened, the basilic vein again may be encountered on the medial portion. The antecubital nerve should be protected if possible. The bicipital aponeurosis is seen in the center of the wound at the fascial level. Once this

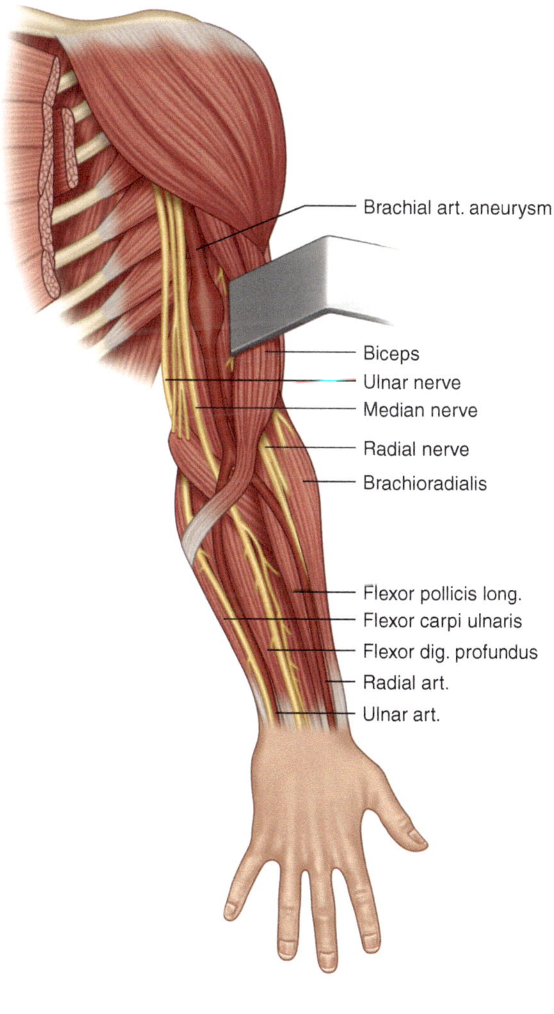

Fig. 16.4 Exposure of left brachial artery, radial and ulnar artery

is divided, the artery can be seen in between two deep brachial veins. Depending on the location and extent of the brachial aneurysm, the artery may be exposed. Aneurysm repair usually involves resection and interposition bypass. Autogenous vein grafts preferably lower extremity veins (great saphenous veins are better) can be harvested. Prosthetic reconstruction may be utilized if there are no adequate vein conduits. The conduit can be tunneled anatomically. In the setting of a pseudoaneurysm, intraoperative assessment of the vessel may be needed to potentially resect the sac and repair the artery primarily or with vein patch angioplasty. If the concern is that the aneurysm is due to an infection and reconstruction is not possible, then the artery may be ligated as long as the deep brachial branch is preserved.

Pearls

Understanding the relation to the artery to the surrounding structures is key to avoiding technical complications. Median nerve is superficial and crosses the artery from lateral to medial position. Injury to the nerve can be devastating. Careful meticulous dissection is necessary to avoid any nerve or venous injuries.

Part II
Open Arterial Reconstructions for Arterial Occlusive Disease

Chapter 17
Carotid Endarterectomy

Sachinder Singh Hans

Surgical Anatomy

Common Carotid and Internal and External Carotid Arteries

The common carotid arteries (CCA) are variable in length and their anatomic origin. The right CCA originates at the bifurcation of the brachiocephalic trunk posterior to the right sternoclavicular joint and continues cephalad in the neck. The left CCA arises from the highest portion of the arch of the aorta to the left and posterior to the brachiocephalic trunk and can be divided into the intrathoracic portion and a cervical portion.

The cervical portion of each CCA passes obliquely cephalad and slightly laterally to the upper border of the thyroid cartilage where it divides into the external and internal carotid arteries. The CCA with the internal jugular vein and vagus nerve are contained in the carotid sheath, the vein coursing lateral to the artery and the vagus nerve lying between the artery and the vein posteriorly; however, in its inferior portion, the vagus nerve tends to cource anteriorly and medial (Fig. 17.1). The upper border of the thyroid cartilage (carotid bifurcation) is usually at the level of the fourth cervical vertebral body. The carotid bifurcation is variable, and bifurcation can be as low as the level of cervical fifth or even cervical sixth vertebral body or high at the level of cervical third vertebral body. At the point of division of the CCA, internal carotid artery (ICA) is slightly dilated into carotid sinus. The adventitial layer of the ICA is thicker in the carotid sinus and contains numerous sensory fibers arising from glossopharyngeal nerve. These nerve fibers respond to changes in the

S. S. Hans (✉)
Vascular and Endovascular Services, Henry Ford Macomb Hospital,
Clinton Twp, MI, USA

S. S. Hans et al. (eds.), *Primary and Repeat Arterial Reconstructions*,
https://doi.org/10.1007/978-3-031-13897-3_17

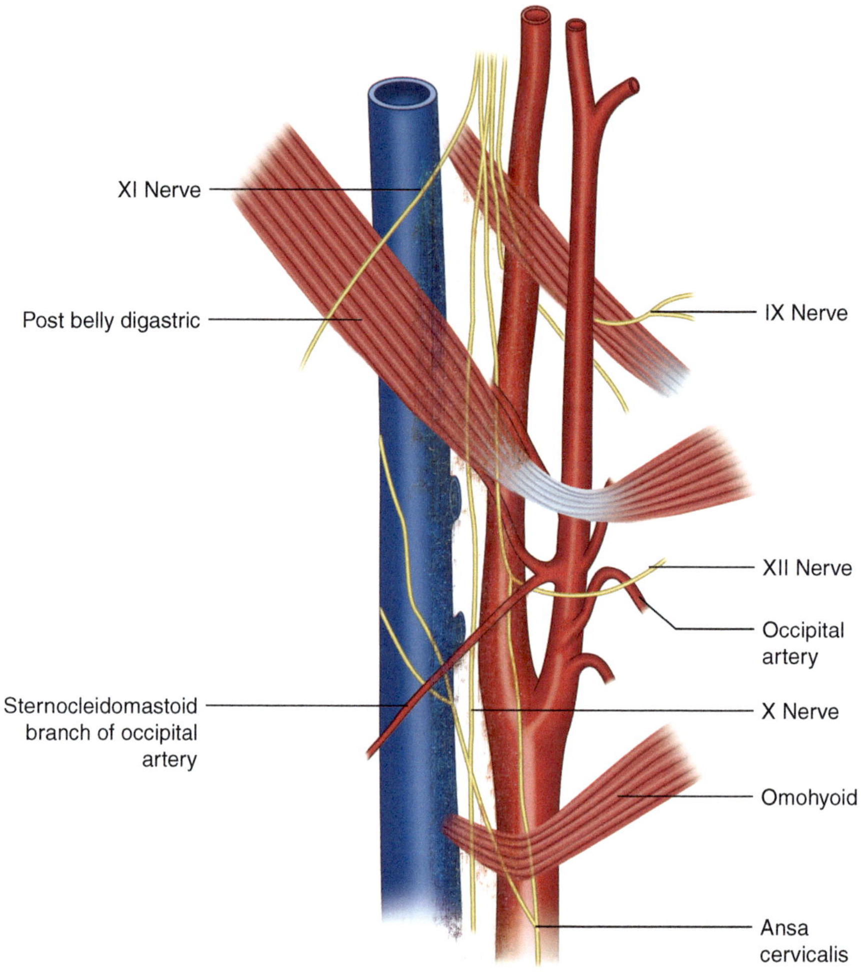

Fig. 17.1 Surgical anatomy of the neck showing carotid bifurcation and surrounding structures (internal jugular vein and nerves)

arterial blood pressure reflexly. The carotid body, which lies behind the point of division of the CCA, is a small brownish red structure which acts as a chemoreceptor.

In most patients, the ICA is posterior or posterolateral to the external carotid artery (ECA).

The External Carotid Artery

The ECA begins opposite to the upper border of the thyroid cartilage between the third and fourth cervical vertebral body and continues cephalad and anteriorly behind the angle of the mandible between the tip of the mastoid process and the angle of the jaw and divides into superficial temporal artery and maxillary arteries. The ECA branches in order are superior thyroid (which may arise from distal CCA), ascending pharyngeal (which may arise from ICA), lingual, facial, occipital, posterior auricular, superficial temporal, and maxillary artery (Fig. 17.1).

The Internal Carotid Artery

The ICA is the primary source of oxygenated blood to anterior portion of the brain and the orbits. The ICA is divided into the following seven segments: cervical (c1), petrous (c2), lacerum (c3), cavernous (c4), clinoid (c5), ophthalmic (c6), and communicating (c7). Internal carotid artery ascends into the skull base and becomes intracranial through the carotid canal of temporal bone. It continues anteriorly through the cavernous sinus and divides into anterior and middle cerebral artery (MCA).

Relationship of Nerves in the Neck to Carotid Arteries

The vagus nerve runs vertically down within the carotid sheath lying between the internal jugular vein (IJV) and the ICA and inferiorly between the same vein and the CCA. On the right side, it descends posterior to IJV and crosses the first part of the subclavian artery. On the left side, vagus nerve enters the thorax between the common carotid and subclavian arteries and posterior to the left brachiocephalic vein. During the performance of carotid endarterectomy (CEA), the vagus nerve in the lower portion of the neck may become more anterior than its usual posterior course and thus may be subject to injury.

At the level of second cervical vertebral body, the vagus nerve gives its superior laryngeal nerve branch which descends along the side of the pharynx first posterior and then medial to the ICA and divides into the internal and external laryngeal nerve.

The Glossopharyngeal Nerve

After its exit from the skull, it courses forward between the IJV and the ICA and descends anterior to the ICA deep to the styloid process and may get injured during the cephalad mobilization of the ICA during CEA for high plaque as it courses deep to the styloid process. Injury to the glossopharyngeal nerve results in loss of sensation to the posterior one-third of the tongue and difficulty swallowing, often requiring PEG tube placement.

The Accessory Spinal Nerve

After its exit from the jugular foramina, it runs posterolaterally behind the IJV in majority of instances but in front of the IJV in some cases and very rarely passes through the vein. It can be damaged in cases where IJV is more anterior in relation to ICA in the upper portion of the neck.

Ramus Mandibularis

Ramus mandibularis or the marginal mandibular branch of the facial nerve runs anteriorly below the angle of the mandible under cover of the platysma and can be injured during CEA if incision is more anteriorly placed. It can also be injured because of overzealous retraction of the tissues (stretch injury).

External Laryngeal Nerve

External laryngeal nerve is smaller than the internal laryngeal nerve and crosses the origin of superior thyroid artery and supplies the cricothyroid muscle. Injury to the external laryngeal nerve results in decreased pitch of the voice.

Hypoglossal Nerve

The hypoglossal nerve is usually posterior or posterosuperior to the common facial vein and is often crossed superiorly by another vein which drains into the IJV. The hypoglossal nerve curves around the sternocleidomastoid branch of the occipital artery, and its division and ligation aid in mobilization of the ICA during CEA. In a few instances, the hypoglossal nerve may be inferior in its course, close to the carotid bifurcation, and, if not carefully dissected, may result in an inadvertent injury.

Ansa Cervicalis

Ansa cervicalis is formed as a loop from the descending branch of the hypoglossal nerve which contains fibers of the C1. The descending branch is joined by the lower root of ansa cervicalis from the second and third cervical nerves, thus forming a loop. One may encounter anatomic variations in the ansa cervicalis with its superior root arising from the vagus, and its division during CEA may result in hoarseness.

Indications

1. Patients with minor to moderate stroke (NIH stroke scale <15) in the distribution of MCA (rarely anterior cerebral artery) in whom the neurological deficit has plateaued. Carotid endarterectomy is rarely performed as an emergency in patients with recent stroke, as medical optimization, and edema around the area of the infarction should improve before undertaking the operation. The risk of perioperative stroke in this group of patients is not increased if CEA is undertaken within 2 weeks of the stroke. Previous published trials reported greatest benefit of CEA within 2 weeks of the neurological event, and after 12 weeks, the benefit of CEA is considerably reduced. MRI brain is essential unless patient has a pacemaker/defibrillator
2. Transient contralateral motor or sensory deficit or speech involvement with spontaneous recovery. Transient loss of vision (amaurosis fugax) which may be complete or partial. Typically, the symptoms last for a few minutes and at the most, 1 h. There is no evidence of infarction on MRI of the brain.
3. Asymptomatic high-grade ICA stenosis (>70%) in selected patients who are otherwise good risk for the procedure and have at least 5 years of life expectancy. Following clinical evaluation, the patient should undergo carotid duplex imaging and non-contrast CT scan of the head, followed by CT angiography of the neck and head. MRI/MRA brain is often necessary for further evaluation in patients who exhibit focal neurological symptoms and/or positive neurological findings.

Anesthesia

The preference of cervical block anesthesia (CBA) over general anesthesia (GA) during performance of CEA has been debated vigorously during the past few decades. Recent results from GALA trial have not shown any superiority in the outcome following CEA for either CBA or GA. We prefer CBA except in patients with a high plaque (cephalad end of the plaque) at the level of second cervical vertebrae, those with anxiety disorder, patients with hearing loss, or patients with poor command of English language for whom general anesthesia is preferred.

Positioning and Incision

A roll is placed between the scapulae to hyperextend the neck with occipital support. The neck is turned laterally to the contralateral side. In patients with "short neck," the shoulder is slightly pulled downward with a wide tape attached to the shoulder with Mastisol adhesive (Eloquest, Ferndale, MI), and tape is then stretched and temporarily attached to the railing on the side of the table near its distal end.

Incision

Three incisions are commonly used:

1. Vertical with slight angulation anteriorly at the lower end.
2. Oblique (starting 2 cm behind the sternocleidomastoid at the upper end and ending 2 cm in front of the muscle). This incision is preferable (Fig. 17.2).
3. Transverse incision.

Vertical incisions leave an unsightly scar, and transverse incisions may limit the exposure in the event the plaque extends for a considerable distance superiorly or inferiorly. The length of incision is determined by the level of carotid bifurcation in relation to the cervical vertebrae, and the extent of the plaque in the ICA and the CCA are determined by preoperative CT angiography. After dividing the platysma, the external jugular vein is ligated and divided. In the upper portion of the incision, the greater auricular nerve is preserved and mobilized posteriorly and superiorly. Division of the greater auricular nerve will result in temporary sensory loss in the corresponding lobule of the ear and angle of the jaw. Dissection plan is continued along the anteromedial border of the sternocleidomastoid muscle. A self-retaining Wheitlaner retractor is applied superiorly and one inferiorly. The dissection plane is developed among the medial border of the IJV and is continued cephalad. Common facial vein is encountered, and ligated and divided, and upper deep cervical lymph nodes are mobilized posteriorly. As the carotid sheath is opened, vagus nerve is visualized posterolaterally between the artery and the vein. Vagus nerve may descend anteriorly as it courses inferiorly. External carotid artery is looped with a silastic loop which is then pulled caudally and held with a hemostat on the drapes at the chest wall. Ansa cervicalis is seen in the upper part of the dissection and is mobilized anteriorly. In the exposed area above the confluence of the common facial vein to the IJV, small unnamed veins joining the IJV are ligated and divided followed by division of the sternocleidomastoid branch of the occipital artery, and this helps to mobilize the hypoglossal nerve cephalad. Local anesthetic (1% lidocaine) is infiltrated around the carotid body to prevent bradycardia. Intravenous heparin (100 units/kg m) is administered by the anesthesia team monitoring of ACT.

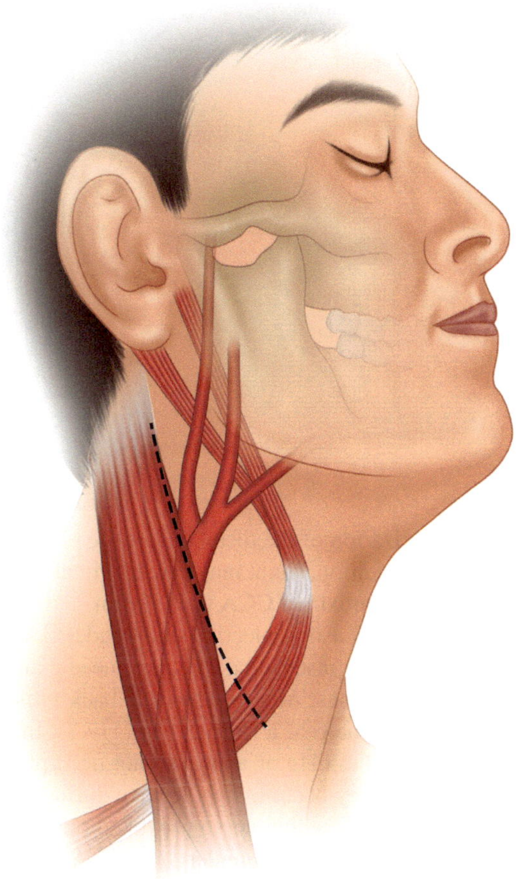

Fig. 17.2 Oblique incision for carotid endarterectomy. The superior part of the incision is 2–3 cm behind the medial border of sternocleidomastoid and inferior part of the incision is 2–3 cm in front of the medial border of sternocleidomastoid

Shunt Placement

There are three approaches regarding the use of shunt to maintain cerebral perfusion during carotid cross clamping:

1. Routine use of shunt
2. Selective use of shunt
3. Carotid endarterectomy without shunt

Surgeons using routine indwelling shunt generally perform the procedure under GA and do not need measurement of stump pressure and EEG monitoring to assess cerebral perfusion, but the flow through the shunt should be documented by the arterial Doppler. The disadvantage of routine use of the shunt is that it may interfere

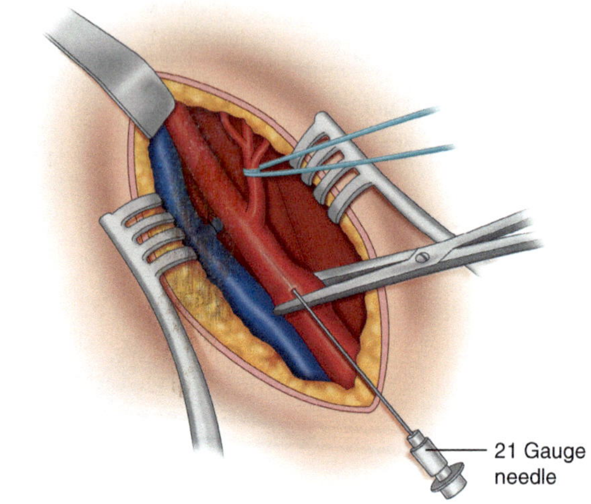

Fig. 17.3 Measurement of stump (back) pressure with proximal clamping of the CCA and occlusion of the ECA with a silastic tape doubled on itself

with visualization of the distal end of the plaque at the termination of the endarterectomy. In addition, shunt may cause intimal injury, dissection and atheroembolization from the proximal CCA to the brain.

For surgeons using selective shunt under GA, the stump pressure monitoring can be performed by inserting a 21-gauge needle and clamping the common and external carotid arteries. Measurement of back pressure (stump pressure) is then performed with a help of a monitor (Fig. 17.3). In general, patients with shunt stump pressure of 40 mmHg or above do not need placement of indwelling shunt during CEA, unless they become hypotensive during the procedure. EEG monitoring with measurement of median nerve provoked potentials is preferable in determining the need for shunt in patients undergoing CEA under GA.

Under CBA, continuous neurological assessment can be performed by having the patient squeeze with his contralateral hand with a toy that makes a "squeaky noise." If patient develops contralateral weakness or becomes unresponsive on clamping of the CCA, a shunt is immediately placed. Carotid endarterectomy without shunt has been proposed by a minority of authors and has shown satisfactory results in small series.

Types of Shunts

One of the original shunts used in carotid artery surgery is Javid™ shunt (Bard, Tempe, AZ). The author prefers Sundt™ shunt (Integra, Plainsboro, NJ) because of its flexibility and ease of insertion. Some surgeons prefer small caliber

Pruitt-Inahara® (LeMaitre Vascular, Burlington, MA) shunt with balloon occlusion proximally and distally. Argyl carotid shunt (Cardinal Health Dublin, OH) is also used by some surgeons.

Shunt Placement

Following placement of an angled vascular clamp to CCA and a Kitzmiller clamp distally into the ICA, an arteriotomy incision is made into the distal CCA which extends into the proximal ICA by angled Potts scissors (Fig. 17.4). The smaller end of the shunt is inserted into the ICA, and a small Javid clamp is applied, and retrograde bleeding occurs through the larger end of the shunt. This end of the shunt is then inserted proximally into the CCA, and large Javid clamp is applied. It is to be noted; silastic vessel loop has already been applied to the CCA and that can be tightened around the CCA along with the larger Javid clamp (Figs. 17.5, 17.6, and 17.7). Unless there are technical difficulties, the cerebral ischemia time during insertion of the shunt should be less than 2–3 min. In patients in whom mid CCA is found to have significant plaque with possibility of ulceration, it is better to insert the larger end of the shunt first into the CCA and to extrude any plaque or debris and then clamp the shunt with a Fogarty softjaw clamp before inserting the distal end into the ICA to prevent plaque embolization.

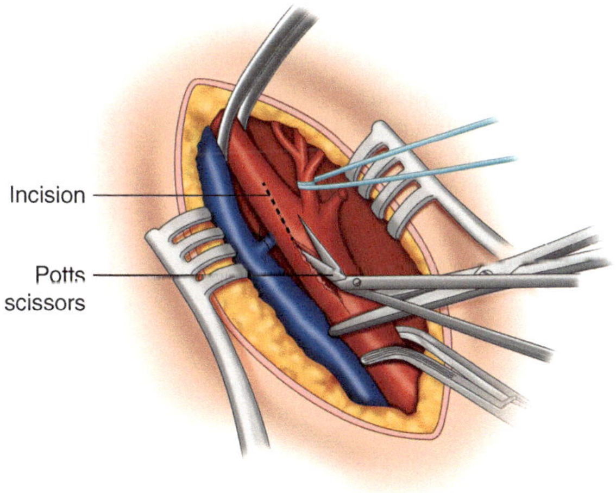

Fig. 17.4 Arteriotomy in the distal CCA and proximal ICA with angled POTTs scissors. Kitzmiller or Yasargil clamp is applied to the ICA

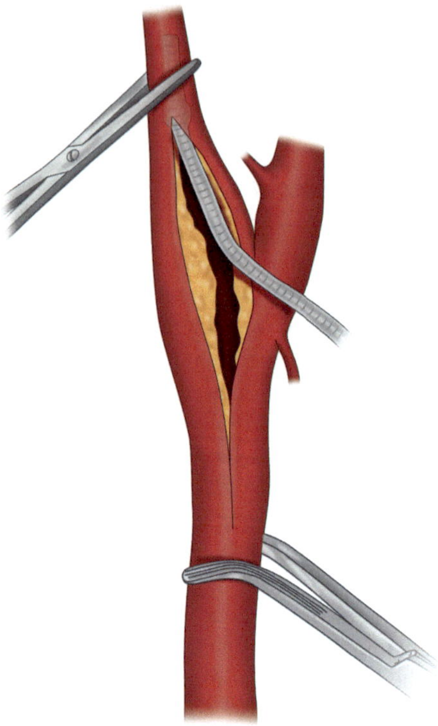

Fig. 17.5 Insertion of shunt with smaller end of the shunt into the ICA upon release of the Kitzmiller or Yasargil clamp

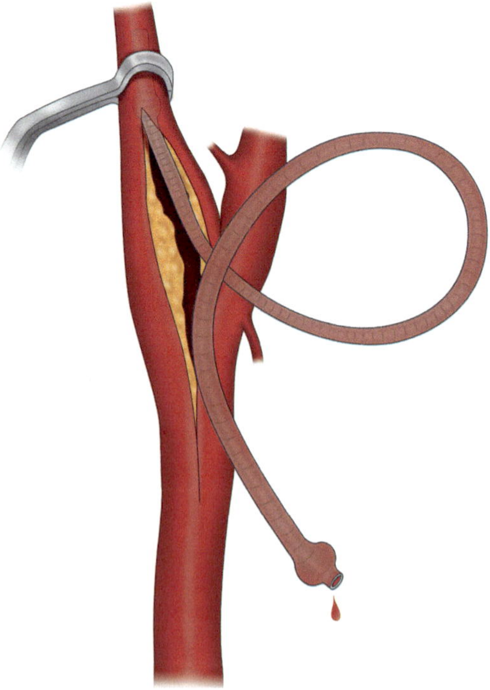

Fig. 17.6 Application of small Javid clamp around the ICA below the bulbous portion of the shunt. Blood from the ICA is filling the shunt and is coming out the larger end of the shunt

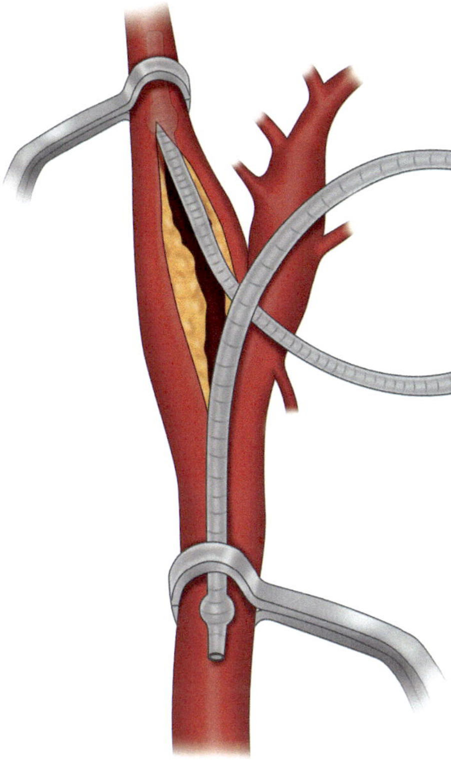

Fig. 17.7 Larger end of the shunt inserted into the CCA after release of the proximal vascular clamp and occlusion with silastic vessel loop. Large Javid clamp is applied around the shunt, proximal to its bulbous portion

Plaque is dissected with a Penfield dissector at the thickest portion of the plaque and continued cephalad until the plaque thins out at its feathery end (Fig. 17.8). Plaque is sharply divided proximally in the CCA. In patients whom the distal end of the plaque is not firmly attached to the arterial wall, a tacking suture is applied in a U-shaped manner (Fig. 17.9). Patch closure is performed by suturing patch to the ICA with a 7-0 cardiovascular polypropylene suture with two needles, and a 6-0 cardiovascular polypropylene for closure of CCA with the patch till shunt prevents further closure. The shunt is removed from CCA first and then from ICA (Figs. 17.10 and 17.11).

Unless the diameter of the distal ICA is greater than 5 mm, arteriotomy should preferably be closed with a patch graft (bovine pericardium patch, PTFE, or Dacron patch). After patch closure is near completed, back bleeding for ICA should occur, and after completion of suture line, CCA clamp is released to ECA first before flow is reestablished into the ICA. Heparin should be reversed with protamine sulfate depending upon the results of the ACT.

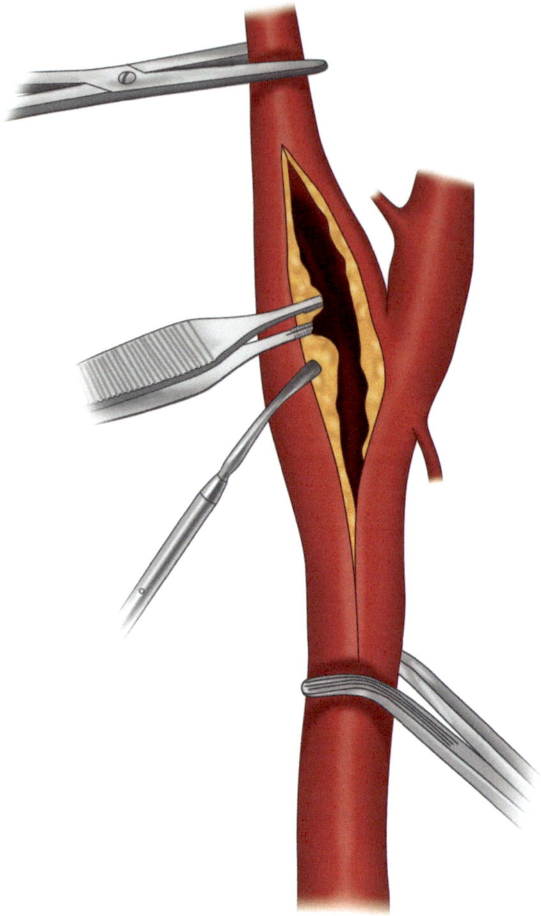

Fig. 17.8 Endarterectomy plane developed at its thickest portion with the use of vascular forceps (DeBankey or Gerald forceps) and dural elevator (dissector)

Eversion Carotid Endarterectomy

Eversion CEA is preferable in patients with elongation of the ICA with tortousity and less than 4 mm diameter. This is an alternative technique to facilitate the removal of plaque isolated to the carotid bulb and proximal ICA. Advantages of eversion technique versus standard CEA include the ability to shorten a redundant ICA, a better visualization of the end point with easier detection of intimal flaps. The use of patch graft is avoided, and a faster closure is achieved by an end-to-end anastomosis of the ICA to the carotid bulb.

In this technique, the ICA is transected obliquely by dividing the crotch of the carotid bulb from the carotid bifurcation to a point more proximal on the lateral side of the CCA (Fig. 17.12). Generally, an opening of 10–15 mm can be obtained without extending the arteriotomy at either end as long as the transection line is beveled enough. Otherwise, the arteriotomy on the lateral wall of the CCA may be extended

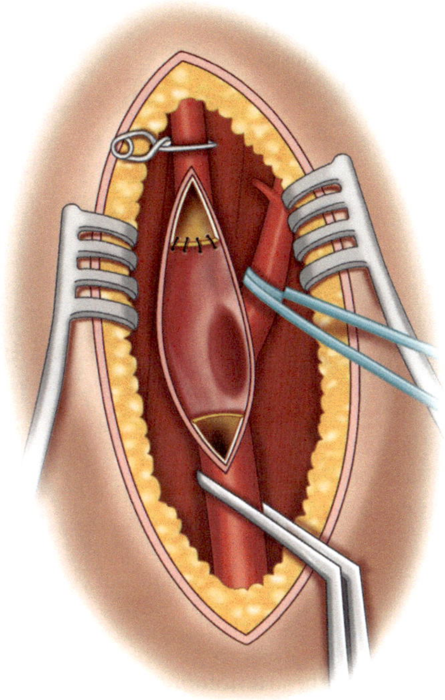

Fig. 17.9 Completion of endarterectomy with sharp transection of the plaque at its proximal end. Two tacking sutures are applied at the distal intima so as to prevent intimal flap. Carotid endarterectomy site with distal tacking suture and proximal sharp transection of the plaque in the CCA

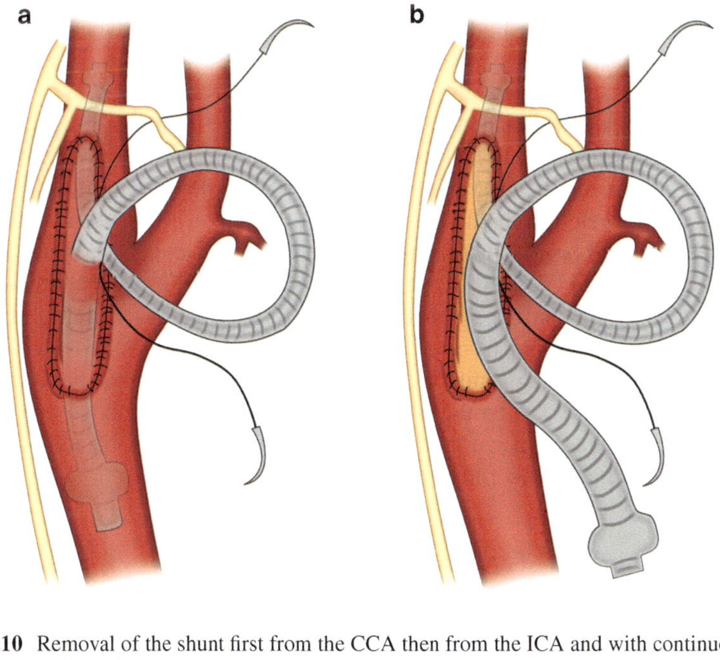

Fig. 17.10 Removal of the shunt first from the CCA then from the ICA and with continuous closure of the patch graft

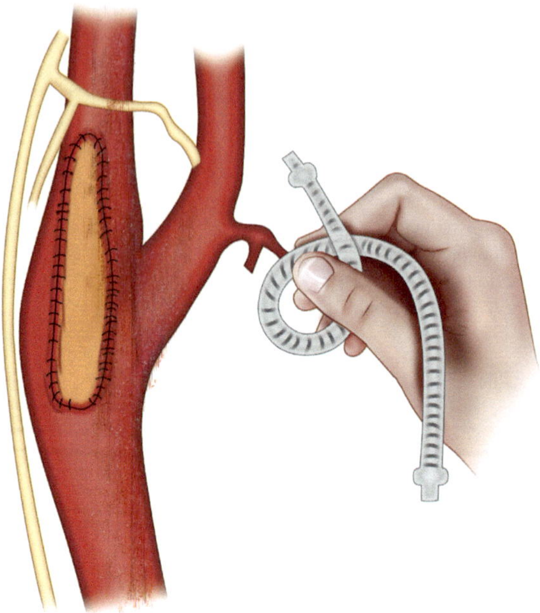

Fig. 17.11 Removal of the shunt first from the CCA then from the ICA and with continuous closure of the patch graft

caudally, and the arteriotomy medial wall of the ICA extended cephalad to a similar length to facilitate later anastomosis of the arteries. An extended arteriotomy into the CCA helps in removal of a more proximal plaque in the CCA. Eversion CEA is performed by circumferentially elevating the plaque with a Penfield dissector from the arterial wall to remove both the intima and the media. The adventitia is grasped with a fine forceps, while the assistant holds the plaque. The adventitia with its outer layer of media is everted, and the atheromatous score is held away in tension until the end of the plaque is reached in the distal ICA. After removal of the plaque, the surgeon may inspect the entire circumference of the end point, remove loose debris, and make certain that the distal intima is adherent to the arterial wall. If a loose intimal flap is detected, it should be peeled off or alternatively "tacked" down using a 7-0 double-armed polypropylene suture from the lumen and tied in the outer wall. Primary anastomosis between ICA and CCA is performed using a continuous 6-0 monofilament suture starting at the most cephalad ICA. The back wall of the anastomosis is usually sutured from the inside of the artery which provides a better visualization. The running suture is completed posteriorly and then brought anteriorly, and finally it is tied. After the completion of anastomosis, blood flow is restored in the usual sequence as performed in standard CEA with back bleeding from the ICA and the antegrade flow filling the ECA.

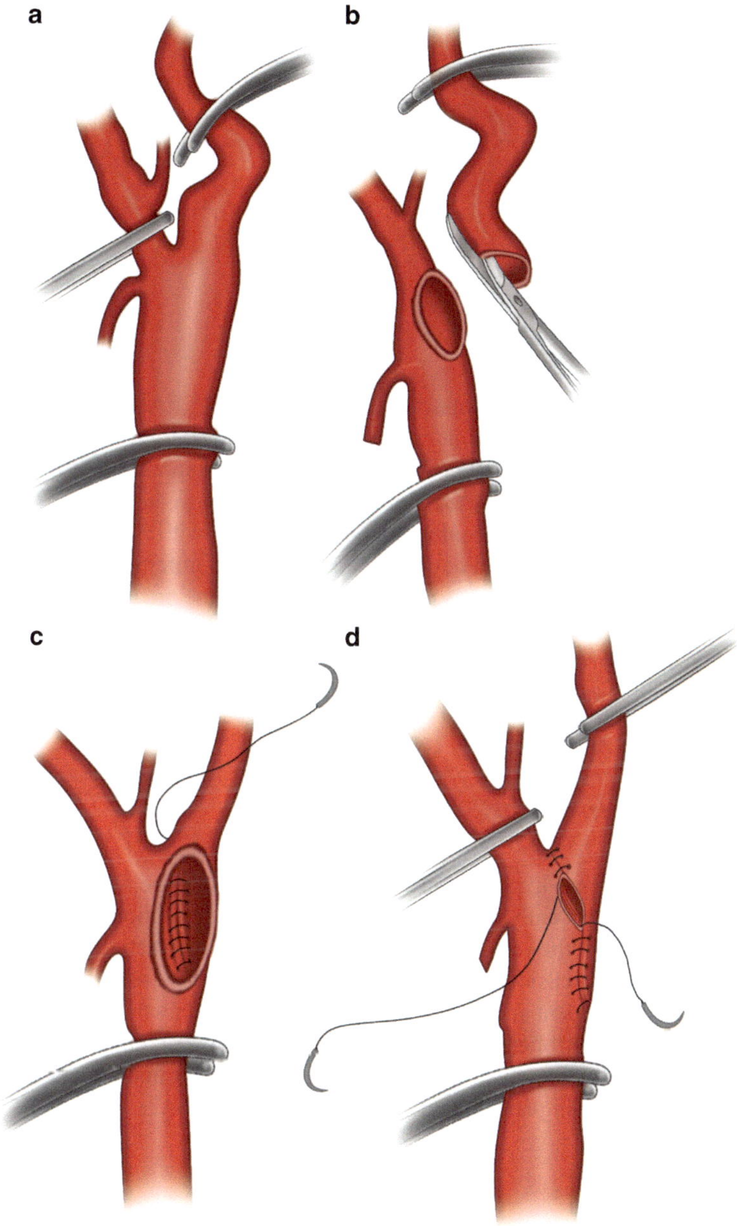

Fig. 17.12 (**a–d**) Steps of eversion CEA. (**a**) Vascular clamp applied to the common internal and external carotid artery. (**b**) Transection of the ICA from its origin and arteriotomy at 9 o'clock position extending superiorly toward ICA. (**c**) Reanastomosis of the ICA to the CCA (posterior layer). (**d**) Near completion of the suture line anteriorly

Postoperative Care

The patient should be kept on antiplatelet medications in the form of aspirin and continue statins and judicious use of antihypertensives unless the patient's blood pressure is low in recovery room.

Complications

Hematoma of the Neck

Hematoma of the neck is the commonest complication of CEA. Usually the hematomas are small and resolve spontaneously in most patients within a few days to 1 week. However, large hematoma is causing extrinsic compression of the trachea, and esophagus should be evacuated in the operating room as an emergency. It may be difficult to perform oral tracheal intubation in a patient with a large hematoma of the neck because of the tracheal deviation, and it is often preferable to evacuate the hematoma by removing the sutures and staples, relieving the pressure on the trachea before attempting intubation. In majority of instances, the bleeding is from the venous branches; however, occasionally the bleeding is from the arterial suture line which may need reinforcement suture placement.

Hemodynamic Instability

Patients may experience hypotension and bradycardia within the first few hours following CEA. This is usually due to carotid sinus nerve stimulation and can be prevented by blocking the carotid body with a local anesthetic. Intraoperative hypertension or hypotension in the recovery room while the patient is waking up from GA is quite frequent and is more common in patients in whom the blood pressure was not well-controlled preoperatively. These patients should be treated with antihypertensive immediately. It has been reported that fewer fluctuations are much less in blood pressure in patients undergoing CEA under CBA.

Cranial Nerve Palsy

Hypoglossal nerve is the most common cranial nerve injured during CEA. Temporary hypoglossal nerve palsy with deviation of the tongue to the ipsilateral side and injury to vagus nerve (causing hoarseness) are not uncommon following CEA. These injuries are more common in redo CEA and in patients who have excessive scarring secondary to radiation. Vagus nerve injury occurs during the application of vascular clamp to the CCA. If there is no recovery in 3 months, permanent damage should be suspected. Hoarseness secondary to vagus nerve injury tends to improve as the opposite vocal cord compensates by its movement to the opposite side. If hoarseness persists following CEA, contralateral CEA, if necessary, should not be performed unless vocal cord function assessment is performed by an ENT surgeon, as bilateral vagus nerve injury though uncommon will necessitate tracheotomy. Injury to the external laryngeal nerve results in the loss of pitch in the voice. Injury to the spinal accessory nerve results in winging of the scapula.

Postoperative Stroke

Postoperative stroke is the most serious complication of the CEA. It usually manifests as a contralateral motor weakness of the upper and lower extremities with speech involvement in right-handed individuals if endarterectomy is performed on the left side. It is often the result of embolization during the operation or in the very early postoperative period. Patient may develop thrombosis at the endarterectomy site usually due to residual intimal flap which may manifest with a neurological deficit following a normal neurological function after the completion of CEA. Cerebral ischemia caused by lack of use of shunt in a patient who has inadequate collateral flow or malfunction of the shunt may be responsible for stroke in a few patients. If the patient wakes up with a neurological deficit in the operating room, the CEA site should be reexplored, and a completion arteriogram should be performed. If patient develops neurological deficit in the recovery room or later (typically 30 min to 12 h after CEA), the patient should undergo emergency noncontrast CT scan of the head to rule out intracerebral hemorrhage which is exceedingly uncommon at this early stage. Once intracerebral hemorrhage is ruled out, the patient should undergo CT angiography of the neck and head as the patient is still in the CT department. If the patient has thrombosis of the ICA associated with MCA (M1 or M2 occlusion), the patient should undergo CEA site thrombectomy and neurovascular intervention for retrieval of the embolic occlusion during the window of 6–8 h following stroke. If there is embolic occlusion in the peripheral branches of MCA, neurovascular intervention is not helpful. Patient should be managed medically and undergo physical, occupational, and speech therapy. Reexploration of the endarterectomy site for suspected thrombosis may be helpful, but in patients with simultaneous occlusion of the MCA, operative thrombectomy at the endarterectomy site will not improve neurological function in majority of instances. Following left CEA, a patient woke up from GA with right-sided weakness and aphasia in the operating room. Neck incision was reopened, and arteriogram was performed which showed occlusion of M1 segment of MCA. Patient underwent neurosurgical retrieval by Solitaire device (EV3 Irvine, CA) and had a complete recovery.

For patients with postoperative intracerebral hemorrhage, neurosurgical consultation should be obtained, and in some instances (hemorrhage in frontal lobe), craniotomy and evacuation of the cerebral hemorrhage may help in neurological recovery. Intracerebral hemorrhage is often due to cerebral hyperperfusion and is often associated with CEA for high-grade ipsilateral carotid stenosis with severe contralateral ICA disease in the form of high-grade stenosis or occlusion. Hyperperfusion syndrome in its mild form presents as post CEA headache and, in its more severe form, as seizures or as intracerebral hemorrhage. It is important to maintain satisfactory blood pressure control following CEA, but this complication is often unavoidable.

Postoperative Myocardial Infarction and Cardiac Arrhythmias

Postoperative myocardial infarction and cardiac arrhythmias may occur following CEA as patients often have associated coronary artery disease. Serum troponin and 12-lead ECG should be performed in patients with unexplained postoperative hypotension, and cardiology consultation should be obtained.

Patch Graft Infection

Patch graft infection following CEA is rare, but a serious complication of CEA requires removal of the patch and autogenous reconstruction using interposition of greater saphenous vein. A myocutaneous flap may be required with consultation from a plastic surgeon. Carotid pseudoaneurysm is an uncommon complication and can be treated with covered stent if underlying infection is ruled out.

Take-Home Points

1. Despite increasing use of trans-carotid artery revascularization (TCAR) and transfemoral carotid stenting, CEA is an extremely useful operation for prevention of stroke in patients with significant extracranial carotid artery stenosis. Optimal imaging, technically satisfactory operation with minimal mobilization of carotid bifurcation, and management of blood pressure fluctuations intraoperatively and postoperatively are key to achieving satisfactory outcomes.

Chapter 18
Carotid Endarterectomy for High Plaque

Sachinder Singh Hans

Occasionally during carotid endarterectomy (CEA), the distal end of the plaque does not remain isolated to within a few centimeters of the carotid bifurcation but continues cephalad requiring additional exposure than is routinely needed. This additional distal exposure can be challenging and may be more difficult in the presence of a high carotid bifurcation or in an obese patients with a "short neck." When the distal extent of the plaque is not able to be determined by duplex ultrasound, high-quality CTA (axial, coronal, and sagittal cuts with reconstruction) often is able to determine the cephalad extent of the plaque in relationship to the body of cervical vertebra.

For practical purposes, the extracranial portion of internal carotid artery (ICA) can be divided into three segments (zones) in planning for CEA. The usual location of carotid bifurcation is at the level of C3–C4 vertebral bodies, and plaque extends to Zone 1 (upper end of C3 vertebral body) in most patients. Zone 2 extends from upper end of C3 vertebral body to upper end of C2 vertebral body, and extent to this level represents a high plaque. Zone 3 is above the level of the C2 vertebral body, and it is extremely uncommon for plaque to extend to this level. In some patients, CTA imaging may fail to detect the distal feathery end of the plaque; high plaque may be an unexpected finding during CEA. In most patients with high plaque, general anesthesia (GA) is required as patient may become uncooperative during distal dissection under cervical block anesthesia (CBA). In the absence of significant calcification in the plaque, carotid artery stenting (CAS): TCAR or Transfemoral should be considered as a more suitable alternative to CEA in cases involving high plaque.

S. S. Hans (✉)
Vascular and Endovascular Services, Henry Ford Macomb Hospital,
Clinton Twp, MI, USA

S. S. Hans et al. (eds.), *Primary and Repeat Arterial Reconstructions*,
https://doi.org/10.1007/978-3-031-13897-3_18

Technical Steps

To obtain additional distal exposure when high plaque is encountered, the sternocleidomastoid branch of the occipital artery and/or the occipital artery itself is ligated and divided freeing up the hypoglossal nerve which then can be retracted cephalad with a silastic vessel loop. In many instances, venous tributaries are crossing this area of dissection and should be carefully ligated and divided. The posterior belly of the digastric muscle is either retracted cephalad after careful mobilization or may have to be divided (Fig. 18.1). If the distal termination of the plaque does not end as a feathery distal end, we place a 3.5 mm or 4.0–4.5 mm arterial dilator (Garrett Dilator, Teleflex Medical, Morrisville, NC) into the ICA to obtain distal control, and this can also help to facilitate the dissection of the plaque with good control of retrograde bleeding while avoiding a distal clamp on the ICA.

In order to facilitate suturing of the patch at the apex of the endarterectomy, two stay sutures of "6-0" cardiovascular polypropylene are placed at the origin of the ICA after removal of the plaque. These sutures are at 3 o'clock and 9 o'clock position. The sutures are retracted caudally to bring "ICA downward" in order to facilitate the exposure at the proximal end of the arteriotomy (Fig. 18.2). Another option

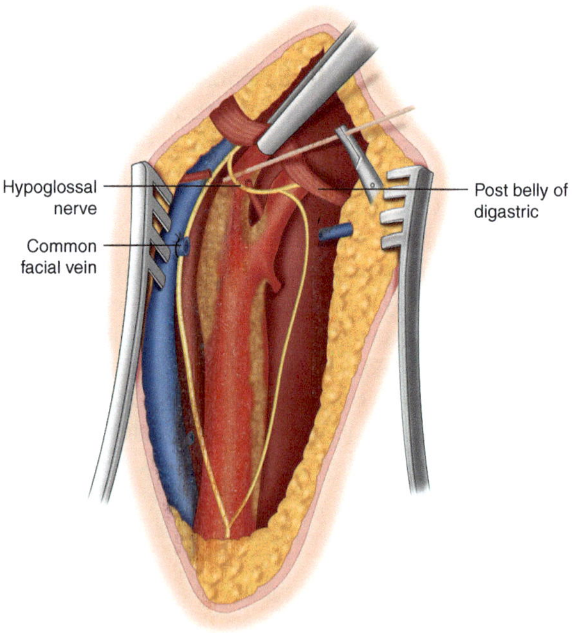

Fig. 18.1 Exposed carotid bifurcation, division and ligation of common facial vein, division of occipital artery, silastic loop around the hypoglossal nerve with retraction of posterior belly of digastric

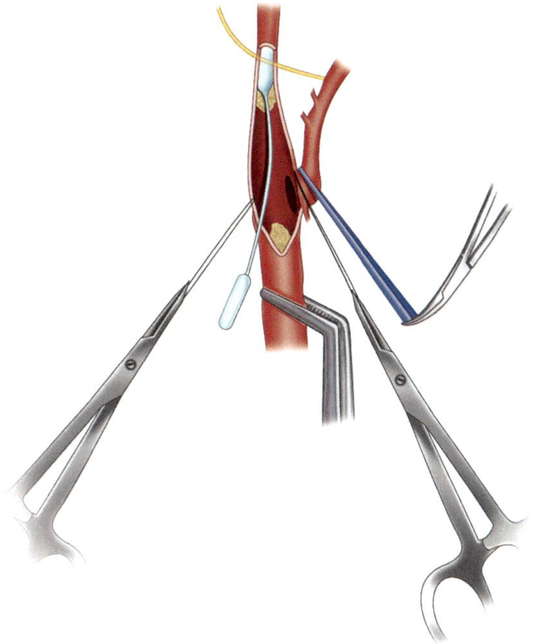

Fig. 18.2 Completed endarterectomy. Arterial dilator in the distal ICA. Two stay sutures retracting the origin of ICA downward. Blue silastic loop around the origin of external carotid artery retracting it downward with a small hemostat

is to place a Pruitt® balloon occlusion catheter (LeMaitre Vascular, Burlington, MA) in the ICA near the base of the skull. The silastic loop around the hypoglossal nerve is gently retracted inferiorly as the suturing at the apex of the patch and the arteriotomy is started. That suture is continued inferiorly, and the two sutures on either side are brought under the hypoglossal nerve, which now is retracted cephalad. At the inferior end of the patch, a 6-0 cardiovascular polypropylene suture is used to suture the distal end of the arteriotomy in the common carotid artery (CCA), and this (suture-line) closure is continued on each side of the patch until dilator prevents further closure. Dilator is then removed, and retrograde flushing from the ICA is done. Yasargil clamp is then applied distally to the ICA, and the vessel loop is tightened around the CCA. Suture line closure is completed. The double vessel loop around the external carotid artery (ECA) is released, and blood is allowed to flow into the ECA before the Yasargil clamp on the ICA is removed (Figs. 18.3 and 18.4). Other maneuvers that may help in exposure at closure of the endarterectomy site are:

1. Transposing the ICA anterior to the XII nerve by dividing the ICA at its origin. This technique is more suitable in patients undergoing eversion CEA when the plaque extends for a long distance cephalad. Following completion of the CEA, the ICA is then sutured to the origin of the ICA near the CCA bifurcation.

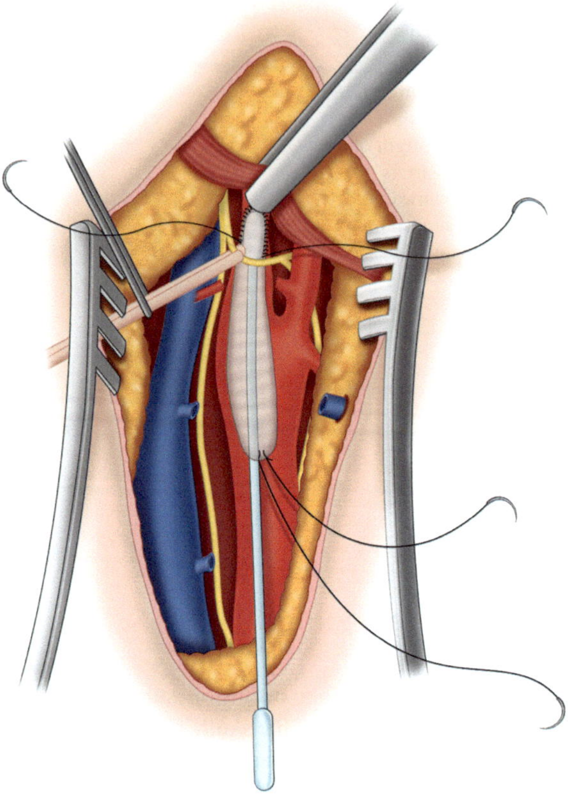

Fig. 18.3 Suturing of the patch started at the apex above the hypoglossal nerve as it is retracted inferiorly by silastic loop. Arterial dilator in the distal ICA controlling bleeding and avoiding the application of vascular clamp to the distal ICA. A suture line is started at the lower end of the patch and opened CCA

2. Retrojugular approach to ICA – The upper end of the incision is extended posteriorly behind the ear, and internal jugular vein is mobilized anteriorly (Fig. 18.4). Spinal accessory nerve is identified, and vagus nerve is mobilized anteriorly. Hypoglossal nerve is not in the operative field with use of retrojugular approach. This enables distal exposure on the ICA.
3. For lesions extending to the junction of upper border of C2 and lower end of C1 (in patients not suitable for carotid stenting due to severe calcification), mandibular subluxation by an ENT surgeon/oral maxillofacial surgeon should be considered. These patients should have a nasotracheal intubation instead of oral-tracheal intubation if mandible subluxation is being planned. The mandible is kept in place by a wire through the anterior nasal spine and through the mandible. In patients with a high plaque extending to the level of the upper portion of the body of the C2 (following division of the posterior belly of the digastric), one can palpate the tip of the styloid process which should be carefully removed by a rongeur as the glossopharyngeal nerve is in close approximation to the styloid process.

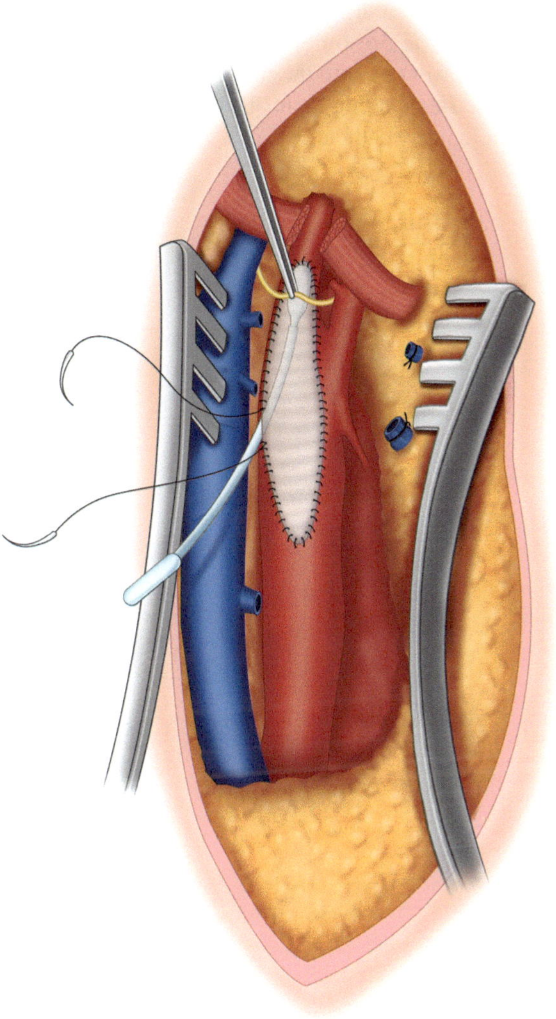

Fig. 18.4 Patch closure is near completion with dilator in place. Division of post belly of digastric or retraction of the posterior belly of digastric and stylohyoid for exposure of distal ICA in patients with high plaque

Intraoperative Carotid Stenting

If one is not certain about the end point of CEA, intraoperative carotid stenting (CAS) should be considered. Some plaques are soft and feathery at its distal end making the determination of their termination difficult during endarterectomy. Intraoperative CAS is performed by extending the lower end of the incision toward the base of the neck with division of the inferior belly of the omohyoid. Using a micropuncture technique 7 Fr. sheath is inserted into CCA just above the base of the neck. A carotid/cerebral arteriogram is performed in the operating room by injecting 8 cc of diluted contrast through the sheath: using a 0.014 mm guidewire (CHOICE™ PT, Boston Scientific Corporation Marlborough, MA) and advancing it under fluoroscopy into the intracranial portion of the ICA and deploying a 6 mm × 4 cm self-expanding stent. Post angioplasty is performed by an appropriately sized angioplasty catheter.

Chapter 19
Carotid Interposition Graft

Sachinder Singh Hans

Indications for carotid interposition grafting include:

(A) Locally advanced head and neck cancer involving the carotid artery
(B) Infected patch graft following carotid endarterectomy (CEA)
(C) Failed endovascular therapy for restenosis following CEA or carotid artery stenting (CAS)
(D) Resection for extracranial carotid aneurysm when end-to-end anastomosis is not feasible
(E) Carotid artery trauma when local repair is not feasible
(F) Carotid stenosis secondary to neck radiation

The conduit used for carotid interposition grafting (CIG) includes either straight or a tapered PTFE graft (WL Gore, Newark DE). In contaminated fields, autogenous reconstruction with a greater saphenous vein (GSV) or superficial femoral artery (SFA) can be used. The SFA should be evaluated by duplex imaging and is preferred in patients undergoing resection of head and neck cancer invading the carotid artery. Failed CAS often occurs in patients with heavy calcified plaque burden or due to structural failure of the stent. Removal of the stent along with the resection of distal common carotid artery (CCA) and proximal internal carotid artery (CIA) is followed by CIG.

S. S. Hans (✉)
Vascular and Endovascular Services, Henry Ford Macomb Hospital, Clinton Twp, MI, USA

S. S. Hans et al. (eds.), *Primary and Repeat Arterial Reconstructions*, https://doi.org/10.1007/978-3-031-13897-3_19

Carotid Interposition Graft for Failed Carotid Stenting

Carotid interposition graft for failed carotid stenting often requires exposure of the distal end of the stent in the ICA. This exposure may be difficult if the cephalad end of the stent extends above the level of the body of the second cervical vertebrae. The operative intervention should be performed under general anesthesia. It is important that any monitoring equipment does not obstruct the potential radiological imaging of the stent in the ICA in the event intraoperative imaging is necessary. The operative dissection is usually more difficult than the standard CEA because of the scar tissue in the area and the inflammatory response due to the presence of the stent. Sharp dissection with a 15-blade scalpel keeping the angle of the blade slightly more horizontal and finding a plane very next to the adventitia of the common and internal carotid artery as well as the external carotid artery (ECA) is necessary (Fig. 19.1). Exposure of the distal ICA is like the one described in the chapter of CEA. We prefer EEG monitoring as well as median nerve-evoked potentials to determine the need for shunt in patients who do not tolerate carotid cross clamping.

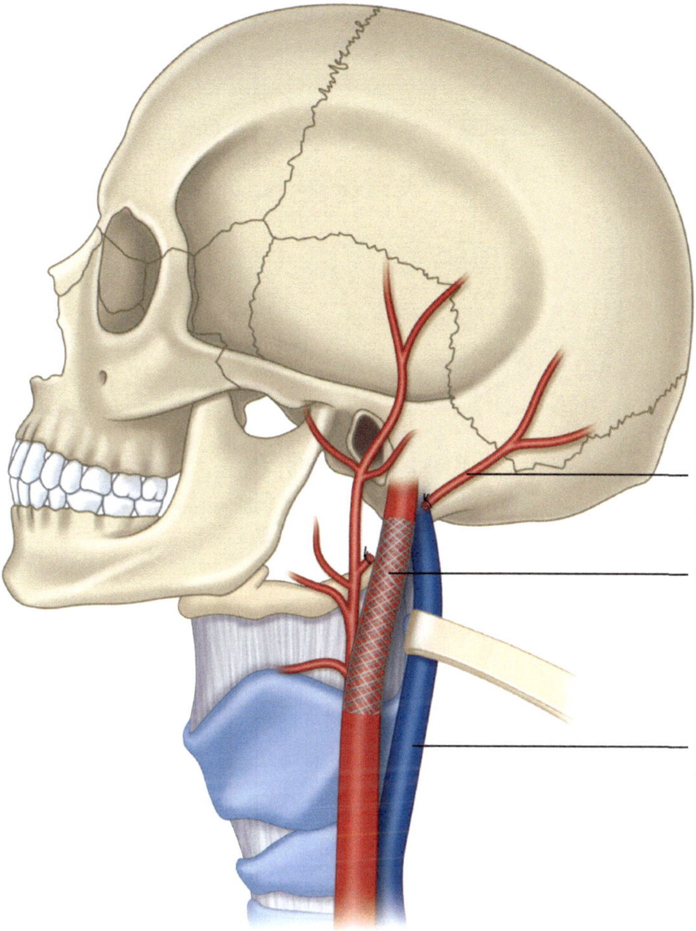

Fig. 19.1 Exposure of distal CCA, ICA and ECA in the neck. ICA has a previous stent

Interposition Graft Without Shunt

If the ephalad end of the stent extends above the second cervical vertebral body, intraoperative balloon occlusion may be necessary to control the retrograde bleeding from the ICA. In systemic heparinization (100 units/kg body weight), the CCA is punctured with a micro puncture needle and using a microcatheter 7F sheath is inserted in the CCA just above the base of the neck, and a 0.014 mm choice PT wire (Boston Scientific, Marlborough MA) is advanced into the ICA toward the base of the skull. A number 3 Fogarty catheter over the wire is inflated using a 50% diluted contrast media (Fig. 19.2). If the upper end of the stent is below the level of the

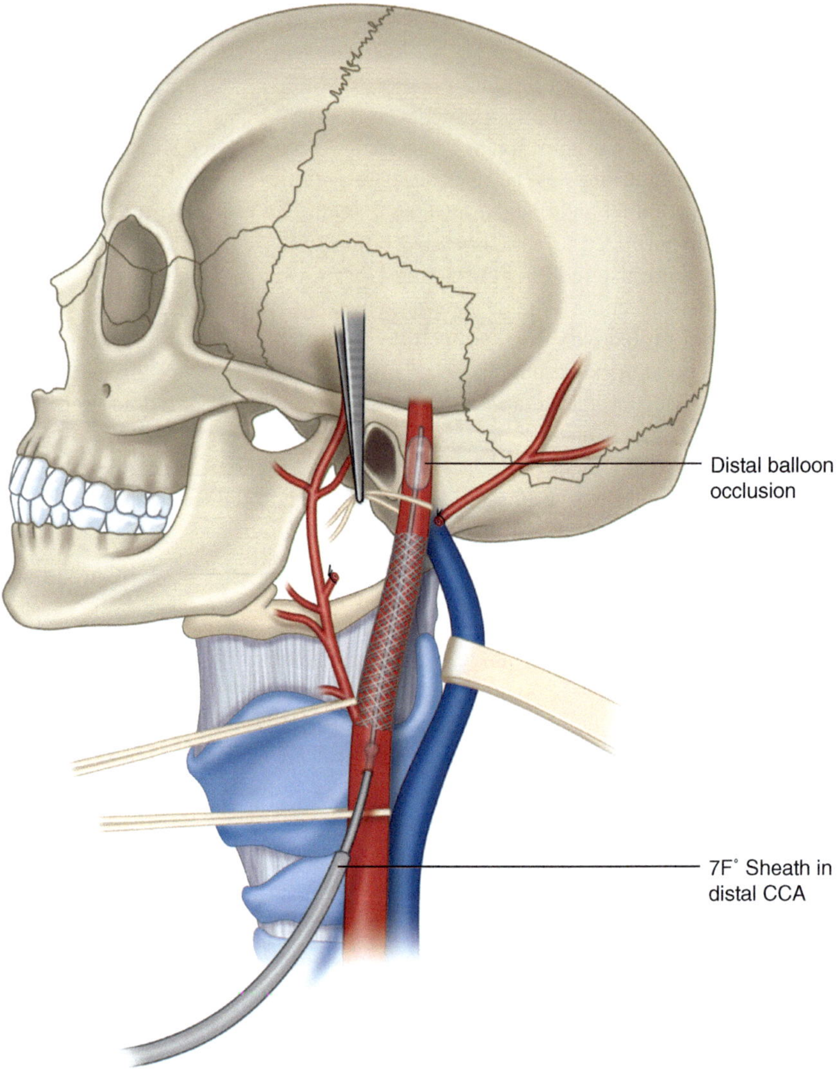

Fig. 19.2 Distal Baloon occlusion of ICA with Baloon filled with contrast to obtain distal control

second cervical vertebral body, balloon occlusion is not necessary. Proximal clamp is applied to CCA a few centimeters below the proximal end of the carotid stent. Distal clamping of the ICA can be performed with careful mobilization of the ICA; applying a vascular clamp, the ICA is divided with a 15-blade scalpel, a few millimeters below the upper end of the stent. The origin of the ECA is also divided, its distal end is suture ligated with a 4-0 cardiovascular polypropylene suture, and the proximal end of the CCA is divided above the proximal clamp. Balloon occlusion catheter is deflated and removed, and soft vascular clamp such as Yasargil clamp (Scanlan Int., St Paul, MN) is applied. The distal anastomosis is performed first, and Yasargil clamp is released so that retrograde blood flow will aid in removing any debris. The vascular clamp is then moved proximally just below the distal anastomosis (Fig. 19.3). Proximal anastomosis is performed in an end-to-end fashion as well with a running 6-0 cardiovascular polypropylene suture (Fig. 19.4). In some patients with discrepancy in the size of the CCA and the graft, an end-to-side proximal anastomosis may be considered.

Fig. 19.3 Distal anastomosis of divided ICA to the interposition graft

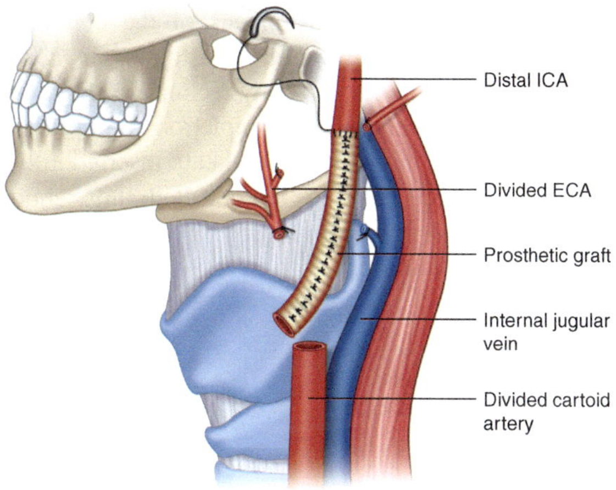

Fig. 19.4 Proximal anastomosis of the interposition graft to divided distal CCA

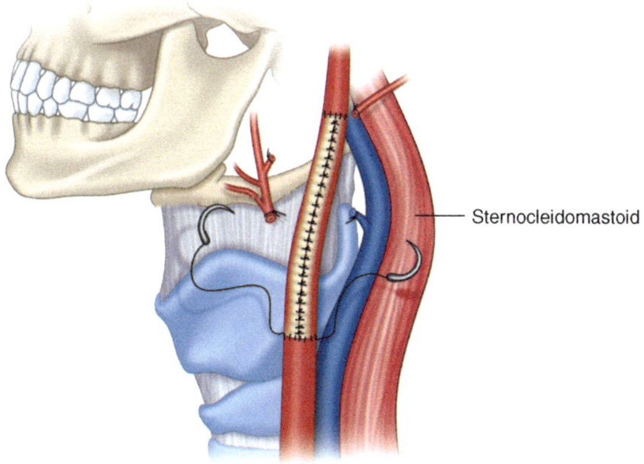

Shunt Placement

If the EEG and somatosensory median nerve-evoked potentials indicate cerebral ischemia or if the stump pressure is less than 40 mmHg (if EEG monitoring is not available), an indwelling shunt should be inserted during the time of carotid cross clamping. The distal end of the shunt is first advanced in to the divided ICA; after back bleeding fills the shunt, the proximal end of the shunt is then inserted into the CCA. The interposition graft is then passed over another shunt (second shunt). The first shunt is removed, and the second shunt with the interposition graft around it is inserted. A distal end to end anastomosis to the conduit (graft) is performed first followed by proximal anastomosis of the conduit (graft) to the divided CCA (Fig. 19.5). Before the proximal anastomosis is completed, the shunt is removed, and suturing is completed. If any technical difficulties are encountered during the interposition graft operation, completion carotid arteriogram should be performed by injecting the contrast via a 5F sheath inserted into the CCA and graft anastomosis. If any abnormal findings are detected, those should be corrected before operation is completed.

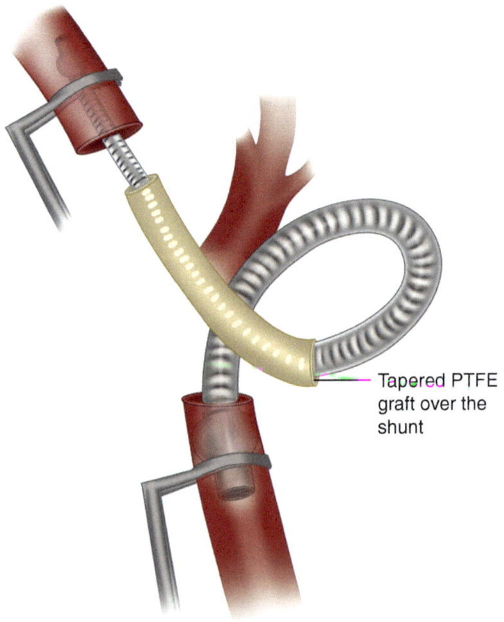

Fig. 19.5 Tapered PTFE graft with Carotid shunt inside the graft in patients showing cerebral ischemia during carotid cross clamping

Complications

Most complications of CIG are like those of CEA. The incidence of cranial nerve injury such as superior laryngeal nerve injury and glossopharyngeal nerve is greater as cephalad exposure of the ICA in the neck is necessary.

Chapter 20
Redo Carotid Endarterectomy

Sachinder Singh Hans

Recurrent carotid disease following carotid endarterectomy (CEA) can be categorized as:

(A) Residual disease
(B) Recurrent stenosis
(C) Late recurrent stenosis

Very early recurrent carotid stenosis is usually due to technical problems with the initial repair. There may be residual disease due to the inadequacy of the endarterectomy at the distal end. It may also result from inadequate removal of the plaque from the common carotid artery (CCA). Carotid restenosis developing within 24 months of endarterectomy is most likely due to myointimal hyperplasia. This is a concentric fibrotic smooth/fibrotic thickening which is firmly adherent to the arterial wall. This type of recurrence is usually apparent by 6 months following endarterectomy, and such lesions usually do not cause embolic stroke and can be diagnosed by duplex ultrasound and confirmed by CT angiography. Recurrent stenosis due to hyperplastic lesions can also be present at the site of clamp application usually at the proximal CCA clamp. After 24 months, late recurrent carotid stenosis is usually due to progressive atherosclerotic disease which may become symptomatic but may remain asymptomatic in most patients. This lesion is most often smooth heterogenous, ulcerated, complex, and usually irregular.

S. S. Hans (✉)
Vascular and Endovascular Services, Henry Ford Macomb Hospital, Clinton Twp, MI, USA

S. S. Hans et al. (eds.), *Primary and Repeat Arterial Reconstructions*, https://doi.org/10.1007/978-3-031-13897-3_20

Indications

Indications for recurrent CEA are similar to those for the index procedure which include asymptomatic severe carotid stenosis (>70%) or symptomatic carotid stenosis greater than 60% stenosis with associated transient ischemic attacks or transient loss of vision (amaurosis fugax) or minor to moderate stroke (NIH stroke <15). Recommendations of repeat CEA should take into consideration the life expectancy and associated comorbidities. Most patients with symptomatic recurrent carotid stenosis or high-grade asymptomatic recurrent stenosis should be treated with CAS.

Preoperative Assessment

Carotid duplex study followed by CT angiography should be performed prior to redo CEA. In some patients catheter-based carotid/cerebral angiography may need to be performed if the quality of CTA is suboptimal.

Procedure

Most redo carotid endarterectomies are performed under general anesthesia with patient positioning similar to as described in the chapter on CEA. The previously placed incision is extended cephalad as well as inferiorly for a distance of 2–3 cm on either side. Common carotid artery is exposed near the base of the neck in a relatively "clean area" which has not been dissected before, and a silastic vessel loop is passed carefully protecting the vagus nerve. Vagus nerve tends to course anteriorly near the base of the neck and should be protected from injury. Internal jugular vein is carefully separated from the common and the proximal ICA after Weitlaner retractors are applied, but the retraction should be gentle as excessive retraction may result in traction injury to the nerves. Sharp dissection is performed with a 15-blade scalpel kept at an angle to separate CCA from surround structures (Fig. 20.1). Hypoglossal nerve is frequently indistinguishable from surround scar tissue above the carotid bifurcation. Invariably posterior belly of the digastric muscle is exposed in the upper portion and is retracted cephalad with a retractor. In few instances, posterior belly of the digastric muscle may need to be divided. Hypoglossal nerve may be intimately adherent to the wall of the ICA and should be carefully separated by sharp dissection and gently retracted with a silastic loop cephalad. Systemic heparinization by anesthesia using unfractionated heparin sulfate at 100 IU/kg with monitoring of

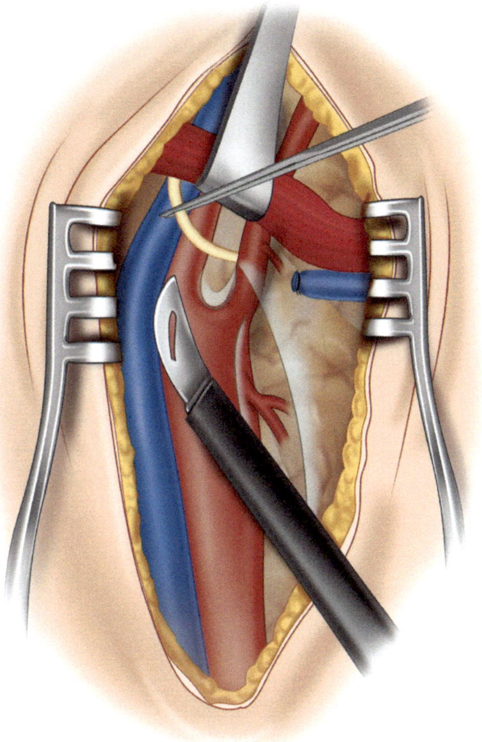

Fig. 20.1 Sharp dissection using 15-blade scalpel separating the adventitia of common and internal carotid artery from surround internal jugular vein. Hypoglossal nerve is looped with vessel loop. Common facial vein is ligated and divided

the ACT between 250 and 300 seconds. The decision to use indwelling shunt is like the one described in the chapter on CEA. In most patients, indwelling shunts are not necessary. Following arteriotomy incision, a 3.5 mm, 4 mm, or 4.5 mm Garrett arterial dilator is inserted in its distal ICA for control of retrograde bleeding (Fig. 20.2). This technique simplifies the suturing at the apex of the patch graft.

Recurrent carotid artery stenosis due to myointimal hyperplasia or atherosclerotic lesion is amenable to re-endarterectomy as the layers of the hyperplastic tissue or the atherosclerotic plaque can be carefully removed; however, the plane is not well defined as in primary endarterectomy. In an occasional patient, hyperplastic lesion may be suitable for patch angioplasty alone. Previously placed patch including old suture material should be preferably be removed. Distal tacking sutures at the end point of endarterectomy may be necessary to tack the distal intima using 6-0 cardiovascular polypropylene suture. In some patients, the quality of the artery following re-endarterectomy is such that interposition patch graft should be performed

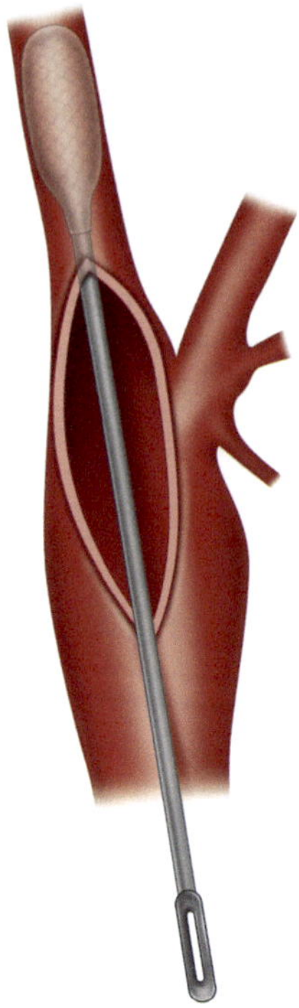

Fig. 20.2 Arteriotomy with control of bleeding with the help of arterial dilator inserted via the arteriotomy

as described in the previous chapter. However, in most cases, a patch graft either using bovine pericardial patch or PTFE patch is preferable. The suture line closure using 6-0 cardiovascular polypropylene for ICA and 5-0 cardiovascular polypropylene for CCA for redo CEA cases should be selected as the arterial wall is relatively thick. In most patients undergoing redo carotid endarterectomy, a Jackson Pratt drain (10 mm flat) should be placed. It should exit through a separate stab incision near the lower neck.

Postoperative Complications

Complications following redo CEA are like those following primary CEA. However, there is increased incidence of cranial nerve palsy.

Take-Home Points

1. Sharp dissection with a 15-blade scalpel is useful in dissecting common and internal carotid artery from surrounding structures.

Chapter 21
Vertebral Artery Reimplantation into the Common Carotid Artery

Sachinder Singh Hans

Surgical Anatomy of Vertebral Artery

The vertebral artery arises from superior and posterior aspect of the first part of the subclavian artery. It ascends to the foramina in the transverse process of all the cervical vertebrae from sixth to the first and then runs laterally entering the skull through the foramen magnum and joins the opposite vertebral artery at the lower border of pons to form the basilar artery. A vertebral artery course is divided into four segments. The first part runs posteriorly and superiorly between the longus colli and the scalenus anticus and posterior to the common carotid artery (CCA). The vertebral vein crosses anterior to the artery; the artery is crossed inferiorly by the inferior thyroid artery. On the left side, the vertebral artery is crossed anteriorly by the thoracic duct. The cervical/dorsal ganglion rests on top of the vertebral artery with medial and lateral rami. The second part of vertebral artery runs cephalad through the transverse foramina of the upper six cervical vertebrae and runs a straight course. The third part exits from the transverse process of the atlas and runs laterally in the suboccipital triangle. The fourth part enters the skull by piercing the dura and arachnoid matter.

Anatomic Variations

Vertebral arteries are often variable (80–85%) in their size. One vertebral artery may be larger and dominant with contralateral vertebral artery hypoplastic or even absent. The origin of vertebral artery can also be variable. They can arise as a

S. S. Hans (✉)
Vascular and Endovascular Services, Henry Ford Macomb Hospital,
Clinton Twp, MI, USA

S. S. Hans et al. (eds.), *Primary and Repeat Arterial Reconstructions*,
https://doi.org/10.1007/978-3-031-13897-3_21

second branch of subclavian artery and may have a duplicate origin. Left vertebral artery may arise from the arch of the aorta between the left CCA and left subclavian artery in 5–7% individuals. Occasionally intracranially branches of the vertebral artery such as posterior inferior cerebellar artery may arise at the level of C1–C2 vertebral body. In rare instances, vertebral artery may end as posterior inferior cerebellar artery.

Indications

Approximately 25% of ischemic strokes occur in the vertebral-basilar territory. The classical symptoms of vertebrobasilar ischemia are usually bilateral and often present as drop attacks, dizziness, vertigo, diplopia, facial numbness, tinnitus, dysphasia, dysarthria, and ataxia. Symptoms occur more commonly secondary to hypoperfusion. Emboli from proximal source may also be responsible for vertebrobasilar ischemia. Surgical reconstruction should not be performed for asymptomatic patients. The surgical requirement is to justify vertebral artery reconstruction for hemodynamic significant stenosis (>70% diameter) in both vertebral arteries and severe stenosis in one and the opposite vertebral artery being hypoplastic. A single vertebral artery is adequate to perfuse the basilar artery. However, patients with symptomatic vertebrobasilar ischemia secondary to emboli may be candidates for open reconstruction regardless of the status of the contralateral vertebral artery.

The vertebral artery origin is better displayed with catheter-based angiography in an oblique projection. Patients with suspected vertebral artery compression should undergo dynamic angiography with provocative positioning.

Technique

The patient is positioned with head elevation (sitting chair position) to decrease the venous pressure. Head extension should be avoided so that the muscles in the neck overlying the vertebral artery may get stretched.

1. The incision is placed transversely just above the clavicle over the sternal and clavicular head of the sternocleidomastoid (Fig. 21.1).
2. The wide subplatysmal skin flaps are created and mobilized.
3. Dissection follows between the two heads of sternocleidomastoid.
4. Inferior belly of the omohyoid is divided.
5. Internal jugular vein is retracted laterally following adequate mobilization.
6. The CCA is reflected medially with the vagus nerve.
7. The dissection is carried between the internal jugular vein and the CCA (Fig. 21.2).

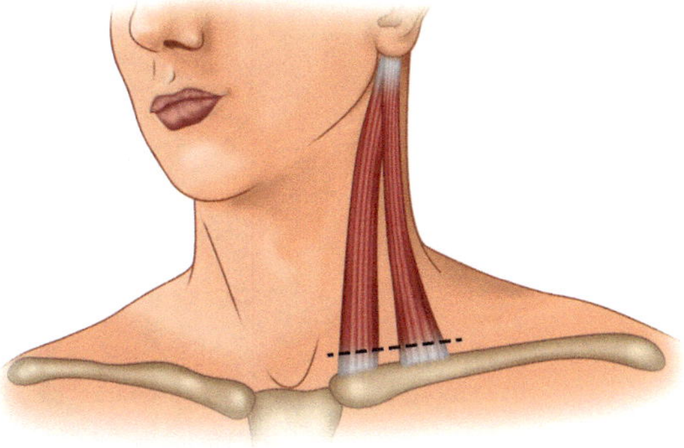

Fig. 21.1 Left Supraclavicular skin incision

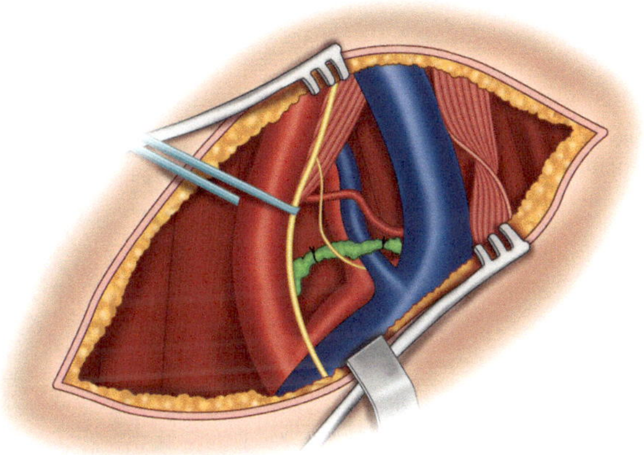

Fig. 21.2 Medial moblization of CCA. Ligation of thoracic duct

8. On the left side, thoracic duct is divided between the suture ligation (Fig. 21.3). On the right side, accessory lymphatic ducts are ligated and divided. The dissection is performed medial to the prescalene fat pad covering the scalenus anticus and Phrenic nerve. The inferior thyroid artery runs transversely in the dissection area and should be ligated and divided. The vertebral vein is identified as it comes out from the angle formed by the longus coli and the scalenus anticus muscle. The vein is anterior to the proximal vertebral artery, and subclavian artery is most inferior. The vertebral vein is ligated and divided (Fig. 21.4). The vertebral and subclavian artery lie deep to vertebral vein. Sympathetic trunk is identified and preserved. The vertebral artery is carefully exposed from its origin (subclavian artery) directly over the tendon of longus colli muscle as it enters the transverse foramina of C6 vertebrae. The vertebral artery is carefully separated from the sympathetic trunk.
9. The appropriate site for vertebral artery transposition is selected. Systemic heparin is administered, and distal end of the vertebral artery is clamped with a

Fig. 21.3 Ligation of vertebral vein

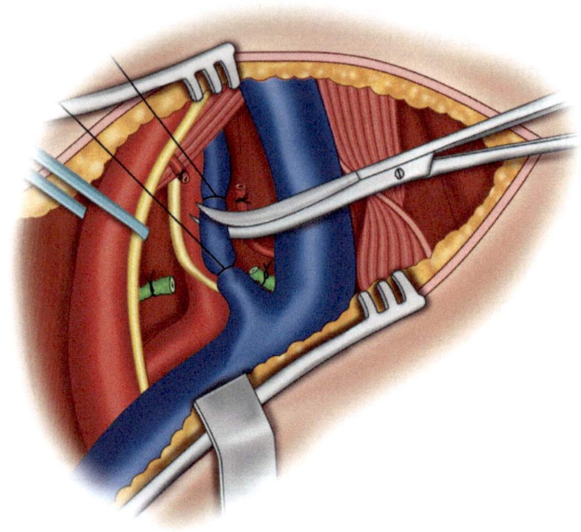

Fig. 21.4 Mobilization of proximal vertebral artery

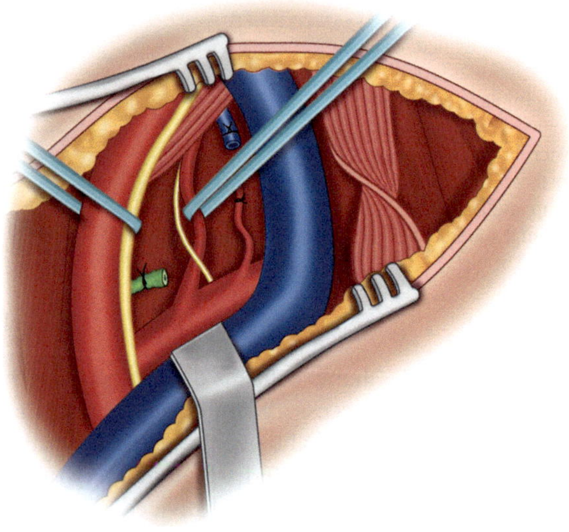

Yasargil clamp. The proximal vertebral artery is ligated with 5-0 or 6-0 CV polypropylene suture. The vertebral artery is divided and brought anterior to sympathetic chain. The proximal end of divided vertebral artery spatulated. The CCA is cross clamped. An elliptical opening is made in the posterolateral wall of the CCA with an aortic punch. The anastomosis of the spatulated vertebral artery is performed in a parachute manner using 7-0 CV polypropylene suture. Once the posterior wall suture line is tightened (parachute suture), anterior suture line is

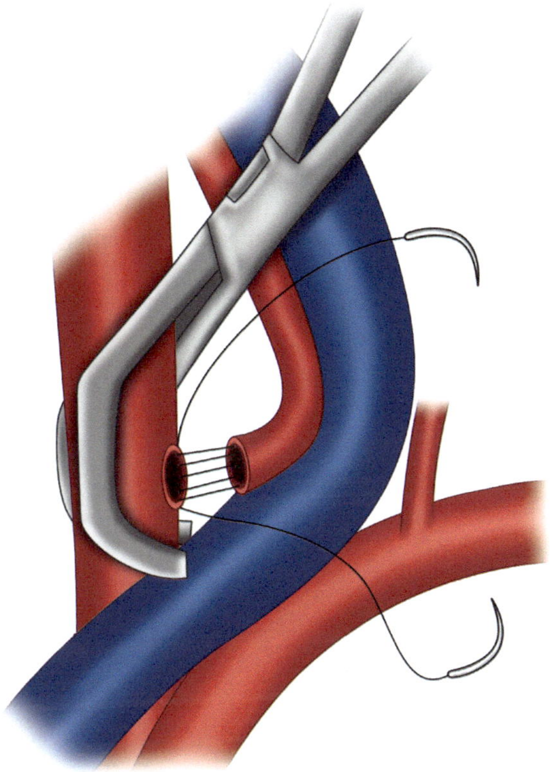

Fig. 21.5 Side biting vascular clamp applied to the CCA and divided vertebral artery is anastomosed end to side to the CCA with 7 "o" cv polypropylene suture

completed (Fig. 21.5). A 10 mm Jackson-Pratt drain is placed and is removed after 24 hours provided there is no chylous leak. Platysma and skin suture line are approximated in layers.

Postoperative Complications

1. Stroke due to immediate thrombosis of the vertebral artery.
2. Vagus and recurrent laryngeal nerve injury may occur in 2% of proximal vertebral reconstructions.
3. Horner Syndrome (8–24%) is far more common. Most patients have resolution of symptoms of Horner Syndrome in 3–4 months' time.
4. Chylous leak should be treated expectedly with local compression, dietary manipulation, and octreotide. If leak persists beyond 3 days, surgical wound

should be reexplored, and direct suture repair of the thoracic or accessory duct should be performed with by placement of a fine monofilament suture. If this technique is unsuccessful, coil embolization of the thoracic duct by intervention radiology should be considered.

Take-Home Points

1. Vertebral artery implantation into CCA for orifical disease of vertebral arteries with symptoms of vertebrobasilar ischemia is a useful operation in carefully selected patients.
2. During dissection, injury to the thoracic duct and sympathetic chain should be carefully avoided.

Chapter 22
Carotid Subclavian Bypass

Timothy J. Nypaver

Carotid subclavian bypass historically was a procedure primarily performed in the management of subclavian stenosis or occlusion. The main indication for carotid subclavian bypass was most commonly for vertebral basilar insufficiency (posterior cerebral circulation) related to reduced perfusion to or retrograde flow (subclavian steal syndrome) in the ipsilateral vertebral artery. Alternately, the procedure could be performed for direct arm perfusion problems with ipsilateral arm exercise fatigue. The common carotid artery (CCA) serves at the donor artery with pulsatile perfusion reestablished to the distal subclavian artery and thereby the vertebral artery. Alternately, in instances of proximal carotid disease, the bypass can be used to restore pulsatile perfusion to the CCA, improving perfusion to the anterior cerebral circulation. In this instance, the subclavian artery serves as the donor artery. One additional indication for the carotid subclavian bypass is the anatomic situation in which the left internal mammary artery (LIMA) has been used (or is going to be used) for the graft for coronary artery bypass in the presence of a proximal subclavian stenosis or occlusion. The bypass functions to maintain perfusion to the left internal mammary which then supplies the coronary circulation.

While carotid subclavian bypass is still used in the setting of subclavian and carotid occlusive disease, the most common indication in the endovascular era has been with debranching procedures in which the subclavian orifice, due to the need to secure a proximal landing zone, is covered by the proximal extent of the thoracic endovascular aneurysm repair (TEVAR) graft. Carotid subclavian bypass is typically performed a few days prior to the TEVAR but can be accomplished concomitantly if necessary. In instances in which upper extremity ischemic symptoms develop post-urgent or emergent TEVAR, bypass is also warranted. Due to concern over the potential of reducing spinal cord perfusion, in the elective situation, an

T. J. Nypaver (✉)
Division of Vascular Surgery, Henry Ford Hospital, Detroit, MI, USA
e-mail: TNYPAVE1@hfhs.org

S. S. Hans et al. (eds.), *Primary and Repeat Arterial Reconstructions*,
https://doi.org/10.1007/978-3-031-13897-3_22

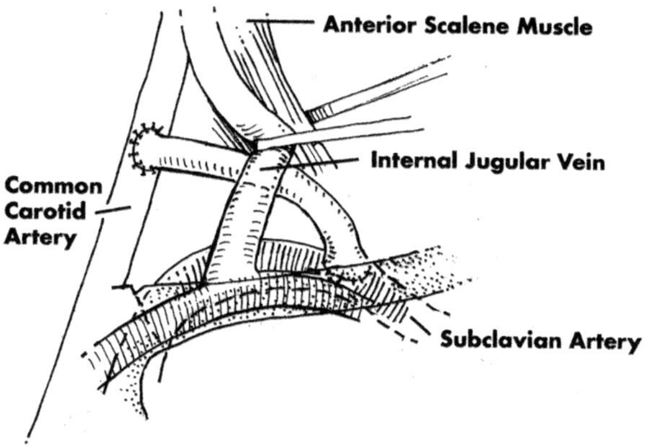

Fig. 22.1 Completed carotid-subclavian bypass with graft placed behind the left Internal Jugular vein

aggressive approach to carotid subclavian bypass prior to TEVAR has been adopted. Absolute indications for this bypass when TEVAR coverage of the left subclavian is anticipated are (1) absent right vertebral artery; (2) small or diseased right vertebral artery; (3) left vertebral artery which terminates in the posterior inferior cerebellar artery (PICA); and (4) history of prior LIMA coronary graft. Carotid subclavian bypass is notable for its excellent patency results and as a procedure which is generally well tolerated by the patient. Except for rare or extenuating circumstances, the bypass is constructed with a prosthetic graft, either Dacron or expanded polytetrafluorethylene (ePTFE) (the author's preference). Finally, the graft, if properly positioned, tends to be very short, usually ≤3 cm in length.

Surgical anatomy: The operation is performed through a single supraclavicular incision and consists of exposure of the common carotid artery in the medial aspect, exposure of the subclavian artery deep to the anterior scalene in the mid-aspect of the wound, and a tunnel created posterior to the internal jugular vein (Fig. 22.1). Important structures which need to be identified and preserved from injury include the vagus nerve (during exposure of the CCA), the phrenic nerve (during the subclavian exposure), and the thoracic duct (empties into the subclavian vein near the confluence of the left internal jugular and the left subclavian vein).

Technical Aspects of the Operation

The patient is positioned supine in a semi-Fowler position, and general anesthesia is used. The arterial line, if utilized, should be placed in the opposite extremity. The patient has a roll placed longitudinally between the shoulder blades with head extension allowing for exposure and access to the supraclavicular area. The neck is rotated to the contralateral side. The incision is made approximately 2 cm lateral to the sternal notch, at the medial border of the sternal head of the sternocleidomastoid muscle (SCM), 1–2 cm above the clavicle proper, and extends approximately 6–8 cm laterally (Fig. 22.2). The platysma is divided linearly, and minimal skin flap is made extending for approximately 2 cm laterally each direction under the

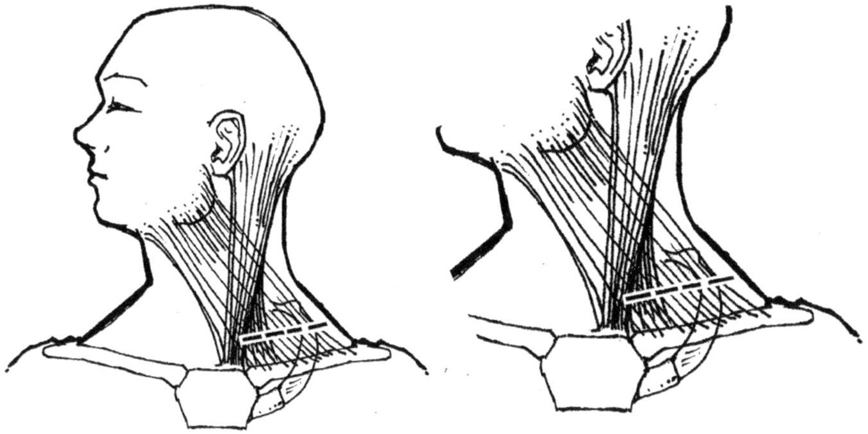

Fig. 22.2 Scalenus anticus is divided a few mm at a time near its insertion into the first rib, carefully protecting the phrenic nerve

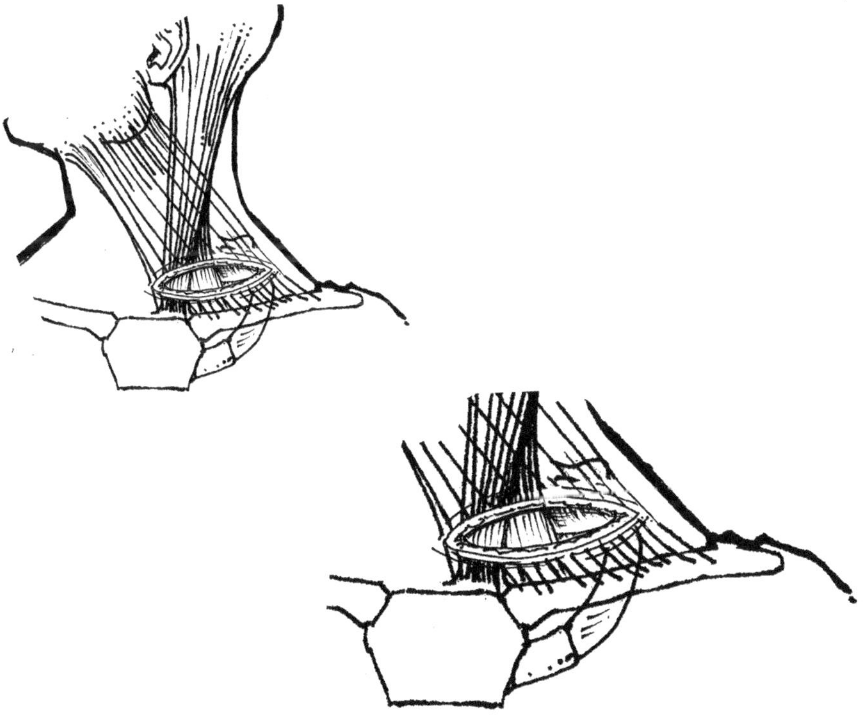

Fig. 22.3 Division of clavicular head of the Sternomastoid with exposure of scalne fat pad

platysma. The external jugular vein and the omohyoid muscle are identified and divided in the mid-wound. The clavicular head of the SCM is identified and divided with cautery to expose the underlying scalene fat pad (Fig. 22.3). Dissection with careful mobilization of the scalene fat pad then ensues with mobilization of the fat pad laterally initiated at the lateral border of the internal jugular. The scalene fat pad is mobilized on its medial, superior, and inferior borders out to the lateral edge of the anterior scalene (Fig. 22.4). The phrenic nerve coursing on the anterior aspect of the anterior scalene (within the investing fascia of the muscle) is identified, notable for its lateral to medial course (Fig. 22.4). The phrenic nerve is gently dissected for a short distance (2–3 cm) to allow for its minimal retraction and protection during the division of the anterior scalene. The phrenic nerve should not be forcibly retracted due to the risk of temporary or permanent diaphragmatic palsy. The thoracic duct is also encountered in this region coursing in the inferomedial corner of the scalene fat pad and, if identified, is simply ligated with polyglactin sutures or monofilament proline (Fig. 22.4). With careful protection of the phrenic nerve, the anterior scalene muscle is dissected on its medial and lateral aspects as close as possible to its insertion on the first rib. The muscle is divided a few millimeters at a time protecting the phrenic nerve throughout this exercise (Fig. 22.5). The author prefers low power cautery; however, sharp division is also utilized, recognizing that the subclavian vein lies just anterior to the anterior scalene muscle in the inferior wound and should be protected. The anterior surface of the subclavian artery should now be visible, and the artery is now dissected out for 3–4 cm and encircled with vessel loops to allow application of distal and proximal vascular clamps. All branches of the subclavian artery are carefully preserved including the thyrocervical trunk; for the purposes of the carotid subclavian bypass, the internal mammary or the vertebral

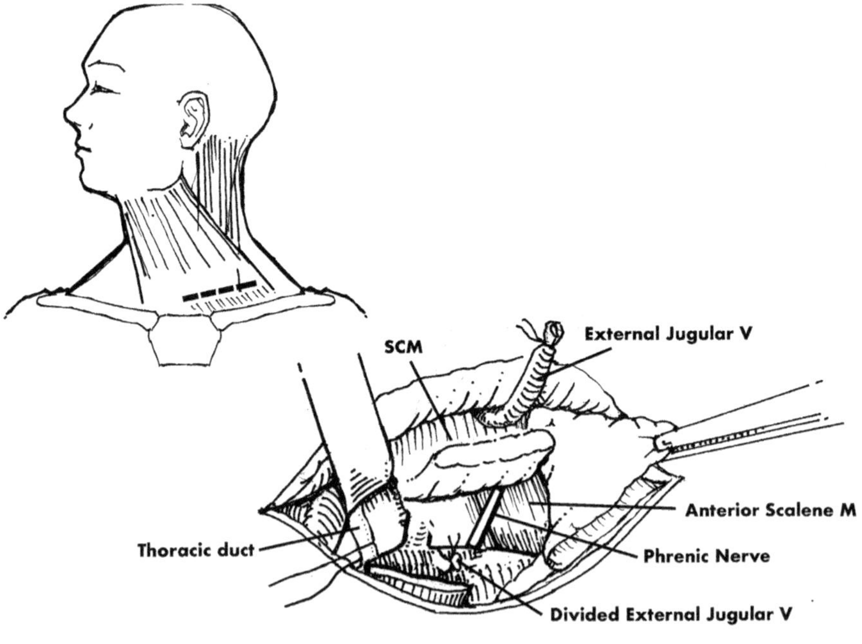

Fig. 22.4 Identification of the phrenic nerve coursing lateral to medially in the investing fascia

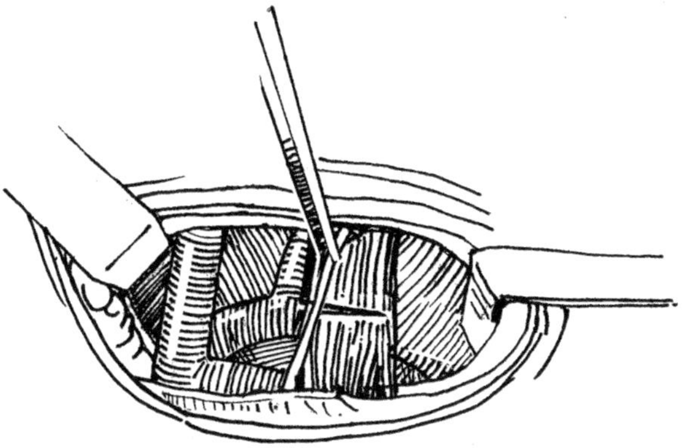

Fig. 22.5 Scalenus anticus is divided a few mm at a time near its insertion into the first rib, carefully protecting the phrenic nerve

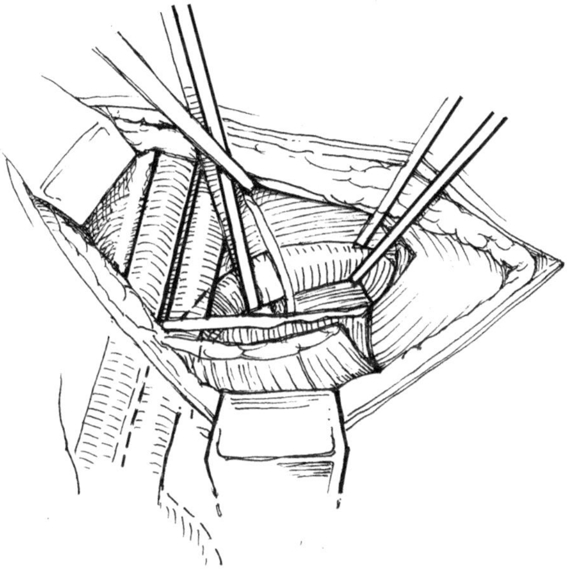

Fig. 22.6 Exposure of the CCA and subclavian artery

artery is infrequently encountered. It is important to keep the dissection close to the artery as the pleurae are frequently just deep to the posterior aspect of the subclavian artery.

Next, the CCA is dissected out with the medial head of the SCM retracted medially—the artery is immediately medial to the jugular vein (Fig. 22.6). The CCA is dissected for 4–5 cm circumferentially. There are no branches in this area, but one needs to be careful to avoid the vagus nerve which lies posterior and in-between the CCA and the internal jugular vein. With the CCA dissected out, the jugular vein is mobilized on its posterior aspect to facilitate the tunnel for the prosthetic graft. Typically, the author has used 6- or 8-mm ePTFE as the graft material, although a similar sized Dacron graft can also be utilized.

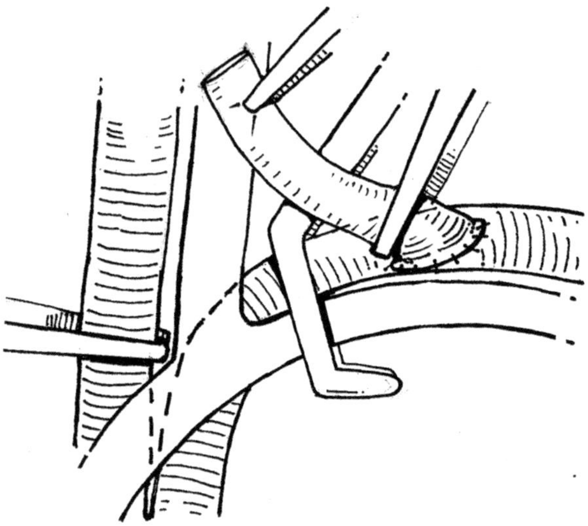

Fig. 22.7 End to side anastomosis to the left subclavian artery following a longitudinal arteriotomy in the subclavian artery

The author prefers to complete the subclavian anastomosis first—the patient receives 70 units/kg of intravenous heparin with an activated clotting time of 200–250 s desirable. The mid and most apical segment of the subclavian artery is used for the site of the anastomosis. The subclavian artery tends to be much more friable than other arteries; superiorly oriented tension on the artery with either forceps, sutures, or vascular clamps is not well tolerated and is to be avoided. Atraumatic vascular clamps are applied typically with an angled Debakey clamp or small Debakey Derra vascular clamp (for the proximal subclavian artery), and the arteriotomy is performed with an 11 blade on the anterior surface (Fig. 22.7). The end of the graft is cut in a beveled Cobra-hood type fashion, and the anastomosis performed with either 5-0 or 6-0 proline, starting on the medial aspect first. The author prefers to do the initial sutures in a parachute fashion, placing a total of five sutures prior to gently pulling and tightening down the sutures. Again, excessive pulling or traction can occur with resultant troublesome tears to the subclavian artery, especially if one is too aggressive. Once the anastomosis is completed, the proximal artery and distal artery are vented through the graft, and the anastomosis is checked for hemostasis. The graft will now be tunneled over to the CCA, and this is performed in a retro-jugular fashion; the graft is positioned superior to the phrenic nerve.

The graft is brought up to the CCA, and a site is selected on the artery that allows the straightest and most direct course of the graft. The CCA is then clamped proximally and distally keeping the planned arteriotomy on the lateral aspect of the common carotid artery—this is facilitated by gentle rotation of the artery when applying the vascular clamps. The bypass graft is anastomosed to the common carotid artery in an end-to-side fashion using a continuous 5-0 or 6-0 monofilament suture (Fig. 22.8). The anastomosis is begun on the center of the back wall, and the suturing continues along the back wall from the inside. Prior to completing the anastomosis, the common carotid artery is vented both proximally and distally. The

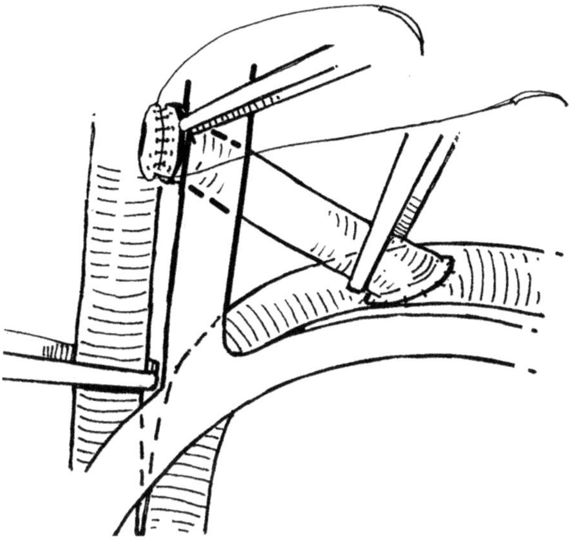

Fig. 22.8 End to side anastomosis of the graft to the CCA

anastomosis is completed, and flow is opened through the graft and through the subclavian anastomosis, prior to restoring flow into the distal CCA. The CCA clamp is well-tolerated, and electroencephalogram monitoring is not routinely used.

Heparin is reversed with protamine, and the wound is carefully observed for any bleeding or any chyle leak. The scalene fat pad is returned to its original position, and the platysma is closed with interrupted 3-0 braided polyglactin suture. The use of a drain in this area is controversial; the author has used a drain frequently especially if any amount of lymph fluid was encountered during the operation.

Carotid Subclavian Transposition

An additional attractive option for proximal subclavian artery occlusive disease is the performance of a carotid subclavian transposition. When extending the landing zone for TEVAR with anticipated coverage of the subclavian origin, carotid subclavian bypass is preferred and has been generally adopted. Carotid subclavian transposition has the advantage of avoiding a prosthetic graft, is performed with a single anastomosis, and has reported superb patency rates. The procedure is slightly more technically challenging due to the need for extensive mobilization of the proximal portion of the subclavian artery with isolation of the internal mammary and vertebral arteries. With carotid subclavian transposition, there is the potential for ligation of the inferior internal memory artery, and thus, this operation is contraindicated in patients who have a left internal mammary artery coronary bypass graft. An adequate length of the subclavian artery proximal to the origin of the vertebral artery is required to allow for mobilization of the subclavian artery (to the common carotid) as well as the requirement for oversewing of the proximal subclavian stump. The mobilized subclavian artery will need to reach the common carotid artery without tension.

Operative details: The operation is initiated in the same fashion as the carotid subclavian bypass as detailed above. The subclavian artery will need to be dissected and mobilized for an additional 3–5 cm proximally, extending down proximal to takeoff of the vertebral artery. If there is inadequate length of the subclavian artery, the procedure can be abandoned in favor of a carotid subclavian bypass. Once the mobilization is completed, the patient is systemically anticoagulated (70 units/kg). The proximal portion of the subclavian artery is clamped with an atraumatic vascular clamp. Once the clamps are secure, the subclavian artery is divided leaving a cuff or 8–10 mm to be oversewn. The proximal stump of this subclavian artery is carefully oversewn expeditiously with 5-0 proline; the author leaves the end sutures long and brought out and attached to rubber shads prior to releasing the clamp to confirm hemostasis and allow for control of the subclavian stump. Once hemostasis has been achieved, the clamp is removed and sutures are cut. This is performed due to the concern that the subclavian stump, once released, can retract into the thoracic cavity and render control problematic. The distal subclavian is brought over to the common carotid artery, again in a retro-jugular position. The anastomosis to the common carotid artery is performed in the same fashion and technique as the carotid anastomosis of the carotid subclavain bypass.

Complications

Complications of carotid subclavian bypass are relatively rare but would include nerve injury (vagus nerve/phrenic nerve), kinking or incorrect positioning of the graft, injury or tearing of the subclavian artery due to its fragility, operative violation of the pleurae, and lymphatic or chyle leak secondary to thoracic duct injury. Injury or excessive traction on the vagus nerve could result in transient vocal cord paralysis/paresis, while injury to the phrenic nerve can result in temporary diaphragmatic palsy. The graft is typically short and with proper positioning of the anastomoses, and appropriate graft length should not have a kink or excessive redundancy. If detected intraoperatively, this finding will mandate operation correction. Injury or tearing of the subclavian artery typically noted with pulling up on sutures or with the inappropriate use of forceps will require patch (bovine pericardium) repair of the artery, maintaining the lumen of the subclavian artery. The subsequent subclavian anastomosis is performed in the middle of the patch. Injury to the thoracic duct can result in troublesome chyle and/or lymphatic drainage; if identified during the operation, duct should be identified and ligated. If chylous drainage is encountered postoperatively, the author has found that early reoperation with ligation or clipping of the chyle leak or the thoracic duct is the most efficient and expeditious manner of handling this complication.

Take-Home Points

1. Carotid subclavian bypass is a durable well-tolerated procedure utilized in the management of symptomatic subclavian or carotid artery occlusive disease. When one is able to cross the subclavian artery stenosis or occlusion successfully, endovascular revascularization is the preferred initial management. Carotid subclavian bypass is reserved for recurrent disease, subclavian artery occlusion (unsuccessful in crossing), or special circumstances related to the vertebral or internal mammary flow. The bypass now is commonly employed in debranching procedures in which the TEVAR graft is expected or anticipated to cover the subclavian orifice.
2. The operation is well tolerated through a single relatively small incision—however, the proximity of important structures including the vagus nerve, phrenic nerve, brachial plexus, venous structures, and the thoracic duct renders this an operation in which one has to be vigilant to avoid excessive traction or injury that can result in nerve palsies or chyle leaks.
3. Prosthetic grafts, either Dacron or ePTFE, are the graft of choice.

Chapter 23
De-branching Operations on Supra-aortic Trunk

Timothy J. Nypaver

1. Carotid-carotid bypass and carotid-carotid-subclavian bypass
2. Ascending aorto-arch vessel debranching

Indications for Carotid-Carotid Bypass and Carotid-Carotid-Subclavian Debranching Procedures and Ascending Aorto-Arch Vessel Debranching Procedures

Carotid-Carotid Bypass and Carotid-Carotid-Subclavian Bypass

The carotid-to-carotid bypass is an infrequent operation which has gained some level of popularity in the setting of debranching procedures to extend the landing zone of thoracic endovascular aneurysm repair (TEVAR) grafts to a level proximal to the origin of the left carotid off of the aortic arch. The complete list of indications for carotid-carotid bypass are as follows: 1. occlusive lesions of the common carotid artery (CCA) or brachiocephalic trunk (innominate artery) not amenable to direct reconstruction or endovascular therapy; and 2. as a procedure to extend the landing zone of TEVARs to a more proximal arch aorta with coverage of the left carotid, often performed concomitantly with a left carotid to left subclavian bypass. In patients with ostial left common carotid lesions, carotid-carotid bypass is typically reserved for those in whom the left subclavian is not suitable as a donor vessel. The indication for the bypass is symptomatic left proximal common carotid artery disease with manifestations of stroke or transient ischemic attack or global reduction

T. J. Nypaver (✉)
Division of Vascular Surgery, Henry Ford Hospital, Detroit, MI, USA
e-mail: TNYPAVE1@hfhs.org

S. S. Hans et al. (eds.), *Primary and Repeat Arterial Reconstructions*,
https://doi.org/10.1007/978-3-031-13897-3_23

in cerebral blood flow. It is important to note that this indication for the carotid-carotid bypass has now been supplanted by endovascular therapy, either transfemoral proximal carotid stenting or with a carotid cutdown and retrograde carotid artery angioplasty and stenting (hybrid procedure). Asymptomatic lesions rarely require intervention. As noted, the major indication for carotid-carotid bypass in the endovascular era has been revascularization of the left CCA to provide a "landing zone" for endovascular repair of aneurysms involving the aortic arch/descending thoracic aorta. This is performed when it is felt that the patient is too high risk, either due to underlying medical comorbidities or prior operations, for the performance of a median sternotomy with direct operative repair involving cardiopulmonary bypass.

Some of the additional clinical considerations include the choice of conduit, whether expanded polytetrafluoroethylene, Dacron, autologous vein, or even the option of transposition, and the tunnel utilized for the bypass. The author favors the retropharyngeal tunnel and graft position, advantageous due to its relatively short distance and direct route. The bypass is located deep, cannot be visualized under the skin, and is routed in the area between the pharynx and the pre-vertebral lamina. The other option would involve making a subcutaneously tunnel which is less desirable, longer, and potentially more prone to infection and kinking. With the carotid-carotid-subclavian bypass, one performs a debranching of the left carotid and left subclavian arteries with TEVAR graft coverage of the left carotid and left subclavian origins. Please refer to the chapter on carotid-subclavian bypass, as this is essentially performed as a separate distinguishable procedure.

Ascending Aorto-Arch Vessel Debranching

When it is necessary to deploy the TEVAR in zone 0 proximal to the origin of the innominate, the debranching procedure now involves the performance of a median sternotomy with an ascending aorto-arch vessel bypass, typically to the innominate and the left carotid (often with pre-performance of a carotid-subclavian bypass) or three vessel bypass reconstruction to the innominate, the left carotid, and the left subclavian. This depends on the position of the left subclavian; in its normal anatomic position, the subclavian artery may be difficult to reach through a median sternotomy. Due to the rotation of the aortic arch in setting of arch pathology, the subclavian artery may be in a more anterior position and therefore more easily reached and dissected for a direct bypass rather than via the indirect carotid-subclavian revascularization. Computed tomographic angiography (CTA), with the study inclusive of the entire ascending aorta, the arch, the cervical and intracranial vessels, is required prior to undertaking this debranching operation. This approach avoids the need to go on cardiopulmonary bypass with its attendant risks and complications.

Preoperative Planning and Surgical Anatomy

Preprocedural imaging involves either CTA or magnetic resonance angiography (MRA). Adequate imaging of the ascending aorta, the aortic arch along with the outflow vessels including the entire cervical and intracranial vasculature and/or proximal vasculature of upper extremities, is required. Evaluation for vocal cord function is routinely carried out preoperatively. Measurement of bilateral upper extremity pressures should be performed to document baseline perfusion. Severe cardiopulmonary diseases, a heavily calcified aortic arch or prior sternotomy are risk factors which render the operation problematic and may even preclude patients as candidates. Due to the greater magnitude of the operation and the need for median sternotomy, a more robust and complete cardiopulmonary workup and evaluation are necessary prior to proceeding with an ascending aorta to arch vessel de-debranching procedure. One would have a lower threshold for obtaining a catheter-based coronary angiogram prior to proceeding with median sternotomy. The anatomic status of the ascending aorta and lack of any significant calcification or pathology are critical to a successful outcome.

Surgical Anatomy: The carotid-carotid bypass operation is performed through bilateral lower cervical incision, whereas the carotid-carotid-subclavian requires the addition of a supraclavicular incision. The CCAs are exposed approximately 2 cm above the sternal notch bilaterally; the graft tunnel is created in a retropharyngeal location immediately anterior to the vertebral body fascia (Figs. 23.1 and

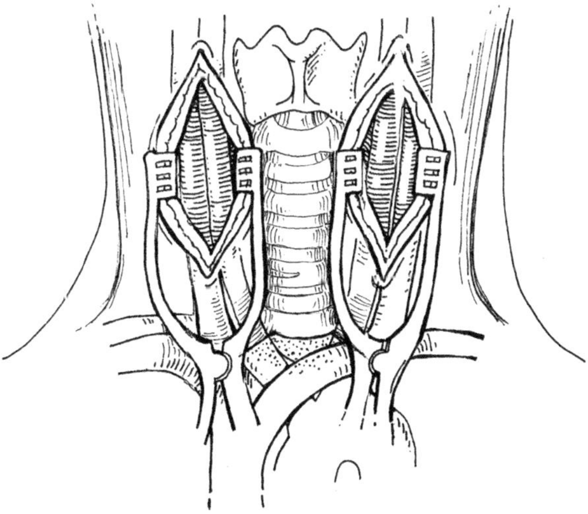

Fig. 23.1 Bilateral vertical cervical incisions centered over the common carotid arteries

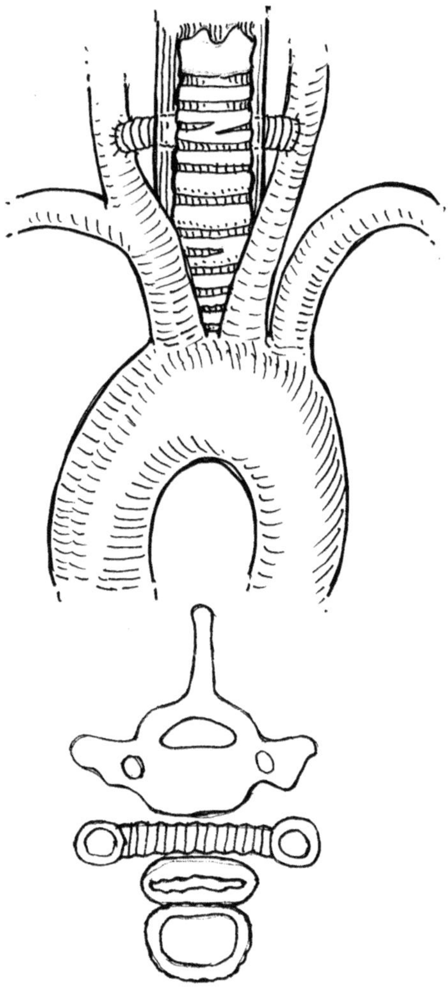

Fig. 23.2 Graft tunnel created in a retropharyngeal location immediately anterior to the vertebral body fascia

23.2). Important structures which need to be identified and preserved from injury include the vagus nerve (during exposure of the CCA), the phrenic nerve (during the subclavian exposure), and the thoracic duct (empties into the subclavian vein near the confluence of the left internal jugular and the left subclavian vein). As this is a bilateral procedure, one needs to be especially vigilant with regard to the vagus nerve.

Operative Steps

Carotid-carotid bypass and carotid-carotid-subclavian bypass

The bypass operations are performed under general anesthesia. The patient is positioned supine in a semi-Fowler position. The arterial line, if utilized, should be placed in the right upper extremity. The patient has a roll placed longitudinally between the shoulder blades with head extension allowing for exposure and access to the sternal notch, the lower neck, and supraclavicular area. The neck is maintained in the midline. The exposure of the CCA ensues with 4–5 cm incisions along the anterior border of the sternocleidomastoid (SCM) (Fig. 23.1) and extends down through the platysma with exposure of the carotid sheath. The jugular vein is kept lateral and typically it is not necessary to dissect out or expose this structure. The CCA is then exposed and dissected out for 3–4 cm. In encircling the CCA, one is careful not to include or injure the vagus nerve. Also, there exists the possibility of an anterior vagus nerve position which can be prone to injury. Likewise, the contralateral incision is carried out exposing the contralateral CCA in a similar fashion. The tunnel is often very short, and it is important to stay on the prevertebral fascia as close as possible with finger dissection in this plane as the tunnel is created. If one is doing a carotid-to-carotid to subclavian bypass, a supraclavicular incision is made with the incision starting and extending more laterally than usual, i.e., 3 cm lateral to the sternal notch. The incision is made 1–2 cm above the clavicle proper and extends approximately 6 cm laterally. Please refer to the chapter on carotid-subclavian bypass. The external jugular vein and the omohyoid muscle are identified and divided in the mid-wound. The clavicular head of the SCM is identified and divided with cautery to expose the underlying scalene fat pad. Dissection with careful mobilization of the scalene fat pad then ensues with mobilization of the fat pad laterally initiated at the lateral border of the internal jugular. The scalene fat pad is mobilized on its medial, superior, and inferior borders out to the lateral edge of the anterior scalene. The phrenic nerve coursing on the anterior aspect of the anterior scalene (within the investing fascia of the muscle) is identified. The thoracic duct is also encountered in this region coursing in the inferomedial corner of the scalene fat pad and, if identified, is simply ligated with polyglactin sutures or monofilament proline. With careful protection of the phrenic nerve, the anterior scalene muscle is dissected on its medial and lateral aspects as close as possible to its insertion on the first rib. The muscle is divided a few millimeters at a time protecting the phrenic nerve throughout this exercise. The anterior surface of the subclavian artery should now be visible, and the artery is now dissected out for 3–4 cm and encircled with vessel loops to allow application of distal and proximal vascular clamps. A tunnel is created in a retro-jugular location from the proximal carotid artery (exposed in the vertical incision) to the subclavian artery (exposed in the supraclavicular incision). Typically, the author has used 6 or 8-mm non-ringed ePTFE as the graft

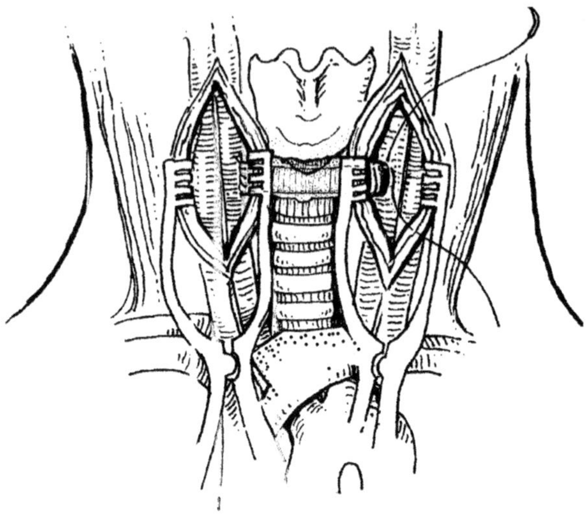

Fig. 23.3 Performance of second common carotid anastomosis after the graft has been tunneled in the retropharyngeal location

material although a similar sized Dacron graft can also be utilized. The patient is then anticoagulated with intravenous heparin at a dose of 70–100 units/kg, maintaining an activated clotting time of 200–250 s. In most instances, the CCA, in the absence of significant carotid bulb or intracranial disease, can be safely clamped. If concern exists over cerebral perfusion, the author has employed electroencephalographic (EEG) monitoring in determining cerebral perfusion. Typically, one proceeds first with the donor CCA (the right), and the graft anastomosis is performed with the arteriotomy performed slightly medially at approximately the 1 or 2 o'clock position. The graft end is then sewn with 5-0 or 6-0 proline suture in a circumferential fashion beginning at the mid posterior portion of the anastomosis. The anastomosis is begun on the center of the back wall and the suturing continues along the back wall from the inside. Prior to completing the anastomosis, the CCA is vented both proximally and distally and flow restored to common carotid prior to initiating anything on the contralateral side. The graft is clamped and with the graft tunneled over to the contralateral carotid, the graft is sized and cut to the appropriate length, and the second anastomosis is performed (Fig. 23.3). Again, the arteriotomy on the left CCA is performed slightly medial, at the 10 or 11 o'clock position. The anastomosis is performed in a similar fashion and flow is restored through the CCA.

The carotid to subclavian bypass, performed as a distinctively separate procedure, is then undertaken, positioning the carotid anastomosis slightly inferior to the carotid-carotid anastomosis (Fig. 23.4). One is referred to the chapter on carotid-subclavian bypass. An alternate and more efficient reconstruction is to sew the distal stump of the divided left CCA directly into the bypass graft, which is being routed from the right carotid over to the left subclavian (Fig. 23.5). This necessitates

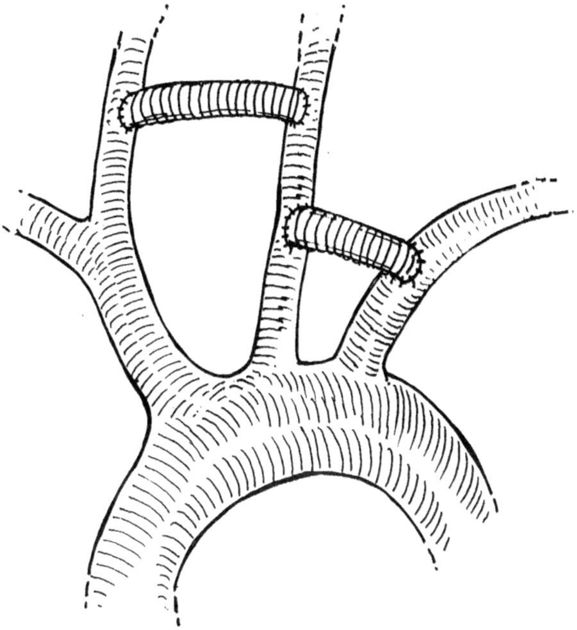

Fig. 23.4 The anatomic positioning of the carotid-carotid and the carotid-subclavian bypass with the carotid anastomosis of the carotid- subclavian bypass inferior to the carotid anastomosis of the carotid-carotid bypass

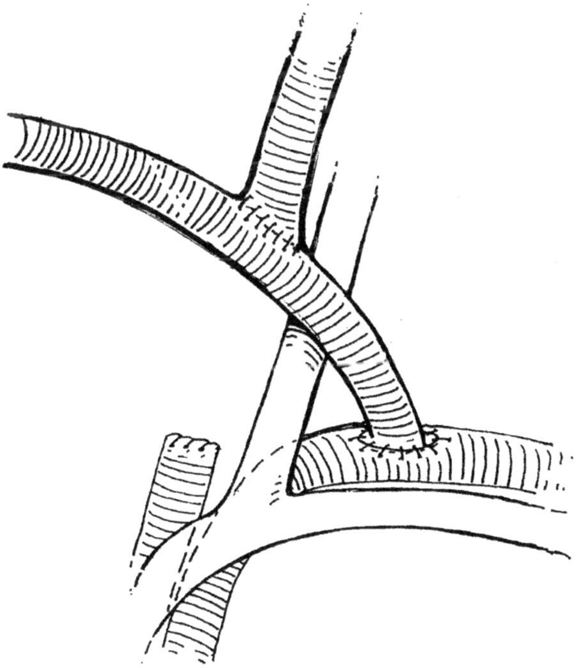

Fig. 23.5 Alternate reconstruction with the distal stump of the divided left CCA implanted directly into the bypass graft, which is then routed from the right carotid over to the left subclavian

performance of an end-to-side anastomosis of the left CCA into the side of the graft and one needs to align this such that there is not excessive redundancy in the left common carotid distally or within the graft itself. The final anastomosis in this configuration is to the left subclavian which is performed with clamping of the graft just beyond the anastomosis to the left carotid. Atraumatic vascular clamps are applied to the subclavian artery with an angled Debakey clamp or small Debakey Derra vascular clamp (for the proximal subclavian artery) and the arteriotomy is performed with an 11 blade on the anterior surface. The end of the graft is cut in a beveled Cobra-hood type fashion and the anastomosis performed with either 5-0 or 6-0 proline, starting on the medial aspect first. The author prefers to do the initial sutures in a parachute fashion, placing a total of 5 sutures prior to gently pulling and tightening down the sutures. Again, excessive pulling or traction is to be avoided as the subclavian artery is notably more fragile than the CCA. Once the anastomosis is completed, the artery is vented through the graft and the anastomosis is checked for hemostasis.

Ascending Aorto-Arch Vessel Debranching Procedure.

The patient is positioned with a posterior shoulder roll to extend the neck and elevate the sternal notch after general anesthesia is induced. The median sternotomy is performed with a slight cervical extension to the right to allow for better expose of the right common carotid and subclavian arteries (Fig. 23.6). The sternum is divided with a sternal saw and a self-retaining retractor is placed. Next the pericardium is divided in the midline and three stay sutures are then placed on both edges of the pericardium to elevate the mediastinal structures and create a pericardial well. The left brachiocephalic vein is dissected circumferentially and encircled with a vessel loop. This loop may be used to retract the vein superiorly or inferiorly. This will allow exposure of the underlying structures. The ascending aorta is exposed, dissecting it free from the main pulmonary trunk laterally and right pulmonary artery inferiorly to allow or additional mobility.

The distal arteries, inclusive of the innominate and the left common carotid, are likewise dissected out. If the innominate is of adequate length (>5 cm) and non-diseased, one may limit the exposure to this vessel in preparation for bypass. With a short or diseased innominate artery, exposure of the right subclavian artery and the right CCA is commonly required, facilitating control and performance of the anastomosis. Importantly, one needs to avoid and protect the recurrent laryngeal nerve as it courses beneath the right subclavian artery and behind the CCA origin before entering the larynx. The left subclavian, if necessary, especially if oriented anteriorly, can also be dissected out in preparation for bypass. As noted previously, if the left subclavian is in a posterior position, the author has performed

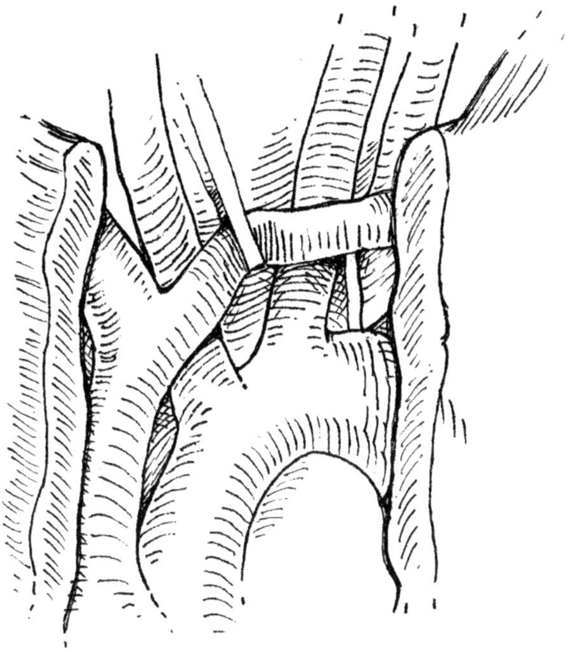

Fig. 23.6 Median sternotomy with exposure of the ascending aorta and the arch vessels

a carotid-subclavian bypass preemptively prior to the median sternotomy and the ascending aortic debranching procedure.

Once the dissection is complete, the patient is systemically heparinized (100 units/kg) with an Activated Clotting Time (ACT) of 200–250 s. The anesthesiology team is then asked to maintain the systolic blood pressure less than 100 mmHg. Once this is achieved, one selects the side-biting aortic clamp site, which needs to be disease-free, and is typically slightly lateral to the right side of the ascending aorta. A side-biting clamp is applied for partial exclusion of the artery (Fig. 23.7). As one is placing a side-biting camp on the ascending aorta, it is imperative that the aorta has been adequately mobilized, and that there is good communication with the anesthesia teams to keep the blood pressure relatively low and controlled. The author favors the use of the Lemole-Strong clamp as the side-biting clamp of choice. The author has greatly benefitted with the assistance of a cardiothoracic/cardiovascular surgeon to facilitate this exposure and subsequent clamp placement.

Once one is confident that the clamp is well-positioned and stable (not sliding off the aorta), the excluded portion is aspirated with a needle and if no bleeding is confirmed, an arteriotomy is then created in the aorta. The author has used the prefabricated Thoracic Arch Graft with radiopaque marker (Terumo, Vascutek) with the size of the graft being sewn to the aorta 12 or 14 mm in diameter and a left carotid

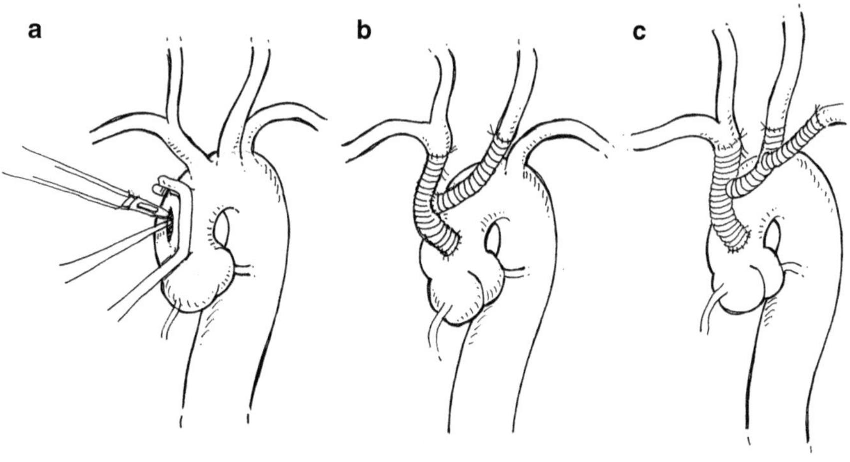

Fig. 23.7 (**a**) Application of side-biting clamp with aortotomy in preparation for proximal anastomosis. (**b**) Completed ascending aorta to innominate and left carotid bypass reconstruction. (**c**) Completed ascending aorta to innominate and left carotid and subclavian bypass reconstruction

branch diameter of 8 or 10 mm (Fig. 23.8). This graft has an accessary branch which will allow for the wire inserted into the thoracic aorta to be directed and exit out the side branch, allowing for dental floss arrangement with the wire secured outside through the median sternotomy and outside the selected femoral artery. While the surgeon in most instances will be passing the thoracic endograft up from the femoral artery to the arch, alternately, one can, over this wire, pass the endograft through this side branch, through the anastomosis (protected with a sheath) and into the arch and descending thoracic aorta. The graft orientation will need to be reversed in this situation. The proximal anastomosis of the graft is beveled appropriately to lay comfortably to the right of the ascending aorta. In using this prefabricated graft, it is important to bevel the anastomosis as close as possible to the accessory side branch (Fig. 23.8). The proximal anastomosis is performed with 4-0 polypropylene suture in a continuous running fashion. One needs to carefully inspect this anastomosis prior to clamp release ensuring that no repair sutures are required and that the suture is appropriately tight. The patient is then temporarily placed in Trendelenburg position as the clamp is released, protecting against air embolization. Flow has been maintained in the innominate, left carotid, and left subclavian system normally up to this point. The innominate is the clamped distally and proximally, and the graft is then positioned and cut to an appropriate length with either the 10 or 12 mm diameter graft then sewn to the innominate artery, the anastomosis performed with 5-0 polypropylene suture in a continuous running fashion. After flow is restored to the innominate, the proximal stump is oversewn with 4-0 proline suture in a Blalock

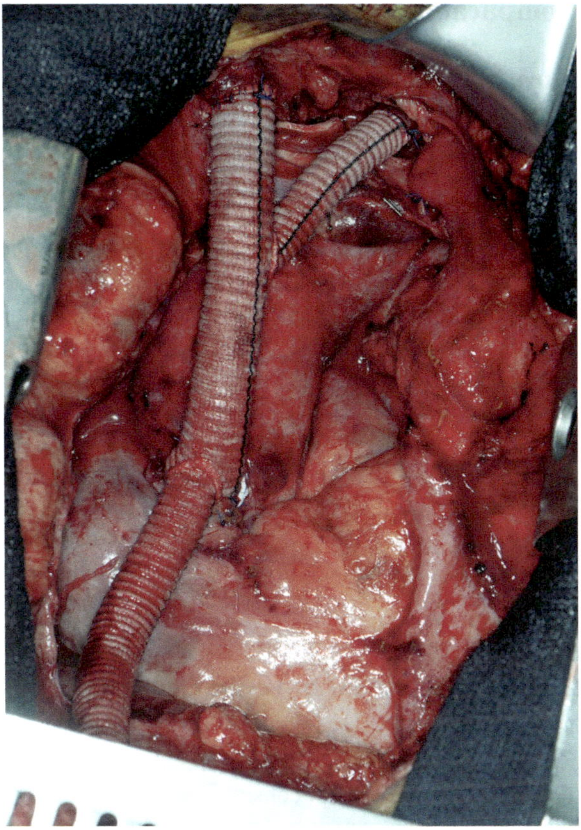

Fig. 23.8 Operative photograph of completed ascending aorta to innominate and left carotid bypass reconstruction (note separate branch just beyond the proximal anastomosis which can be used for retrograde delivery of endograft or alternately wire exit and control for delivery of endograft from below

fashion securing the innominate stump. Then one proceeds with the left carotid and, if necessary, the left subclavian, in a similar fashion (Fig. 23.7). Graft redundancy is not well tolerated. The graft is typically positioned underneath the innominate vein. The subclavian anastomosis, when using the prefabricated graft, will require the sewing in of a jump graft off the left carotid branch segment and can be performed prior to the left carotid anastomosis (Fig. 23.7). The jump graft selected is 8 mm in diameter.

Once the bypass procedures are all completed and each arch vessel stump has been oversewn and secured, the heparin effect is reversed with protamine. Hemostasis is ensured. One large bore drainage tube is used to drain the mediastinum. It is exteriorized inferiorly and sutured to the skin. The sternal incision is closed in the standard fashion.

Complications:

Carotid-Carotid Bypass and Carotid-Carotid-Subclavian Bypass.

The carotid-carotid bypass is typically well-tolerated. It is beneficial to use careful finger dissection in creating the tunnel, noting that is imperative that the tunnel is created immediately anterior to the prevertebral fascia. This avoids any undue tension on or issues with the esophagus. Clamping of calcified or diseased arteries can easily lead to stroke. Vagus nerve injury, through retraction or misidentification, is relatively rare. Preoperative determination of vocal cord function is mandatory to avoid the potential of injuring the nerve supply to the only mobile vocal cord. When the carotid-subclavian operation is added, additional complications include diaphragmatic palsy (phrenic nerve injury), chyle leak (thoracic duct injury), brachial plexus palsy (clamping or excessive traction on the brachial plexus) and entrance into the pleural space. The author advocates for early return to the OR in cases of identified chyle leaks as this remains the most direct and successful means of treating this annoying problem. Potential issue and complications may arise out of the deployment of the TEVAR in the arch and include stroke (3–5%) and endoleaks.

Ascending Aorto-Arch Vessel Debranching Procedure

Mediastinal drainage should be minimal, and any sudden increase in mediastinal tube output should prompt consideration for return to the operating room. The debranching procedure in zone 0 with median sternotomy and ascending aorta to innominate, carotid, and subclavian bypass, while avoiding the perils of cardiopulmonary bypass, is recognized as a major operative procedure with a substantial cardiac event rate (myocardial infarction; major adverse cardiovascular events) and pulmonary (pneumonia, prolonged intubation) complications. This underscores the importance of preoperative cardiopulmonary risk assessment. Stroke remains a significant problem, occurring in 3–5% of patients, likely related to calcification or atheromatous debris within the aorta which embolizes at the time of clamp placement, or alternately, during TEVAR device insertion and deployment. Likewise, the second half of the full anticipated operation, the insertion of the TEVAR, is associated with inherent risks related to endovascular aortic manipulation (dissection, embolization) and aortic stent graft insertion (endoleak).

Take Home Points
It is important to note that these operations are performed as a preliminary procedure to allow for an endovascular procedure (TEVAR) to hopefully successfully treat the underlying aneurysm disease that involves the arch and the descending thoracic aorta. These procedures are meant to be less invasive than direct revascularization options.

Key summation points of the operative procedure are as follows: (1) carotid-carotid bypass is tolerated very well by the patient; it is important to pay specific attention to the tunneling in a retropharyngeal position; (2) carotid-carotid-subclavian bypass allows for complete debranching of the thoracic aorta up to the innominate vessel which allows for significant extension of the landing zone: this procedure can be relatively easily performed through small incisions with minimal hemodynamic consequence; and (3) the ascending aorto to arch vessel bypass is a very specific operation that entails a significant cardio-pulmonary risk, is best performed with a team approach, and does allow extension of the endograft into zone 0 without the requirement of cardio-pulmonary bypass.

Chapter 24
Brachiocephalic Reconstruction

Mitchell R. Weaver

Indications

The most common indications for intervention on the supra-aortic trunk vessels are neurologic symptoms such as stroke and vertebral basilar insufficiency, severe lifestyle-limiting upper extremity effort fatigue, or evidence of upper extremity atheroembolism. In the current practice of vascular surgery, with the advancement of endovascular techniques, and the availability of extra-thoracic/nonanatomic arterial reconstructions, transthoracic supra-aortic trunk reconstructions are relatively uncommon. However, clinic situations are encountered such as when multiple arch branch vessels are diseased or cases in which complete arch debranching is required in order to prepare a landing zone for a thoracic endograft, or repair of an isolated innominate artery aneurysm, where an anatomic transthoracic arterial reconstruction may be the preferred or only option.

In common with most other vascular beds, atherosclerotic arterial occlusive disease is the most common etiology of supra-aortic trunk lesions. Patients presenting with supra-aortic trunk arterial disease should be thoroughly evaluated for associated arterial atherosclerotic risk factors (i.e., tobacco abuse, dyslipidemia, hypertension, diabetes mellitus, renal insufficiency, and family history), as well as for symptoms or history of arterial occlusive disease in other vascular beds including the coronary arteries and lower extremities (claudication) which should be sought.

M. R. Weaver (✉)
Henry Ford Hospital, Detroit, MI, USA

Wayne State University School of Medicine, Detroit, MI, USA
e-mail: mweaver1@hfhs.org

S. S. Hans et al. (eds.), *Primary and Repeat Arterial Reconstructions*,
https://doi.org/10.1007/978-3-031-13897-3_24

Preoperative Planning and Anatomy

Preoperative studies should include noninvasive bilateral upper extremity arterial segmental pressures which will identify fixed obstructive lesions, quantify degree of arterial insufficiency, and provide for a baseline to compare to post-intervention results in order to evaluate the effectiveness of the intervention. The normal pressure differential between arms should not exceed 15 mmHg, and a pressure drop of 20 mmHg or more between levels indicates an intervening hemodynamically significant lesion. Blunted or monophasic Doppler waveforms should prompt high thigh pressure measurements for comparison to upper extremity pressures to exclude the possibility of bilateral proximal upper extremity arterial disease.

Imaging studies are required to confirm diagnosis and plan operative intervention. Adequate imaging requires imaging of the aortic arch along with the outflow vessels including the entire cervical and intracranial vasculature and/or upper extremities. Imaging must assess the ascending aorta locating an appropriate and safe site for clamping the aorta and creation of the proximal anastomosis with the graft. Sites to serve as distal targets for the bypass whether that is the distal innominate artery, right subclavian artery, or carotid arteries must be defined. Also, concurrent carotid artery bifurcation arterial occlusive disease that may require intervention should be defined. Cross-sectional imaging with computed tomography angiography (CTA) is the most common imaging modality used to define this anatomy. Additional imaging studies that may be of use include magnetic resonance angiography (MRA), transthoracic and transesophageal echocardiogram, carotid duplex ultrasound, and trans-arterial catheter-directed digital subtraction angiography.

Preoperative cardiopulmonary assessment is important prior to proceeding with aortic arch reconstruction. It is important to evaluate for any cardiac dysfunction, valvular disease, or coronary ischemia. Noninvasive studies such as transthoracic echo and myocardial perfusion scans are useful in this evaluation. There is a low threshold for obtaining catheter-based coronary angiography prior to proceeding with a transthoracic aortic arch arterial reconstruction given the need for sternotomy. Severe cardiopulmonary disease, a heavily calcified aortic arch or prior sternotomy, places patients at higher risk, makes the operation more difficult, and may preclude them as candidates for the operation.

Details of Procedure

Preparation

Procedures are performed under general anesthesia. Appropriate preoperative antibiotics are administered within 1 h prior to incision. Preoperative discussion with the anesthesiology team in regards to arterial line placement and venous access is important. Pre operative considerations include which arteries with be bypassed, planned sites for arterial clamping, planned site for performance of arterial anastomosis, and whether any concomitant procedures such as carotid endarterectomy is appropriate.

The patient is position with a posterior shoulder roll to extend the neck and elevate the sternal notch. Median sternotomy or in some cases hemisternotomy is performed often with a slight cervical extension to the right to better expose the right common carotid and subclavian arteries as the innominate bifurcation is often the site of distal anastomosis, or if left carotid artery or subclavian artery exposure required incisions that may be extended to the left (Fig. 24.1). Having divided the sternum, a self-retaining retractor is place. Next the pericardium is divided in the midline, and three stay sutures are then placed on both edges of the pericardium to elevate the mediastinal structures and create a pericardial well (Fig. 24.2). The thymus is typically incised along the intralobar cleft, and the left brachiocephalic vein is the dissected circumferentially and encircled with a vessel loop. This loop may be used to retract the vein superiorly or inferiorly to provide exposure to the underlying structures (Figs. 24.3 and 24.4). The ascending aorta is exposed dissecting it free from the main pulmonary trunk laterally and right pulmonary artery inferiorly in order to provide additional mobility and proximal control.

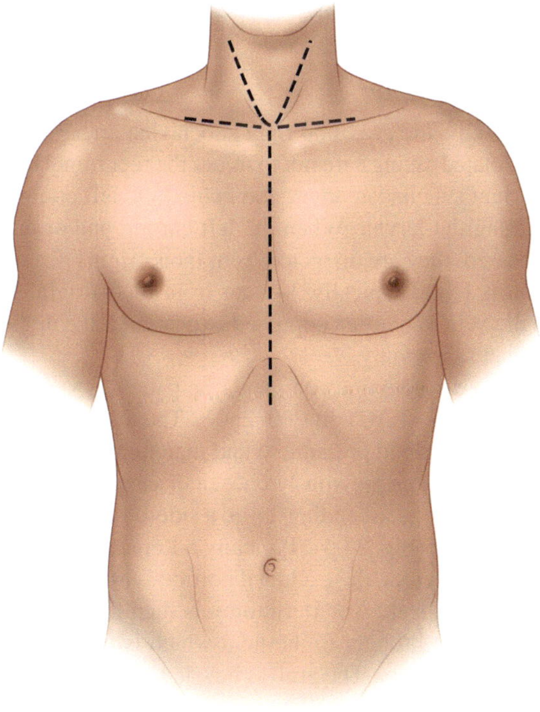

Fig. 24.1 Median sternotomy incision site with optional cervical (along anterior border of sternocleidomastoid muscle) or supraclavicular extension incisions for exposure of ascending aorta and aortic trunk vessels

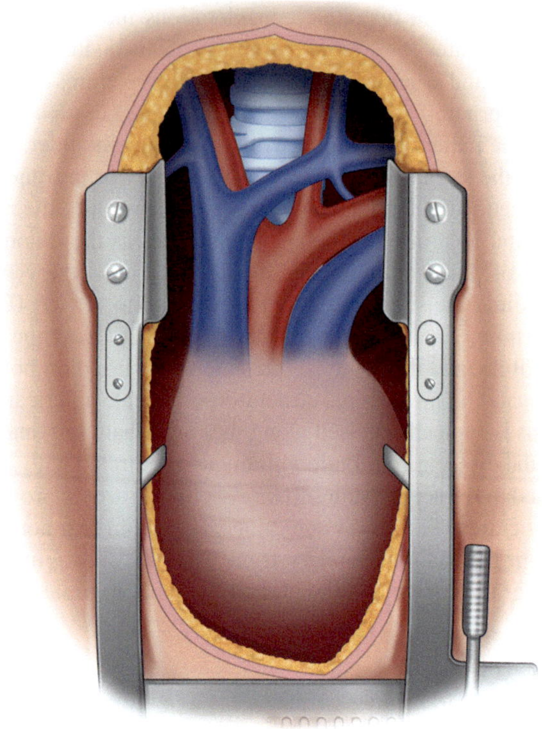

Fig. 24.2 Exposure via median sternotomy incision (with thymus excised)

Distally, the proximal right subclavian artery and right common carotid arteries are isolated taking care not to injure the recurrent laryngeal nerve as it courses under the right subclavian artery and behind the left common carotid artery origin before entering the larynx. When the left carotid and/or left subclavian arteries are to be bypassed, they are dissected from their origins distally until a non-disease soft segment is found typically 3–5 cm from their origin. Division of the left brachiocephalic vein may offer improved exposure of the left subclavian vein via an anterior median sternotomy.

Once dissection is complete, the patient is systemically heparinized (100 units/kg) with a goal ACT of 200–250 s. The anesthesiology team is then asked to drop the systolic blood pressure to and maintain at approximately 100 mmHg. Once this is achieved, to a previously chosen disease free site usually slightly laterally to the right side of the ascending aorta, a side-biting clamp is applied for partial exclusion of the artery (Fig. 24.5). Typically a Lemole-Strong clamp is used for this. Prior to incising the aorta, the excluded portion is aspirated with a needle to insure that there is no clamp leak. An arteriotomy is then created in the aorta. An appropriate size graft is then brought to the field which is typically 10–12 mm for a bypass to the innominate artery. The graft is beveled appropriately to lay comfortably to the right of the ascending aorta. The proximal anastomosis is performed with 4-0 polypropylene in a continuous running fashion.

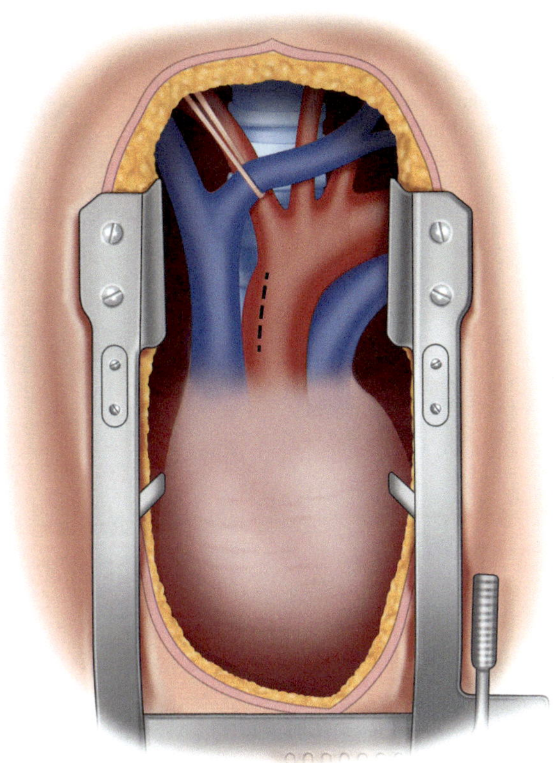

Fig. 24.3 Image demonstrating exposure of the ascending aorta with mobilization of left brachiocephalic vein. Dashed line demonstrates planned site for aortic anastomosis

Once completed, any slack within the suture line is removed and the suture tied. The patient is then temporarily placed in Trendelenburg position as the clamp is released to check for bleeding. The Trendelenburg position is to protect against air trapped in the anastomosis embolizing into the carotid system. Side branches to the left carotid artery or subclavian artery should come off the main graft as proximal as possible (3–4 cm) from the graft origin so as to exit the chest from the left side of the trachea as opposed to in front of it. Inverted bifurcated grafts are typically not used as the main bodies when cut tangentially for end to-side anastomosis require larger aortotomy and when the graft is distended and the chest is closed occupying too much space and can lead to compression and kinking.

Distal anastomoses are then performed. For bypass of the innominate artery, the site of anastomosis is typical to the bifurcation of the artery or separately to the subclavian and common carotid arteries. Ideally, the right subclavian and common carotid arteries are controlled separately as opposed to clamping the distal innominate artery as plaque may extend to this area, and there also may lead to great chance of injuring the recurrent laryngeal nerve. The proximal ends of the arteries are oversewn. The graft is beveled appropriately in order to lay comfortably under the innominate vein without causing compression. The anastomosis is then performed with 5-0 polypropylene suture in a continuous running fashion (Fig. 24.6).

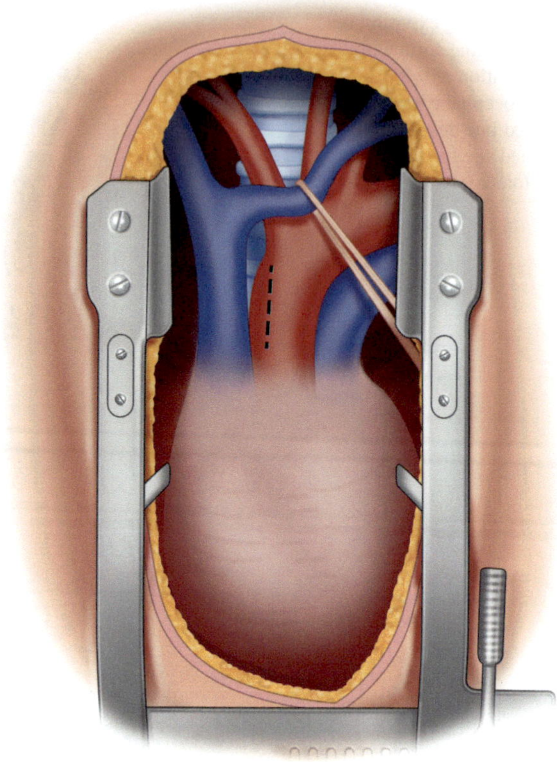

Fig. 24.4 Image demonstrating exposure and control of proximal right subclavian and common carotid arteries

The same technique can be applied to bypass the left carotid artery or the left subclavian artery when they are involved. If more than one artery is involved, then side branch grafts can be anastomosed to the larger main graft ideally prior to starting the bypass. Commercially available branded grafts are available that are designed for bypassing more than one arch vessel. Depending on the anatomy of the left subclavian artery, specifically how lateral and posterior it is positioned, adequate exposure for performing arterial reconstruction via a median sternotomy may not be possible. If revascularization of this vessel is required, an extra anatomic reconstruction may be considered after direct revascularization of the left carotid artery.

Having completed the bypass, the heparin effect is reversed with protamine. Hemostasis is insured. Typically one large bore drainage tube is used to drain the mediastinum. It is exteriorized inferiorly and sutured to the skin. The sternal incision is closed in the standard fashion.

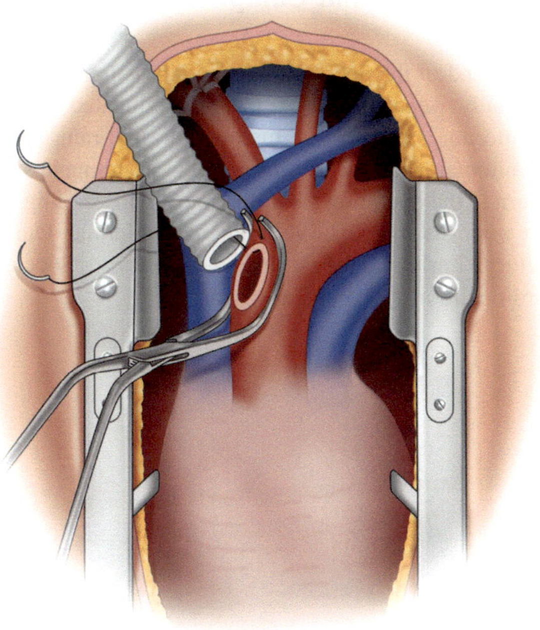

Fig. 24.5 Image demonstrating side-biting clamp placed on ascending aorta with performance of end of graft to side of aorta anastomosis

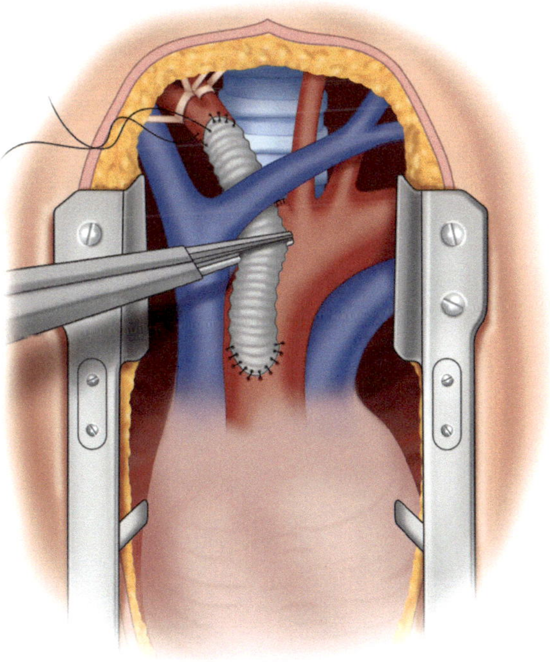

Fig. 24.6 Image demonstrating graft having been anatomosed to ascending aorta, tunneled under left brachiocephalic vein and being sewn to the distal end of the innominate artery

Post-Op Care and Complications

At the end of the operation, the patient is transferred to the intensive care unit and gradually weaned off sedation and extubated when fully awake. Hemodynamic monitoring is provided to maintain normal-range BP. Mediastinal drainage should be minimal, and any sudden increase in drainage should prompt consideration for return to the operating room for control of bleeding. The mediastinal tubes are usually removed the next day if output is minimal. Outcomes are typically very satisfactory. Early complications when they do occur typically involve bleeding, cardiopulmonary events, or stroke.

Chapter 25
Aortofemoral Bypass

Alexander D. Shepard

Endoluminal techniques have supplanted open bypass as the primary operative therapy for aortoiliac occlusive disease (AIOD). In contemporary practice, only patients with the most advanced disease are candidates for aortofemoral bypass (AFB). This population includes patients who have frequently undergone previous aortoiliac stenting and often have significant inflammatory changes associated with indwelling stents and prior femoral artery punctures which can greatly increase the difficulty of arterial dissection and graft tunneling for these procedures. These challenges are compounded by the fact that AFB is infrequently performed today because of the success of endoluminal procedures.

Indications for this procedure are the same as for any peripheral artery disease procedure – lifestyle-limiting claudication and chronic limb-threatening ischemia. That said, in our experience, AFB patients usually have severe multilevel involvement with TASC D disease in the aortoiliac segment. Juxtarenal aortic occlusion is a clear indication in symptomatic patients. Heavily calcified aortoiliac segments or aortoiliac hypoplasia are other circumstances frequently mandating AFB over stenting. Disease in the femoral arteries is the rule, and concomitant femoral endarterectomy is frequently necessary.

As with any open aortic reconstruction, careful preoperative assessment of the patient's cardiac, pulmonary, and renal function is necessary. Preoperative imaging can be performed with angiography or more commonly in our practice, a thin-cut, high-quality computed tomographic angiogram (CTA) of the abdomen/pelvis and bilateral lower extremities (LE). Attention should be focused on the degree of aortoiliac calcification, concomitant renal and/or visceral artery occlusive disease (with particular attention to the patency of the inferior mesenteric artery), the presence of juxtarenal aortic plaque, and any vascular anomalies (e.g., accessory renal arteries,

A. D. Shepard (✉)
Division of Vascular Surgery, Henry Ford Hospital, Detroit, MI, USA
e-mail: ASHEPAR2@hfhs.org

S. S. Hans et al. (eds.), *Primary and Repeat Arterial Reconstructions*,
https://doi.org/10.1007/978-3-031-13897-3_25

retroaortic left renal vein). A good imaging study is critical to proper planning for the procedure – selection of clamp site, need for concomitant proximal or distal endarterectomy(ies), etc. Anesthetic monitoring consists of an arterial line and a central line except for high-risk patients where transesophageal 2-D echocardiography can be helpful. Foley catheter is routine.

Operative Steps

These procedures are usually performed through a midline celiotomy with a transperitoneal (TP), infra-mesocolic approach to the aorta. The patient is placed on the table supine with the right arm tucked at the side to create a space for anchoring a mechanical retraction system (e.g., Thompson or Omni Tract) to the table. There is controversy as to whether to expose the femoral arteries first or open the abdomen first with AFB. We prefer to start in the groins so that the abdomen is open for less time with less evaporative fluid losses and risk for hypothermia.

Groin Exposure: Groin dissection can be carried out through either a transverse or longitudinal incision. We rarely use transverse incisions because of the limited exposure available. However, in obese patients with limited or no femoral artery disease, a transverse incision can reduce the risk of wound complications. Prior to beginning the procedure, duplex ultrasound is used to determine the level of the femoral bifurcations. This allows precise placement of groin incisions tailored to the disease location and is particularly helpful in patients with absent femoral pulses where dissection in false planes in search of the artery can increase the risk of lymphatic complications. Dissection of the femoral vessels can be quite challenging if the patient has undergone multiple prior endoluminal procedures particularly if closure devices have been used. Such scarring often requires sharp scalpel dissection with a #15 blade. We have found an ultrasonic scalpel helpful for reducing lymph leaks and use ties only for lymph nodes and large crossing vessels. With heavily scarred and redo groin procedures, identification and dissection of a diseased superficial femoral artery (SFA) is sometimes easiest for getting one's landmarks. This vessel can be palpated as a firm cord just below the femoral bifurcation. After identifying this artery, dissection can proceed proximally to the common femoral artery (CFA). Following circumferential control of these arteries, the profunda femoris artery (PFA) is dissected out last taking care to watch for a posterior branch of the distal-most CFA which originates at the level of the bifurcation in a large percentage of patients. Failure to control this branch prior to making a femoral arteriotomy can result in troublesome backbleeding.

The extent of femoral dissection is determined by the level of disease, but even with a normal CFA, at least 4 cm of mobilized artery is needed to provide a spot for a femoral anastomosis. With an occluded SFA, there is usually disease within the origin of the PFA which must be addressed to ensure an optimal outcome. If this can be corrected with an eversion endarterectomy of the PFA, then only a cm or two of this artery needs to be mobilized. Not infrequently, however, the disease extends further distally and requires more extensive exposure. Blind endarterectomy of the PFA is to be avoided, but failure to correct such disease will compromise outflow and jeopardize long-term patency. More distal PFA exposure usually requires division of at least one and often two crossing veins; if large, these should be suture ligated to avoid subsequent tie dislodgment during arterial reconstruction.

After completing the groin dissections, the distal portions of the retroperitoneal tunnels into the abdomen are created. When starting these tunnels, it is important to visualize the distal-most external iliac artery (EIA) by dividing a small portion of the inguinal ligament. This maneuver also prevents postoperative graft limb compression by the taut, undivided ligament. During this exposure, a large crossing vein (the lateral iliac circumflex vein) is invariably visualized on the anterior surface of the distal EIA. This venous branch (also known as the "vein of pain") should always be carefully looked for and divided between ligatures to avoid an avulsion injury during graft tunneling. Once this vein has been divided, the operator's index finger, fingernail down, is passed along the surface of the EIA proximally to start the retroperitoneal tunnel for the graft limb.

Abdominal Exposure: One has several choices in terms of abdominal incisions for AFB. Most surgeons prefer a midline celiotomy with a TP, infra-mesocolic approach to the IR aorta. A transverse incision can be used for patients with severe pulmonary disease, but this approach sacrifices thoraco-epigastric collaterals which are often an important source of LE perfusion in these patients. A left flank retroperitoneal approach can also be used (see section later in chapter). The abdomen is opened from xiphoid to midway between the umbilicus and symphysis pubis. Abdominal exploration is rarely necessary because of the accuracy of preoperative CTA. A table-mounted mechanical retraction system (i.e., Thompson or Omni Tract) provides excellent exposure without the need for a second assistant. The transverse colon and greater omentum are pulled cephalad, out of the abdomen, while the small bowel is retracted to the patient's right. We believe that packing the small bowel into the right side of the abdomen, rather than retracting it out of the abdomen, reduces the amount of bowel edema by the end of the procedure. Division of the ligament of Treitz allows mobilization of the duodenum off the aortic neck with better mobility of the small bowel (Fig. 25.1). The posterior retroperitoneum overlying the aorta in the midline is incised from below the reflected duodenum to just below the inferior mesenteric artery (IMA). Cephalad dissection reveals the left renal vein (LRV) which marks the proximal extent of exposure (Fig. 25.2). The inferior mesenteric vein runs in a more superficial plane and can be ligated/divided as necessary. The anterior surface of the aorta is cleared of overlying RP fat from the lower border of the LRV to just below the IMA using an ultrasonic scalpel. Lymphatics along the LRV should be ligated to decrease the risk of a chyle leak.

In most situations, the aorta immediately distal to the LRV is suitable for proximal anastomosis. The aorta at this level can be controlled circumferentially if desired, although we usually mobilize just enough to allow placement of a vertically oriented cross clamp to avoid injury to adjacent lumbar arteries. Distally,

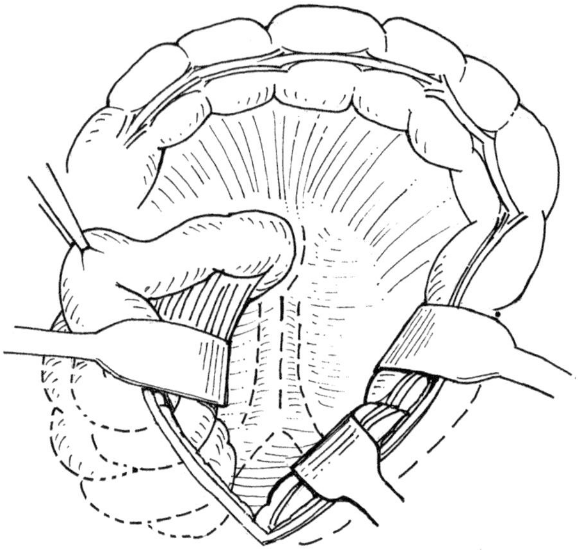

Fig. 25.1 Infra-mesocolic exposure of the IR aorta with transverse colon reflected superiorly, small bowel retracted to the right and descending/sigmoid colon retracted to the left

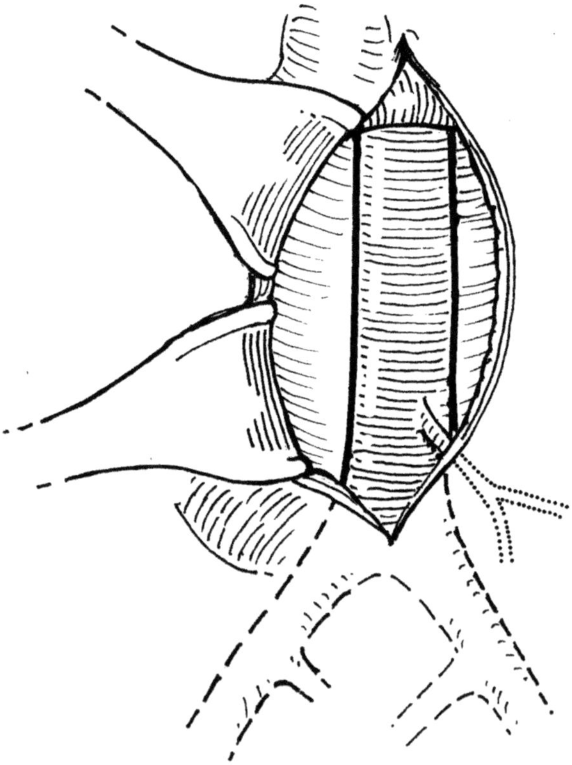

Fig. 25.2 Incision through retroperitoneum to expose the IR aorta from the crossing LRV superiorly to just above the bifurcation distally. The IMA is the only major branch originating anteriorly

circumferential control of the aorta is obtained just below the IMA taking care to avoid damage to the hypogastric plexus and the presacral nerves, which course anterior to the aorta and travel caudally over the origin of the left common iliac artery. Injury can lead to erectile dysfunction in men. Retroperitoneal tunnels from the exposed aorta to the groins are then completed by means of blunt index finger dissection (again fingernail down) taking care to pass posterior to the ureters (Fig. 25.3). Tunneling of a graft limb anterior to the ureter can lead to ureteral entrapment between the limb and native iliac artery risking postoperative ureteral obstruction. A long aortic clamp is passed from the groin into the aortic retroperitoneal space, guided by the surgeon's index fingers from above and below, and an umbilical tape pulled through to mark these tunnels.

Reconstruction: Following heparinization to a therapeutic ACT (>250 s), the IR aorta is clamped just below the renal arteries after clamping the IMA, if it is patent. A TA-30 stapler (with 2.5 mm staples) is then passed around the aorta just below the IMA and fired. We perform end-to-end proximal anastomoses almost universally, so

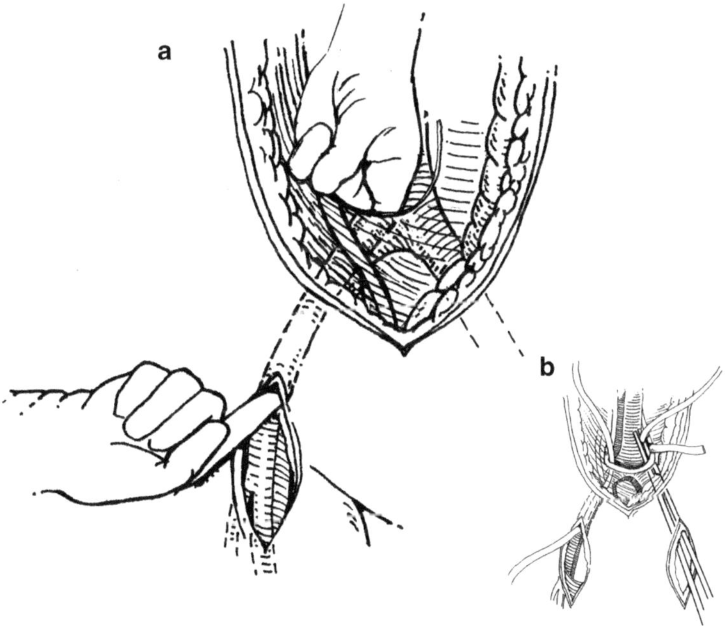

Fig. 25.3 Creating retroperitoneal tunnels from the aorta to both groins by blunt index finger dissection from above and below. These tunnels run along the anterior surfaces of the iliac arteries and *behind* the ureters. (**a**) Index fingers creating the retroperitonesl tunnel on the right side from the abdominal aorta to the right groin. (**b**) Umbilical tape or silastic tubing being pulled through the created tunnel to mark its course

the aorta is next transected at the proposed proximal anastomotic site. This is placed close to the renal arteries to reduce the risk of future graft compromise from progression of atherosclerotic disease in the residual aorta. The aorta a few centimeters distal to the transection line is clamped to prevent backbleeding. A segment of aorta is then resected to just below the IMA taking care to leave a small piece of aortic wall attached to the IMA, if patent. Backbleeding lumbar arteries are ligated as they are encountered. Excising a piece of aorta creates "a trough" for the graft to lie in and makes graft coverage at the end of the case much easier.

A bifurcated vascular prosthesis of appropriate size is selected – typically a 16 × 8 mm for men and a 14 × 7 mm for women; we prefer a polytetrafluoroethylene (PTFE) graft because of our perception of better patency. The main shaft of the graft is trimmed to a length of 3–4 cm – a short main shaft is believed to enhance graft patency. After preparing the proximal aortic cuff by removing any adherent debris or thrombus, and occasionally endarterectomizing it, an end-to-end anastomosis is performed with a running 3-0 or 4-0 polypropylene stitch using the parachute technique (Fig. 25.4). After ensuring a hemostatic anastomosis, the graft limbs are gently delivered into the groins through the retroperitoneal tunnels.

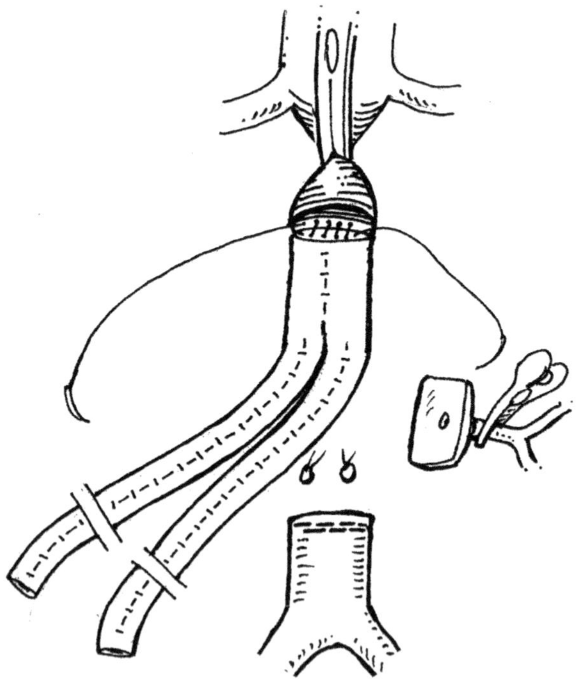

Fig. 25.4 IR aorta clamped and divided. A segment of aorta from the infrarenal cuff to just below the IMA is resected. If the IMA is patent, a small cuff of aortic wall containing the origin of the IMA is excised. Intervening lumbar arteries are ligated, and the distal aorta is stapled closed. End-to-end anastomosis is performed to a bifurcated aortic prosthesis using a "parachute" technique

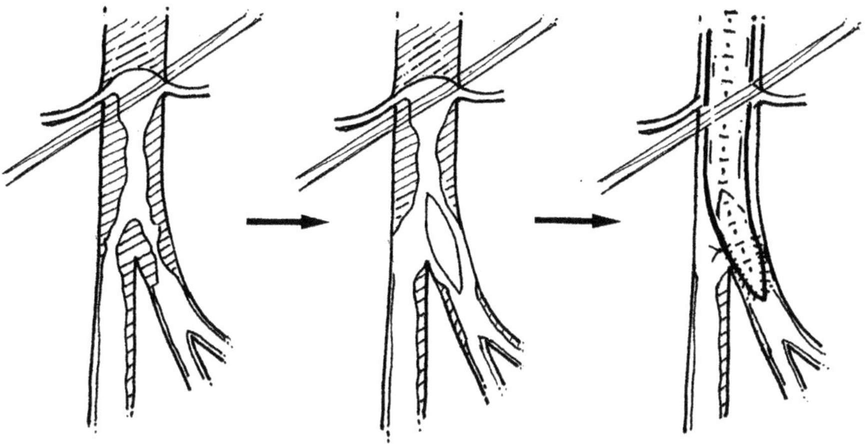

Fig. 25.5 Left femoral artery exposed and a short segment across the profunda femoris origin endarterectomized in preparation for an end-to-side graft limb to femoral artery anastomosis

Distal anastomoses are performed on the CFAs and, if necessary, carried through the origins of the PFAs in the presence of bifurcation disease. The CFA, SFA, and PFA are clamped, as well as the posterior branch artery at the bifurcation. A 2.5–3 cm (longer if necessary) longitudinal arteriotomy is performed on the CFA and extended into the PFA or less frequently the SFA as needed. Concomitant endarterectomy may be needed prior to performing the distal anastomosis. Clearing disease from the proximal PFA is critical as this artery is often the dominant outflow vessel in patients with significant SFA disease and failure to do so can compromise long-term graft patency. Ostial disease in the PFA can frequently be treated with an eversion endarterectomy, though one must be certain that the vessel distal to the plaque is normal or risk raising a distal flap which leads to luminal compromise (Fig. 25.5). After preparation of the distal anastomotic site, the graft is distended by temporary removal of the proximal clamp, trimmed to length and appropriately beveled to fit the arteriotomy. An end-to-side anastomosis is then created in "parachute" fashion beginning with the "heel" of the graft. After venting, the anastomosis is secured and flow restored to the lower extremity while carefully communicating with the anesthesia team. Following completion of the second side, the feet are checked for Doppler flow signals to ensure technical adequacy of the reconstruction. Before reversing the heparin anticoagulation, backbleeding from a patent IMA is checked. In most ases of AIOD, a patent IMA has served as a collateral channel to the lower extremities so that restoration of pulsatile femoral flow is usually sufficient to ensure adequate IMA backbleeding. In the rare circumstance where such backbleeding is deemed inadequate, the IMA should be reimplanted into the left limb of the graft (Fig. 25.6). Otherwise, it can be ligated.

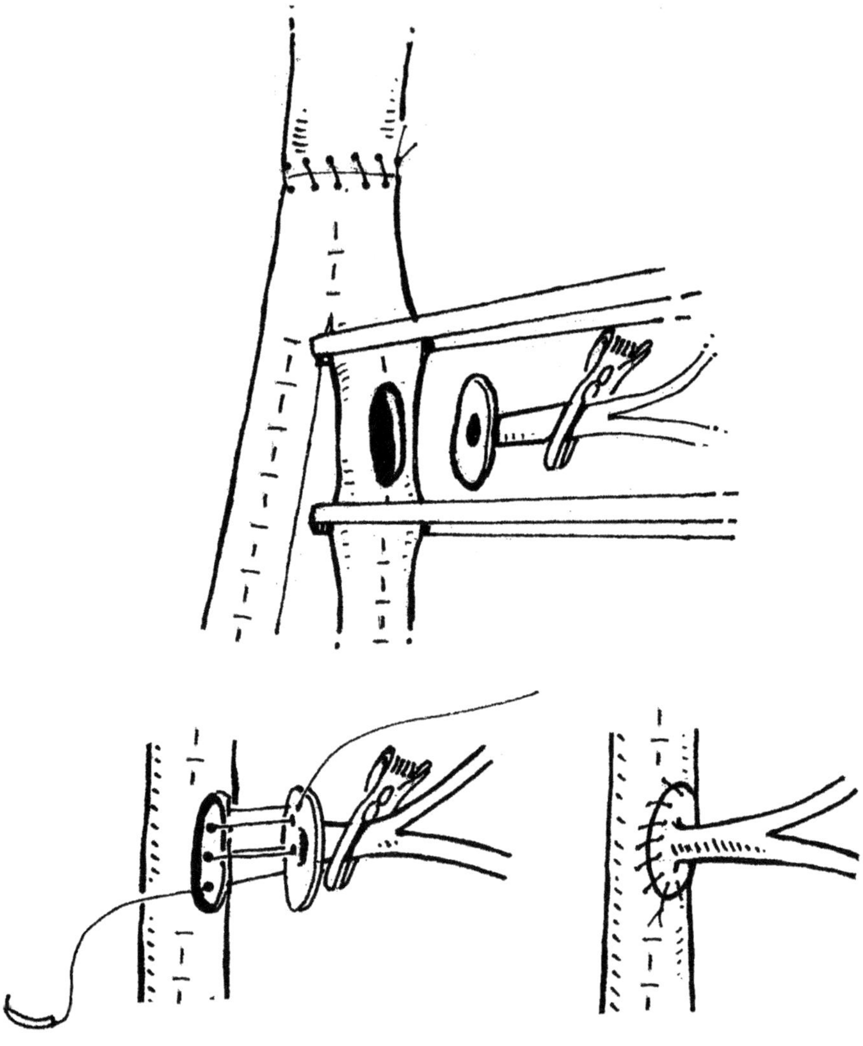

Fig. 25.6 IMA reconstruction: Left limb of aortofemoral graft controlled proximally/distally and a small graftotomy made. The IMA is sewn on as a Carrel patch of endarterectomized aortic wall

Protamine is used to reverse anticoagulation, and after assuring hemostasis, closure is affected. The retroperitoneum is closed over the graft in two layers and the groins in three layers (Fig. 25.7). Incisional negative pressure dressings are routinely placed on the groin incisions.

Special circumstances: Juxtarenal aortic occlusion requires suprarenal (SR) aortic clamping in order to safely remove the thrombotic plug. When more proximal aortic exposure is required, the LRV may be either mobilized or ligated/divided.

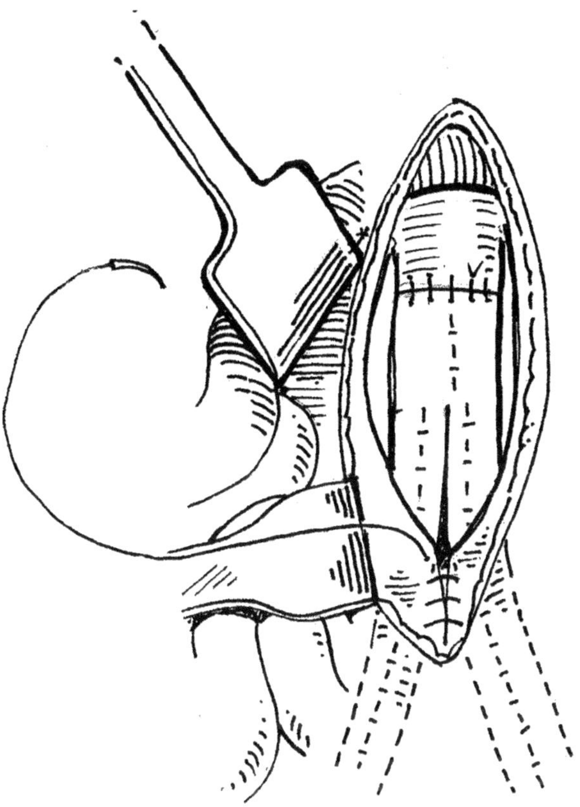

Fig. 25.7 Retroperitoneal closure over aortic graft in two layers. This is critical to avoid a graft entericl erosion/fistula

Mobilization requires freeing up the vein from the inferior vena cava back toward the left kidney with division of the three intervening branches distal to the kidney (lumbar branch, gonadal, and adrenal veins) (Fig. 25.8). It is important to decide which technique (mobilization or division) to use because preservation of these branches is critical to providing collateral outflow to the kidney if the LRV is divided. Following SR clamping, the thrombotic plug can usually be carefully removed through the transected IR aorta. A long enough aortic cuff should be left to allow placement of an IR clamp once the occlusive plug is removed. Severe calcification of the IR aorta ("porcelain aorta") is another circumstance that may require temporary SR or more proximal aortic clamping. In this setting, a calcified core of plaque is removed to create an aortic cuff soft enough to accept stitches. This endarterectomy must be performed very carefully to avoid full thickness injury to the aortic wall. When sewing to an endarterectomized aortic cuff, we use 4-0 polypropylene on a small needle.

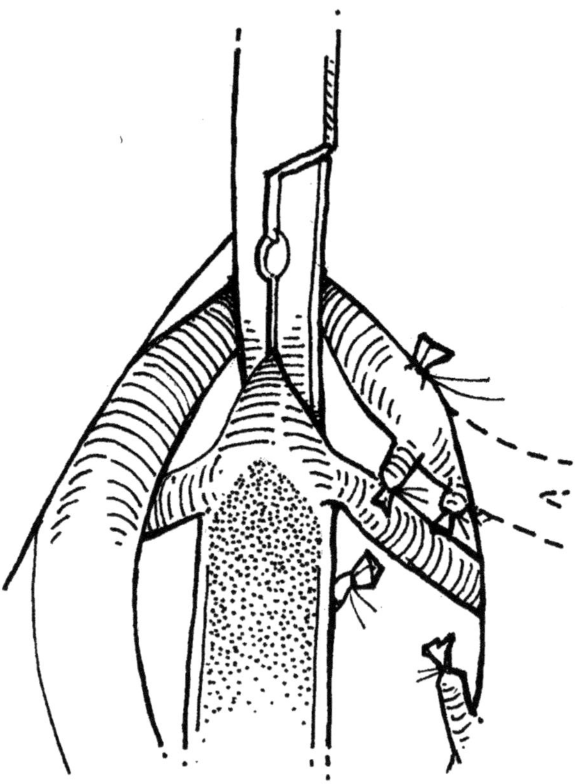

Fig. 25.8 Mobilization of the LRV following division of adrenal, gonadal, and lumbar branches to expose the pararenal aorta and allow placement of a SR aortic cross-clamp

Retroperitoneal Approach to the Aorta

A left flank retroperitoneal (RP) approach to the aorta can very helpful in certain situations. The patient is placed in a modified right lateral decubitus position with the shoulders positioned at 60–70° to the table, and the hips rotated as far posteriorly as possible. The primary operator stands on the patient's left, and the table is rotated to the left to flatten out the hips as much as possible for groin exposure and all the way to the right for abdominal exposure. It is important to mark the groin incisions when the patient has been properly positioned as these incisions will be shifted to the patient's left than when s/he is supine. An overhanging panniculus can make right femoral exposure challenging in obese patients.

For IR aortic exposure, the flank incision begins midway between the umbilicus and symphysis pubis and extends from the lateral margin of the left rectus into the 11th intercostal space for 8–10 cm. The abdominal wall and intercostal musculature are divided, and the RP space entered at the tip of the 12th rib. The peritoneum is stripped away anteriorly as far as the rectus and a RP plane developed posterolaterally behind the left kidney and ureter which are reflected anteriorly. The IR aorta and more distally the left iliac artery are exposed in the base of the wound by retracting the peritoneal sac and its contents to the patient's right. Proximally, the left renal artery (LRA) is identified during the early stages of dissection. The lumbar branch of the LRV crosses over the aorta proximally and is a reliable landmark to the origin of the LRA. This vein is ligated and divided to provide exposure of the IR aortic neck; a much larger than normal lumbar branch should prompt concern for a retro-aortic left RV. In this situation, the aorta should be exposed anterior to the kidney to avoid ligating the LRV. The left posterolateral wall of the aorta is exposed to the bifurcation by dividing overlying periaortic fat and lymphatics with an ultrasonic scalpel. The aorta just below the LRA is mobilized for clamping. When SR control is required, the left diaphragmatic crus (a firm tendinous band crossing the aorta just proximal to the origin of the LRA) is divided 2–3 cm along the axis of the aorta and the underlying aorta exposed. The origin of the LRA is cleared off, and index finger dissection anterior and posterior to the aorta creates planes for clamp placement.

The IMA is identified a few centimeters above the bifurcation and if patent preserved; if not, it is ligated and divided to improve exposure for the right RP tunnel. The tunnel to the left groin is easily made from this approach, but the right side is much more difficult and requires great care to avoid inadvertent entry into the peritoneal cavity.

Following vascular reconstruction and hemostasis, any incision made in the left diaphragm is oversewn and pleural air evacuated through a temporary 16 Fr red-rubber catheter with lung insufflation. The ribs are reapproximated with looped #1 PDS, while the muscle layers of the abdominal wall and chest are closed separately with running 0 or 2-0 PDS suture.

This RP approach takes more time than a standard midline celiotomy but is associated with reduced evaporative fluid losses, ileus, and incisional pain. It is ideal for patients with significant pulmonary dysfunction or a "hostile abdomen" from multiple prior celiotomies and those requiring aortic clamping above the renals.

Redo AFB

Redo AFB is fortunately a rare procedure in the endovascular era. Scar tissue greatly complicates exposure and tunnel creation. We usually place ureteral stents preoperatively to aid in ureteral identification. Although a RP approach can aid proximal exposure particularly if SR clamping is necessary, it can make redo groin exposure much more challenging. Creating a new tunnel to the right groin is undoubtedly the most difficult part of the procedure with this approach and must be done with great care to avoid a right ureteral injury or inadvertent entry into the abdomen. In certain situations where this is not possible to do safely, an aorto-unifemoral bypass to the left groin can be performed with a femoral-femoral bypass to the right groin. A descending thoracic aorta to femoral bypass is another option when severe scarring precludes IR aortic exposure. A two-team approach to redo groin dissections is beneficial. Sharp dissection with a #15 blade avoids dulling multiple pairs of scissors, and debulking segments of thrombosed graft can help create a space for the new graft. This operation is quite challenging and should only be undertaken in reasonable risk patients by the most experienced surgeons.

Though uncommonly performed in the modern era of endovascular interventions, AFB remains a very good operation for AIOD with excellent long-term patency. Commonly encountered complications including groin lymphatic leaks, venous injury, and ischemic colitis can be avoided by careful preoperative planning and precise operative execution.

Further Reading

Szilagyi DE, Elliott JP, Smith RF, Reddy DJ, McPharlin M. A thirty-year survey of the reconstructive surgical treatment of aortoiliac occlusive disease. J Vasc Surg. 1986;3(3):421–36.

Kakkos SK, Haurani MJ, Shepard AD, Nypaver TJ, Reddy DJ, Weaver MR, Lin JC, Haddad GK. Patterns and outcomes of aortofemoral bypass grafting in the era of endovascular interventions. Eur J Vasc Endovasc Surg. 2011;42:658–66.

Chiu KWH, Davies PG, Nightingale AW, Bradbury AW, Adam DJ. Review of direct anatomical open surgical management of atherosclerotic aorto-iliac occlusive disease. Eur J Vasc Endovasc Surg. 2010;39(4):460–71.

Shepard AD, Tollefson DFJ, Reddy DJ, Evans JR, Elliott JP, Smith RF, Ernst CB. Left flank retroperitoneal exposure: a technical aid to complex aortic reconstruction. J Vasc Surg. 1991;14(3):283–91.

Chapter 26
Thoraco Femoral Bypass for Aorto Iliac Occlusive Disease

Iraklis I. Pipinos and Sachinder Singh Hans

Indications

Bypass from the descending thoracic aorta to femoral artery is an uncommon primary procedure and should be considered only in good risk patients with a satisfactory cardiopulmonary status in the presence of juxtarenal aortic occlusion with symptoms of chronic functional claudication or critical limb ischemia. This procedure should be considered only if conventional aortofemoral reconstruction is not feasible or in patients who have a prior history of multiple abdominal operations, extensive intra-abdominal scarring, failed prior infrarenal aortic reconstruction, infected aortic prosthesis, or other retroperitoneal pathology.

Preoperative Evaluation

Risk stratification with noninvasive cardiac stress test, 2D echocardiogram, and pulmonary functional test should be performed prior to the operation. Evaluation of the descending thoracic aorta using thin section CTA of the chest/abdomen/pelvis and bilateral lower extremity should be performed. Contraindications include aneurysmal disease or extensive calcification of descending thoracic aorta or inability to tolerate single lung ventilation. Relative contraindications include advanced chronic obstructive pulmonary disease and prior thoracotomy.

I. I. Pipinos
Department of Surgery, University of Nebraska Medical Center, Omaha, NE, USA
e-mail: ipipinos@unmc.edu

S. S. Hans (✉)
Vascular and Endovascular Services, Henry Ford Macomb Hospital,
Clinton Twp, MI, USA

S. S. Hans et al. (eds.), *Primary and Repeat Arterial Reconstructions*,
https://doi.org/10.1007/978-3-031-13897-3_26

Positioning

The patient is positioned on the operating table with a vacuum bean bag extending from the shoulders to the proximal thigh. Following induction of general anesthesia and placement of a double lumen endotracheal tube, the left hemithorax is placed at an angle of 45°–65° on the operating table while maintaining the pelvis as flat as possible to allow access to both groin areas. The left arm is supported on an arm rest. And a silicone roll is placed under the right axilla to prevent brachial plexus injury (Fig. 26.1). Air is evacuated from the bean bag. Pillow rests are placed under the knees and between the legs to prevent hyperextension with the patient's legs secured to the operating table with a safety strap. In the event full thoracotomy becomes necessary, left scapula and thoracic spine should be included in the operative field.

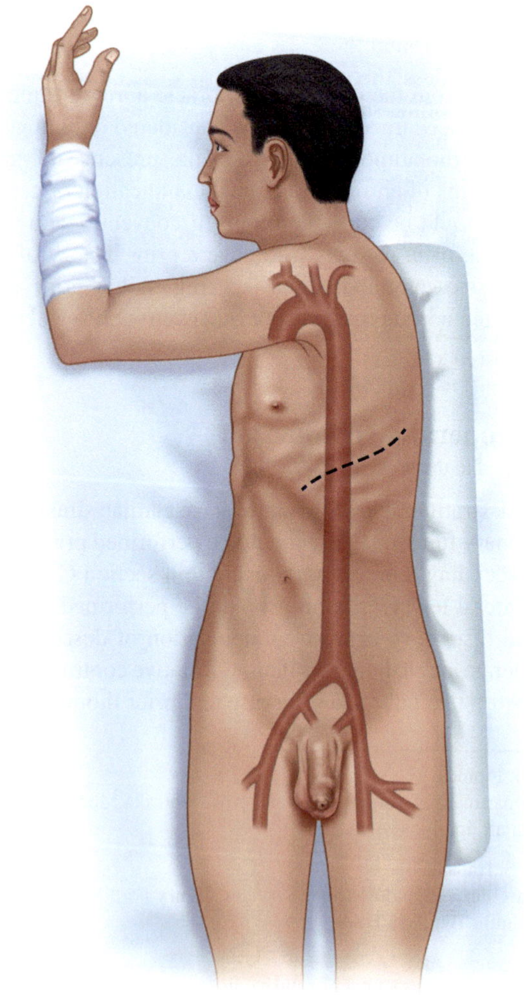

Fig. 26.1 Patient positioned after double lumen endotracheal intubation in a 45°–60° right lateral decubitus position, with the left arm secured over an arm rest. The pelvis is placed as flat as possible to allow access of both groins for exposure of the femoral vessels. The left thorax is exposed sufficiently to allow a posterolateral mini-thoracotomy

Groin Incisions and Retroperitoneal Tunnels

The femoral arteries are dissected first in both groins to reduce the length of time, and the left chest cavities open thereby reducing the heat loss. The right femoral artery is exposed through a standard vertical incision extending to just above the inguinal ligament (groin crease). As the pelvis is tilted to the right, the femoral exposure is facilitated by rotating the operating table slightly toward the left. The left groin incision is extended approximately 8–10 cm cephalad above the inguinal ligament (inguinal crease). At the cephalad end of the left groin incision, the retroperitoneum is accessed, thus helping the creation of the tunnel, connecting the left groin to the left chest. An 8–10 cm long incision is carried to the aponeurosis of the external oblique and the internal oblique muscles on the left extending parallel to the inguinal ligament and 2–3 cm cephalad to its caudal border. The internal oblique muscles are divided, and transverse muscle and transverse fascia are opened in the lateral aspect of the incision (Fig. 26.2). The retroperitoneal space is then entered medial to the iliac crest and anterior superior iliac spine making this the caudal portion of the retroperitoneal tunnel for the passage of the graft.

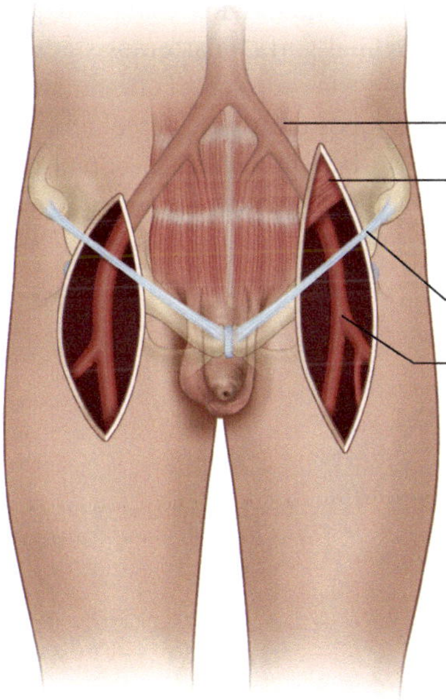

Fig. 26.2 Exposure of femoral artery is carried out first. On the left side, the excision is extended 10 cm above the inguinal ligament and an additional 10 cm incision through the aponeurosis of the external oblique and internal oblique muscles on the left extending parallel to the inguinal ligament and approximately 2 cm cephalad to its caudal border. The internal oblique muscles are divided in the direction of their fibers, and transverse abdominis muscle and transverse fascia are opened to the lateral aspect of the incision. This incision is used for the creation of the retroperitoneal tunnel to the left chest. When bifurcated graft is used, this incision is also used to route the right limb of the graft from its retroperitoneal location to a preperitoneal channel and into the right groin

Exposure of the Thoracic Aorta

The operating table is tilted to the patient's right side and a limited posterolateral thoracotomy (mini thoracotomy) through the eight intercostal space to expose the descending thoracic aorta. The exposure can also be obtained from the seventh or ninth intercostal space depending on the position of the patient and body habitus. The latissimus dorsi muscle is spared by developing superior and inferior skin flaps to allow posterior retraction of the muscle thus reducing postoperative pain. The intercostal muscles are incised along the superior of the border of the inferior rib of the selected rib, and the pleural cavities entered carefully avoiding injury to the underlying lung parenchyma. A rib spreader is inserted and opened gradually to prevent fracture of the ribs. Additional exposure if required can be obtained by resection of the cephalad rib or transecting it at the posterior aspect of the incision. The left lung is deflated, and inferior pulmonary ligament is taken down to the level of inferior pulmonary vein. The lung is retracted into upper thorax, and 2-0 silk sutures are placed and tied using "figure-of-eight" technique at the center of the diaphragm and are brought through the anterior and inferior chest wall and secured to retract the diaphragm to aid in satisfactory exposure of the distal descending thoracic aorta. The visceral pleura covering the distal descending thoracic aorta is incised, and approximately a 6 cm segment of the thoracic aorta is exposed above the diaphragm (Fig. 26.3). The site of proximal aortic anastomosis is selected in a segment free of atherosclerotic disease. The aorta is dissected circumferentially, and both proximally and distally and umbilical tapes or silastic vessel loops are passed to help place the proximal clamp in the aorta. The site of proximal anastomosis should be high enough above the crus of the diaphragm to avoid kinking of the proximal graft following tunneling of the graft.

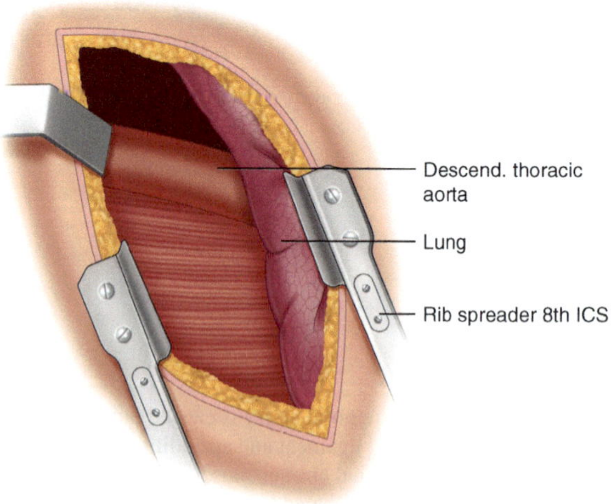

Fig. 26.3 An eight intercostal space thoracotomy is performed sparing the sartorius and latissimus dorsi muscle. The left lung is deflated, and the distal aorta is exposed by dividing the overlying the pleura for 3–4 in

Tunneling of the Graft

A retroperitoneal tunnel is created to facilitate the passage of the graft from the thorax to the groins. A 2 cm incision is made in the posteromedial aspect of the left hemidiaphragm over the ribs through the open chest cavity. The site of aortotomy and the exit site of the graft are aligned carefully so that thoracic portion of graft curves smoothly without any kink. The left hand is placed through the left retroperitoneal tunnel incision, and the dissection proceeds cephalad along the left retroperitoneal plane in a slow and deliberate manner. The dissection plane proceeds cephalad and medially anterior to the external iliac vessels and the psoas major muscles posterior to the left kidney and posteromedial to the spleen and meets the right hand as its fingers slide posterior to the spleen starting from the left hemithorax. A large tunneler (DeBakey, Gore, or Garrett) is then guided through the tunnel, and an umbilical tape is laid to facilitate the passage of the graft. In a patient necessitating the use of bifurcated graft, the shaft and its two limbs are tunneled through the retroperitoneal channel and are tunneled through the left retroperitoneal channel and brought through through the left retroperitoneal incision. Following this, a preperitoneal channel is made that enables the right limb of the graft to reach the right groin incision. A simultaneous blunt finger dissection is utilized to create this second tunnel between the left suprainguinal area, retroperitoneal space, and the groin. This tunnel courses immediately posterior to the rectus abdominis muscle in an anterior and cephalad plane to the urinary bladder in the preperitoneal space. The right inguinal ligament is partially divided in its medial aspect to allow the passage of the right limb of the graft without compression. Another option is to first perform the thoracic aorta to left femoral bypass using a straight tube graft (8–10 mm in diameter) and then perform a standard crossover femoral-femoral graft using an 8 mm in diameter conduit from the hood of the first graft and anastomosed to the common femoral artery with the tunnel in a subcutaneous location.

Choice of Graft

A partially occluding side-biting clamp such as Cobra (Savantia Medical, Sialkot Pakistan) or Lemole-Strong clamp (Becton Dickinson Franklin Lakes, NJ USA) can be applied to distal thoracic aorta as it helps maintain antegrade blood flow through the aorta during performance of the proximal anastomosis. This limits the severity of ischemia to lower torso, anterior spinal artery, and visceral arteries. If a partially occluding side-biting clamp is not feasible due to the small size of the aorta, the aorta may be clamped completely by a vertically placed angled vascular clamp superiorly (complete occlusion) and an angled vascular clamp inferiorly to control the intercostal artery bleeding. Prior to aortic clamping, systemic heparin (100 units IU/kg) is administered intravenously by the anesthesia team, and ACT is monitored between the range of 250 and 300s. An appropriately sized graft is selected to match the size of the aorta and femoral arteries. A 16 × 8 mm or 14 × 7 mm bifurcated graft is most commonly used. In patients with a straight graft from the aorta to femoral artery, 8–10 mm graft is selected, and from left to right crossover femoral-femoral graft, an 8 mm graft is preferred.

Graft material such as Dacron or PTFE is equally suitable as conduits. The aortotomy is created, and the body of the graft is sized accordingly and divided. When a bifurcated graft is used for reconstruction, the body of the graft is kept as long as possible to make certain that the limbs of the graft can reach the right femoral artery without tension. If the graft cannot reach the right groin, excess graft from the contralateral limb can be divided and used to construct a composite right limb (graft-graft composite). A tension-free aortic anastomosis performed using 2-0 or 3-0 CV polypropylene suture in a continuous fashion (Fig. 26.4). Following completion of proximal anastomosis, vascular clamp is applied to the body of the graft, and aortic clamps are released to check for any leaks.

Tunneling of the graft from the left chest to the left groin is carefully performed with a help of a tunneler. The opening of the diaphragm should be adequate so that the graft is not compressed during its passage. The correct orientation and tension of the graft limb should be maintained to prevent graft kinking or twisting. When a

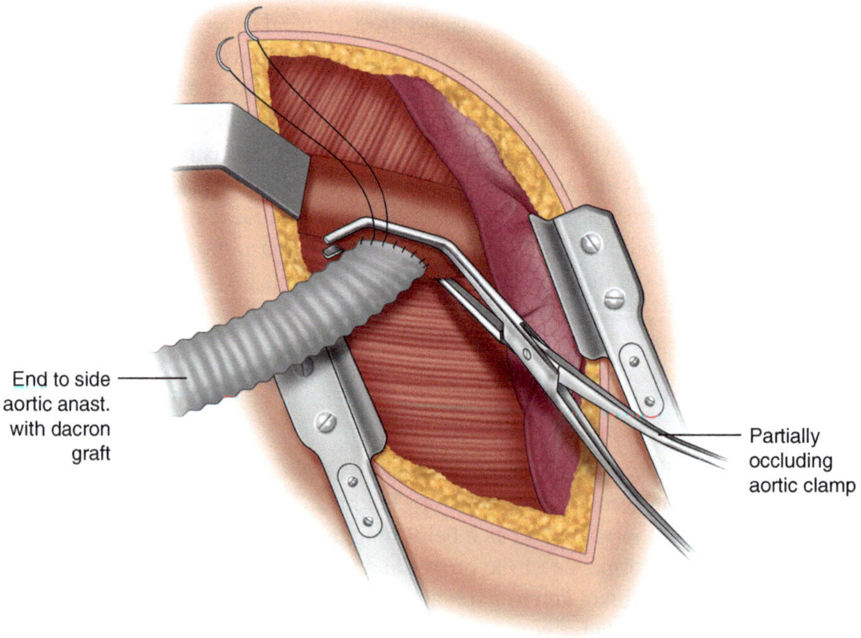

Fig. 26.4 The proximal anastomosis is performed using a partially occluding clamp. A running suture is acceptable if the quality of the aorta is satisfactory. Interrupted sutures with Teflon pledgets can be used to control bleeding if aorta is not optimal for a continuous suture anastomosis

bifurcated graft is required the right limb of the graft is brought around the left retroperitoneum with a gentle curve into the preperitoneal space behind the rectus abdominis muscle anterior to the urinary bladder (retropubic space). The right femoral anastomosis is then completed. In patients with a previously failed axillo-bifemoral or aorto-bifemoral graft, the distal anastomosis is thoracic aorto-femoral graft which may require anastomosis to the profunda femoral arteries (deep femoral artery) or anastomosis to the most distal limbs of the remote graft. Profunda femoris artery (deep femoral artery) is the most suitable artery as an outflow for performance of the thoracic aorta to femoral bypass as external iliac artery and superficial femoral arteries are frequently diseased in this group of patients. Occasionally, common femoral endarterectomy and extensive profundo plasty with patch angioplasty may be necessary to perform a satisfactory distal anastomosis.

Heparin is reversed with protamine sulfate depending upon the results of ACT. The thoracic and femoral incisions are closed in layers. A large chest tube (36 F) is placed through the incision caudal to the thoracotomy incision, and its tip is positioned to the apex of the chest cavity. The lung is reinflated, and the ribs are approximated with using absorbable sutures in a figure-of-eight configuration. The chest wall muscles are closed in layers, and the skin is closed with sutures and staples.

Complications

Reoperation for bleeding, respiratory failure, postoperative MI, and uncommonly renal failure and paraplegia may develop. In patients in whom total clamping of the aorta is required because of its small size for performance of proximal anastomosis, the incidence of ischemia to the torso and spinal cord ischemia is quite low as proximal anastomosis can be completed in about 8 to 10 min.

Chapter 27
Mesenteric Artery Bypass and Reconstruction

Timothy J. Nypaver

Indications for Mesenteric Artery Bypass

Chronic Mesenteric Ischemia

Open mesenteric bypasses or reconstructions are procedures performed in the management of chronic mesenteric ischemia (CMI), symptomatic with manifestations of postprandial abdominal pain, weight loss, food fear, early satiety, or diarrhea in association with significant mesenteric artery occlusive disease. The diagnosis requires a high index of suspicion as there is typically a significant delay (greater than 10 months) from onset of symptoms to definitive diagnosis and treatment. The mesenteric circulation is a high-resistance vascular bed which typically requires multivessel involvement for symptom development. Occasionally, single-vessel disease, specifically of the superior mesenteric artery (SMA), may be severe enough for patients to develop chronic mesenteric symptoms related to CMI. Atherosclerosis is the primary etiology in 95–98% of cases with the remaining including fibromuscular dysplasia, aortic dissection, or trauma. It has been demonstrated that asymptomatic disease rarely progresses to symptomatic disease; thus, the indications for intervention exist only for symptomatic mesenteric artery occlusive disease. The goals of treatment are as follows: relief of pain, restoration of normal weight, and improvement in survival with the reduction in risk of bowel ischemia. Like many other vascular disease beds, the management of symptomatic mesenteric artery occlusive disease is primarily performed employing endovascular means of treatment. Approximately 77% of overall cases are now treated endovascularly, with open operations reserved for an anatomic disease pattern not amenable to

T. J. Nypaver (✉)
Division of Vascular Surgery, Henry Ford Hospital, Detroit, MI, USA
e-mail: TNYPAVE1@hfhs.org

S. S. Hans et al. (eds.), *Primary and Repeat Arterial Reconstructions*,
https://doi.org/10.1007/978-3-031-13897-3_27

endovascular intervention, or one in which endovascular intervention is thought to have limited durability. Additionally, open operations are performed for recurrent symptoms and recurrent disease following a previous endovascular intervention. Some of the unfavorable anatomic criteria for endovascular intervention would include extensive occlusions, severe calcification, tandem lesions, small size blood vessels, or occluded stents or stent-grafts. When the surgeon is encountering one of these clinical situations, the options for revascularization are primarily three: antegrade mesenteric revascularization, retrograde mesenteric revascularization, and local mesenteric endarterectomy/trapdoor aortic endarterectomy. Each of these operations has specific indications with disadvantages and advantages in their use and selection for the patient with CMI. Additionally, when one is considering open mesenteric revascularization, the following operative axioms apply: (1) multivessel revascularization is favored over single-vessel revascularization, and (2) prosthetic grafts fare better than venous grafts when bypass is performed.

Acute Mesenteric Ischemia

Acute mesenteric ischemia (AMI) is a distinctly different clinical entity which necessitates a different algorithmic approach. However, the management of AMI may require a similar open operation as to that performed for CMI. Most AMI is managed in an endovascular fashion with a combination of thrombolysis, mechanical thrombectomy, and catheter-based angioplasty with stent or stent-graft insertion. A hybrid intervention is also an attractive method of revascularization which entails open SMA exposure and retrograde endovascular angioplasty or stenting. Lastly, in AMI, it may become necessary to avoid prosthetic grafts due to the presence of bowel infarction or contamination, in which case a venous bypass would be preferred.

Preoperative Planning and Surgical Anatomy

Preoperative Planning

Preprocedural imaging involves either computed tomographic arteriography (CTA) or magnetic resonance angiography (MRA) with adequate imaging of the thoracic aorta, perivisceral aorta, infrarenal aorta, and pelvis along with high-quality imaging of all mesenteric vessels (celiac axis, SMA, and inferior mesenteric artery) and their branches. Severe cardiopulmonary disease, a heavily calcified supraceliac (SC) aorta or infrarenal aorta, and prior abdominal operations are risk factors which increase overall morbidity. The SC aorta to mesenteric antegrade bypass has the advantages of excellent patency, anatomic flow direction, and reduced risk of graft redundancy or kinking. However, it does usually require a prosthetic graft and has a risk of significant physiologic insult to the patient with the potential for increased cardiopulmonary complications. The retrograde bypass is a less invasive procedure which may be ideal for a high-risk patient. Disadvantages include the possibility of graft kinking and reduced patency when compared to antegrade bypass. Lastly, the trapdoor aortic endarterectomy is a complex procedure with longer SC aortic cross-clamp times and should be reserved for the good risk patient who has severe local anatomic disease with perivisceral aortic disease and disease confined to or within 2–3 cm of the celiac and SMA origins. It is advantageous in that no prosthetic graft is required and patency rates are excellent.

Surgical Anatomy

The SC Aorto-mesenteric Bypass (Antegrade Bypass)

The SC aorto-mesenteric bypass can be performed through two separate distinct surgical approaches and exposures. The first is a transperitoneal approach which entails an anterior exposure of the SC aorta through the lesser sac with a division of the gastrohepatic ligament (Fig. 27.1) and the diaphragmatic crus (Fig. 27.2). This exposure is preferred in patients who have significant weight loss, a low body mass index (BMI), and no prior abdominal operations. However, it does require discordant exposure of the SMA below the inferior border of the pancreas, performed through a separate plane of dissection to that of the SC aorta. Alternately, the left flank retroperitoneal exposure through the ninth intercostal space allows for complete exposure of the SC aorta as well as all mesenteric vessels, all within the same plane. This approach may be problematic if the occlusive disease extends out to a significant degree, greater than 6 cm on the SMA, as it may be more difficult to

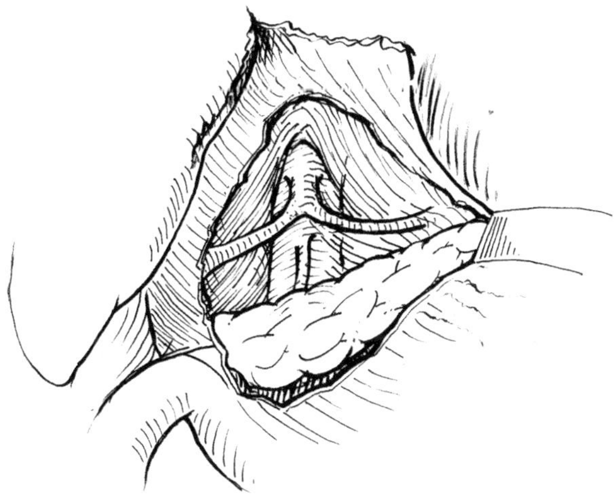

Fig. 27.1 Anterior exposure of supraceliac aorta using an incision in gastrohepatic omentum

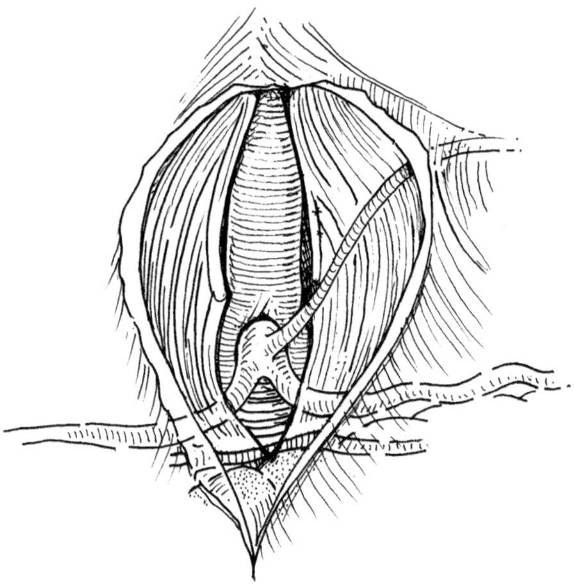

Fig. 27.2 Opening of the diaphragmatic crus

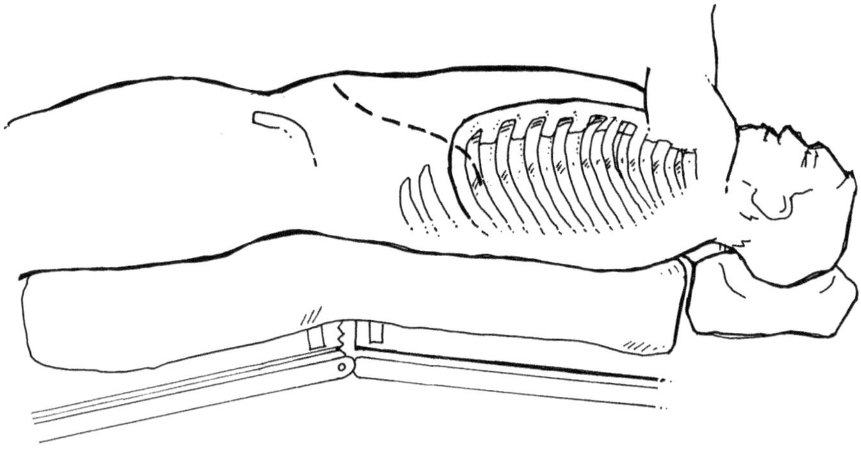

Fig. 27.3 Skin incision for retroperitoneal exposure

expose the SMA distally via this approach. In general, we have preferred the left flank retroperitoneal approach as patients tolerate this well, and the operative procedure can be performed through a single plane exposure. This is accomplished through a left flank incision in the ninth intercostal space extending from the intercostal space to the lateral rectus sheath with division of the musculature of the abdominal wall and entry into the retroperitoneal space (Fig. 27.3). Mobilization of the peritoneum and intraperitoneal contents to the midline ensues, maintaining the psoas muscle on the posterior aspect of the exposure and then developing a plane anterior to the left kidney. The kidney remains in an anatomic position with identification of the left renal artery and then the vein coursing over the aorta (Figs. 27.4 and 27.5). The dissection continues superiorly to the level of the diaphragmatic crus which is then divided allowing exposure of the SC aorta. The crus can be divided slowly with Bovie cauterization with a right-angle clamp protecting the underlying aorta. The celiac axis is then identified and circumferentially dissected with vessel loop control. Likewise, the SMA at the site of the anticipated distal anastomosis is dissected free. The patient is systemically anticoagulated, and the graft is chosen; typically, a 12 × 6, 14 × 7, or 16 × 8 bifurcated Dacron graft is selected. The proximal anastomosis is performed first. The author favors complete cross clamping of

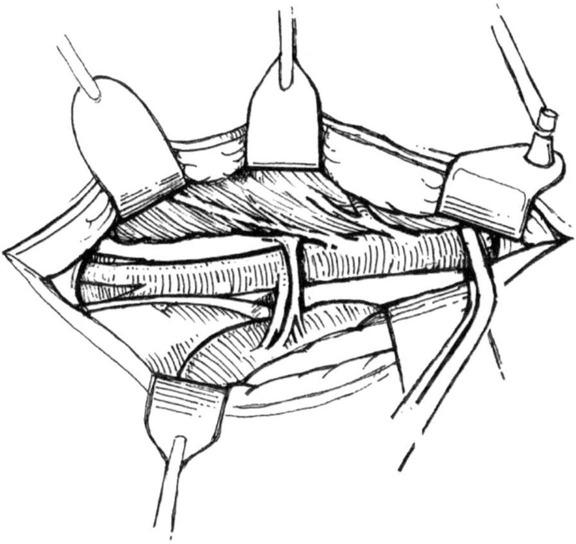

Fig. 27.4 Retroperitoneal exposure with the kidney in anatomical position

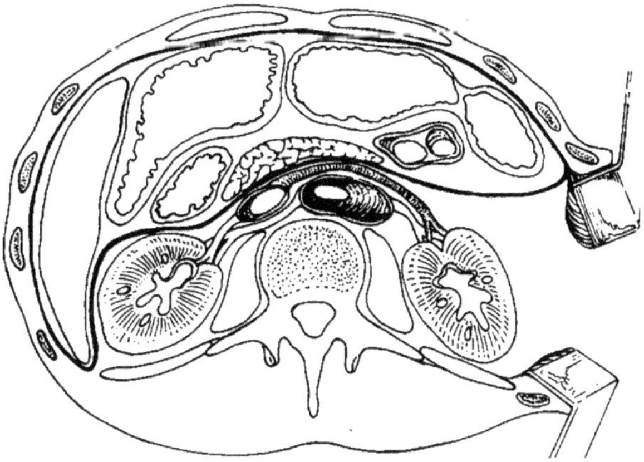

Fig. 27.5 Diagrammatic representation of dissection plane for retroperitoneal exposure with left kidney in anatomical position

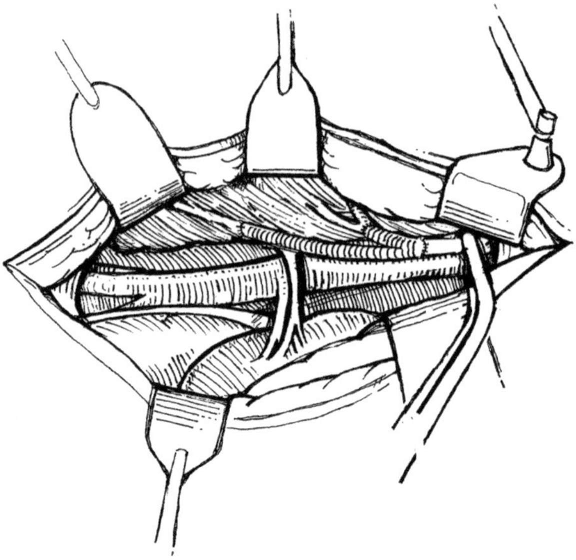

Fig. 27.6 Exposure of SMA with bifurcation graft to the celiac and SMA

the SC aorta (as opposed to a side biting clamp) (Fig. 27.6). An aortotomy is made extending slightly medially distally, and the anastomosis is performed in a parachute fashion starting at the heel of the anastomosis, using 4-0 proline suture. The clamps are released, and the anastomosis is checked for hemostasis. A graft clamp (Fogarty Hydragrip Clamp) has been placed on the graft main body, and then the right limb is cut appropriately for the celiac axis anastomosis. An end-to-end anastomosis to the distal celiac axis is accomplished with 4-0 proline suture. This graft limb is relatively short. The proximal celiac axis is ligated and oversewn. Lastly, the SMA anastomosis is performed with the graft lying in the retroperitoneal space extending down to the intended SMA anastomotic site, anterior to the left renal artery and vein. In general, this is performed in an end-to-end fashion. If there are branches more proximal to the desired anastomotic site, then an end-to-side anastomosis should be considered (Fig. 27.6). Flow is reestablished into the SMA, and hemostasis is achieved. The tissues are allowed to fall back into the retroperitoneal space, and the abdominal musculature layers are closed together with PDS. The remaining incision is closed in the usual fashion. As the pleural cavity has been entered, a thoracostomy tube is placed, typically a 20 French chest tube.

Alternately, if a transperitoneal approach has been chosen, a midline incision is made. The left lobe of the liver is mobilized and retracted to the patient's right (Fig. 27.1). A nasogastric tube is in place which allows identification of the esophagus which is retracted to the patient's left. The gastrohepatic ligament is divided as are the crura tissues exposing the anterior surface of the SC aorta which is dissected in a nearly circumferentially fashion to allow for complete cross clamp application (Fig. 27.2). The celiac axis is dissected with exposure of the proximal portion of the celiac. In general, an end-to-end anastomosis is attempted (Fig. 27.7); if the disease extends significantly beyond the orifice of the celiac, then the anastomosis can be

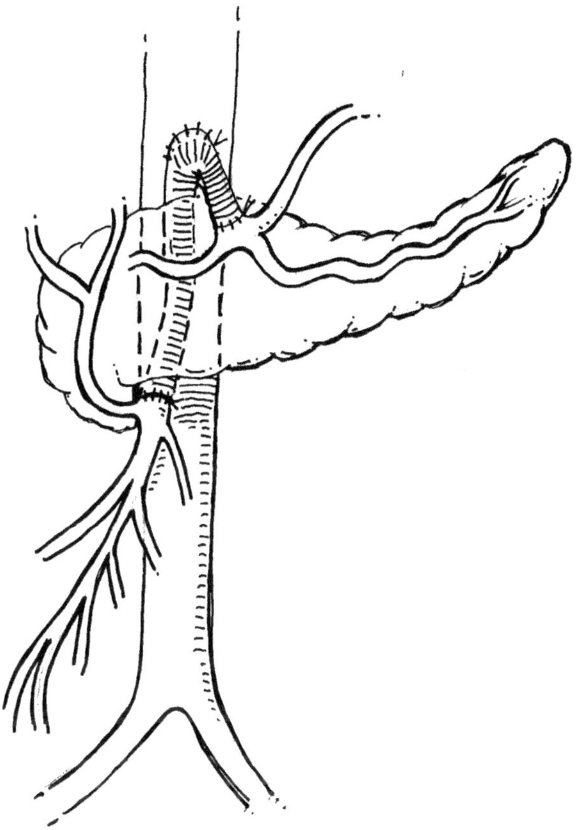

Fig. 27.7 Completed aortoceliac and mesenteric bypass in relationship to pancreas

performed to the hepatic artery. The SMA will need to be exposed in a separate plane. This is accomplished by tracing the transverse mesocolon back with identification of the middle colic artery. A transverse incision near the origin of the middle colic artery is undertaken with exposure of the SMA at the inferior border of the pancreas just medial to the superior mesenteric artery vein. The bypass will need to be a tunneled in an infra-pancreatic position connecting the two surgical planes with the bypass extending in the retro-pancreatic position to the SMA (Fig. 27.7). Otherwise, the procedure is performed identical to the retroperitoneal exposure.

Retrograde Bypass

The retrograde bypass from the iliac to the SMA is selected in high-risk patients for whom an endovascular option does not exist. Additional indications include patient with calcific disease involving the SC aorta or those high-risk patients who have failed prior endovascular revascularization. The operation is performed transperitoneally, and the author has adopted the C-shaped graft configuration. The inflow artery is either one of the common iliac arteries (the right iliac is favored with better configuration of the graft), whereas the distal anastomosis is most often constructed to a single vessel, that being the SMA. The author has favored the use of 8 mm external supported PTFE. The SMA is exposed via a lateral approach with mobilization of the duodenum to the patient's right and dissection immediately cephalad to the duodenum with exposure and mobilization of the SMA up to the level of the left renal vein (Fig. 27.8). Importantly, the tunnel created is on the left side of the retroperitoneum and follows a gentle curve over to the SMA. The distal anastomosis (the SMA anastomosis) is created first in an end-to-side fashion with 5-0 proline suture. The bowel contents are allowed to fall back, and a gentle curve without excessive redundancy is fashioned with the graft coursing under the retroperitoneum to the right common iliac artery. The aorta can also be chosen as the inflow site, useful in the setting of calcific disease involving both iliacs. An end of graft to side of iliac is created with the common iliac arteriotomy positioned slightly medially. As the possibility of graft kinking is one of the potential drawbacks to this

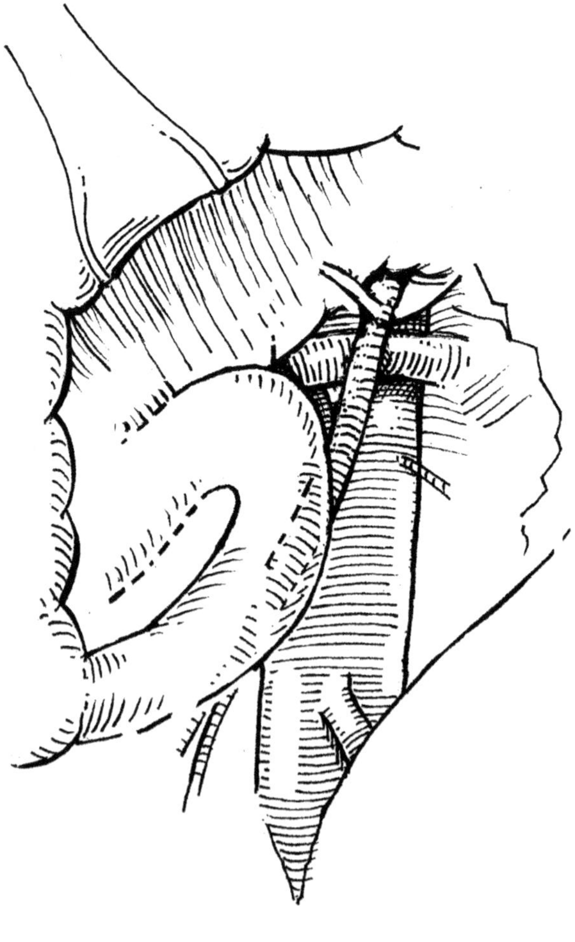

Fig. 27.8 Exposure of SMA cephalad to left renal vein

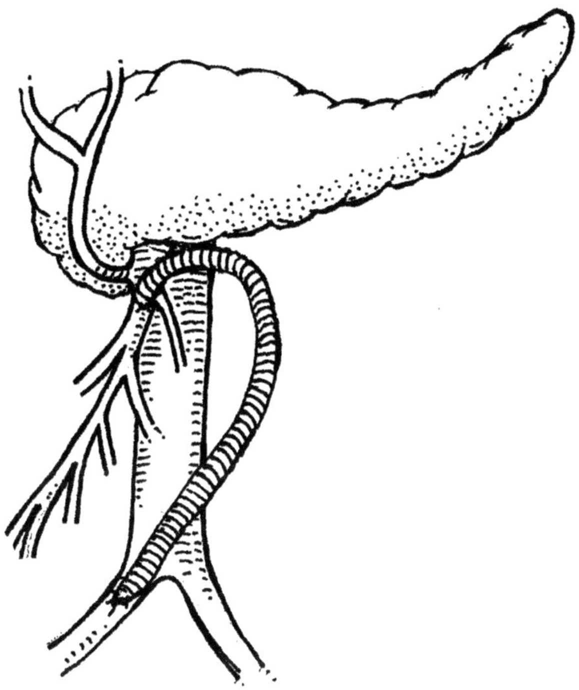

Fig. 27.9 Retrograde bypass from common iliac artery to SMA

procedure, attention to the appropriate length and course of the graft is essential (Fig. 27.9). Routine post bypass reconstruction assessment with intraoperative Doppler is accomplished, and the retroperitoneum is closed over the graft.

Trapdoor Aortic Endarterectomy

The trapdoor aortic endarterectomy is a well-established means of revascularization in the setting of chronic mesenteric ischemia associated with a significant component of the perivisceral aortic disease. It is most useful in instances where the occlusive disease is confined to or within 2–3 cm of the origins of the SMA and celiac axis. It is major operation indicated in low-risk patients with suitable anatomic pattern of disease. This operation is generally not used in the setting of acute mesenteric ischemia.

The patient's aorta is approached through the left flank retroperitoneal approach with the incision made in the ninth intercostal space (Fig. 27.3). The abdominal musculature is divided sequentially with Bovie cauterization taking care to maintain the retroperitoneal position and not violate the peritoneal cavity. The lumber vein off the left renal vein is identified and divided to enhance mobilization the left kidney anteriorly. Dissection in the retroperitoneum proceeds cautiously with the division of retroperitoneal tissue using a combination of Bovie cauterization, hemoclips, ties, or the harmonic scalpel. The diaphragmatic crus is identified and divided, exposing the underlying SC aorta. The SC aorta is dissected circumferentially as are the origins of the visceral vessels, i.e., the celiac axis and the SMA. The aorta below the SMA is dissected circumferentially. It is the preference of the author to either include the lumbar vessels within the aortic cross clamp (preferential) or individually control each of the lumbar vessel. Once the patient is anticoagulated, the aorta proximally is clamped as is the aorta below the SMA; typically, the clamps are positioned 2–4 cm above the celiac axis and 2–3 cm below the SMA. The clamp may be positioned below the left renal artery dependent upon its positioning and origin in relation to the SMA. The patient routinely receives intravenous mannitol, 25 g (or 0.5 g/kg). The celiac axis and the SMA are controlled with double-looped vessel loops. The aortotomy is performed extending below the SMA to above the origin of the celiac. A plaque elevator is required to initiate a plane, and one needs to be certain that the aortic wall being left behind is not too thin. The plaque is divided superiorly in a circumferential fashion with a stepdown from the diseased aorta proximally to the endarterectomized aorta. This rarely requires tacking sutures. The same is performed for the distal site, and one frequently can allow this to feather out circumferentially; occasionally tacking sutures are required. Finally, the eversion endarterectomy of the celiac and SMA is performed with gentle traction and an eversion technique employed ensuring a clean distal endpoint (Fig. 27.10). The aortotomy is rapidly closed with a running suture of 4-0 proline suture on a small needle. Prior to completing the anastomosis, the distal camp is released, and flow

Fig. 27.10 Trapdoor aortic endarterectomy

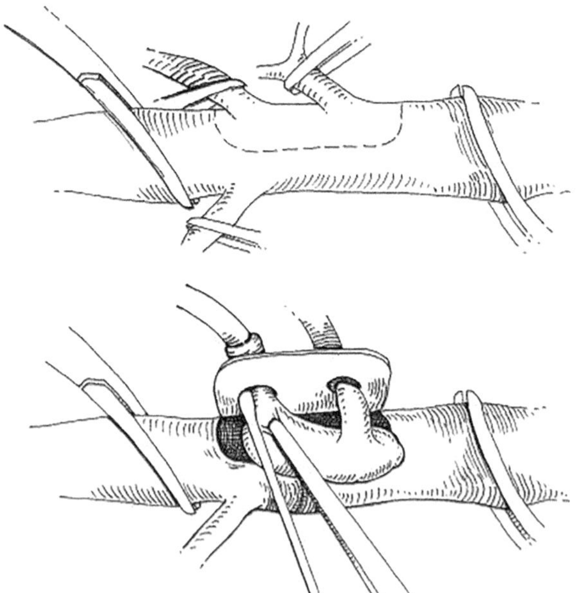

restored distally into the aorta then into the celiac and finally the SMA. Hemostasis is confirmed, and then the flank incision is closed as delineated above.

Complications

If bowel ischemia is in question (AMI), one should strongly consider autogenous vein reconstruction. Although this is more time consuming and can be fraught with kinking, redundancy, or twisting, autogenous grafts are more resistant to infection. This is especially the case when one encounters bowel contamination and an endovascular or hybrid approach cannot be performed successfully. One needs to be aware of the course of the graft as any redundancy or kinking of the graft is not well tolerated and can lead to graft occlusion. This applies to both prosthetic graft and vein bypasses. This is especially true as the graft is frequently sewn to the mesenteric vessels in a position which will be different once the bowel is able to return to its anatomical position. Graft patency results are excellent with secondary patency of 97% achievable. Mortality is not inconsequential, in the range of 5–8%. Ischemia-reperfusion with open bypass or reconstructions for CMI is a factor which influences outcome as postoperative pathophysiologic derangements are common including respiratory failure, renal insufficiency, hyperbilirubinemia, coagulopathy, and thrombocytopenia.

Take-Home Points

1. Endovascular revascularization is the preferred method of initial mesenteric revascularization.
2. Open mesenteric revascularization is utilized in instances of recurrent disease not amenable to repeat intervention, failure of attempted endovascular intervention, and anatomic pattern of disease which does not render itself to endovascular intervention.
3. The bypass selected is tailored to the patient's anatomy, comorbid conditions, acuity of presentation, and whether there is any issue with infarcted bowel.
4. The key to avoid graft elongation, angulation, or kinking of the graft is to cut the graft to length with the SMA in a nearly anatomic position.
5. Antegrade SC aorta to mesenteric bypass is overall the preferred method of revascularization; however, one needs to be aware of other open surgical options to optimize patient care and outcome. This can be performed through either a retroperitoneal or transperitoneal approach.
6. Two-vessel reconstruction is preferred over single-vessel revascularization. Open bypass or endarterectomy do have superior patency when compared to endovascular operations. A preoperative plan involving a detailed review of the anatomy, an evaluation of the patient's cardiopulmonary reserve, and selection of the appropriate revascularization method are integral to a successful patient outcome.

Chapter 28
Aortorenal Bypass and Renal Artery Reconstruction

Kaitlyn Dobesh and Timothy J. Nypaver

Indications

Open operations for renal artery occlusive disease (RAOD) with renal artery repair (endarterectomy) and bypass have largely been replaced by endovascular techniques, including renal artery balloon angioplasty and stenting. Randomized controlled studies, including the CORAL trial, although heavily criticized, have not provided evidence in favor of revascularization. The ASTRAL trial failed to show any improvement in systolic blood pressure, creatinine, or glomerular filtration rate (GFR) when compared to medical therapy, while the CORAL study demonstrated a modest blood pressure improvement and no difference in creatinine or GFR. Thus, the indications for intervention into renal artery stenosis (renovascular hypertension and ischemic nephropathy) have been heavily scrutinized and are now restricted to very specific indications. In this context, correction of renal arterial inflow stenosis is reserved for very select patients with resistant hypertensive patients who have failed maximal medical therapy, have worsening renal function, and/or unexplained congestive heart failure. Expectantly, the number of renal artery interventions has decreased, and the performance of a surgically isolated renal artery bypass, for occlusive lesions, is now relatively rare. While uncommonly performed in isolation, the practicing vascular surgeon still needs to be familiar with the techniques and conduct of renal artery revascularization procedures, especially in the setting of concomitant open aortic reconstructions or aortic pathology involving the renal branches.

K. Dobesh
Henry Ford Hospital, Detroit, MI, USA

T. J. Nypaver (✉)
Division of Vascular Surgery, Henry Ford Hospital, Detroit, MI, USA
e-mail: TNYPAVE1@hfhs.org

S. S. Hans et al. (eds.), *Primary and Repeat Arterial Reconstructions*,
https://doi.org/10.1007/978-3-031-13897-3_28

The primary indication for open aortorenal bypass in modern vascular surgery continues to be needed for renal artery reconstruction during open aortic repair. This would include those patients with suprarenal abdominal aortic aneurysm (AAA) that require bypass, patients with infrarenal AAAs with significant RAOD, and those patients with aortoiliac occlusive disease (AIOD) requiring aortofemoral bypass who also have RAOD. Patients with bilateral moderate severe (60–80% stenosis) or severe disease (>80% stenosis) in the setting of severe hypertension, especially with evidence of excretory renal function impairment like azotemia, should be considered for concomitant bypass at the time of their aortic reconstruction. Performing simultaneous renal reconstruction during AAA and AIOD repair has not been shown to increase mortality, but there is a notable increase in morbidity and postoperative dialysis rates, seen more so in AIOD than with AAA. For combined renal artery stenosis and AAA, preoperative percutaneous transluminal renal artery angioplasty (plus stenting), prior to the open repair, remains an option; however, there is no outcome advantage compared to those with combined open renal artery reconstruction and AAA repair.

Additional indications for renal artery reconstruction also exist. There continues to be a need for open aortorenal bypass in select patients with renal artery aneurysms (different chapter), mid-aortic syndrome, and pediatric patients with hypoplastic renal artery lesions. These latter procedures should be performed at specialized centers. Also, renal artery bypass will be required in debranching abdominal operations performed very selectively for high-risk patients with suprarenal aneurysms or thoracoabdominal aneurysms. Lastly, isolated renal artery reconstruction may be required in the setting of failed endovascular interactions, particularly if there is an isolated solo kidney.

Preoperative Planning

Initial determination of the extent of renal artery stenosis is performed with renal Duplex ultrasound. Peak systolic velocity (PSV) of >200 cm/s is associated with >50% stenosis, and the ratio of >3.5 of renal artery to aorta PSV correlates with >60% stenosis. If unable to perform renal artery duplex, computed tomography angiography (CTA) or magnetic resonance angiography (MRA) may also be of use, although CTA does require iodinated contrast and should be used cautiously in the setting of renal dysfunction. CTA and MRA can also aid in identifying anatomy, including orientation of the arteries, as well as the presence and location of renal artery branches and accessory vessels. Renal artery duplex with measurement of a resistive index can be a surrogate for determining the amount of intraparenchymal renal disease present, which may assist in determining who may improve from surgical revascularization.

Preoperative Decision-Making

In the adult patient, two graft options are typically used for renal bypass: autologous saphenous vein and synthetic polytetrafluoroethylene (PTFE) graft. The selection of conduit depends upon the indication for the procedure and if the bypass is being performed in the setting of a concomitant operation. Saphenous vein may be utilized in isolated renal artery reconstruction; however, PTFE is generally used for cases of combined aortic reconstruction. The inflow is typically the infrarenal aorta or the aortic graft; however, there may be instances in which the bypass may originate from the iliac artery. This includes those patients with advanced aortic arteriosclerosis, patients with prior aorto-aortic reconstructions, congenital aortic coarctations, and debranching operations in the treatment of thoracoabdominal or suprarenal aneurysm disease.

In general, the authors favor a bypass procedure (as opposed to endarterectomy) when the need for renal artery revascularization exists; nevertheless, there are times in which renal artery endarterectomy, either direct or via an eversion technique, may be preferred. Overall, equivalent outcomes have been reported.

Surgical Anatomy and Exposure

Two main approaches are used for exposure of the origins of the renal arteries in the context of bypass, the medial visceral rotation (MVR) and the infra-mesocolic approach. Selection of approach will depend on the extent of the suprarenal aorta that needs to be exposed and whether the distal aspect of the main renal artery will require exposure. The infra-mesocolic approach is suitable for the majority of renal artery reconstructions with the medial visceral rotation reserved for those instances with which very distal reconstructions are being contemplated, most commonly on the right.

Infra-mesocolic Approach: (Left and Proximal Right)

The abdomen and peritoneal cavity can be opened via a midline incision extending up to xiphoid process. A supraumbilical transverse incision is also possible. In the infra-mesocolic approach, the small bowel is retracted to the patient's right, and the colon retracted superiorly, allowing a midline exposure of the retroperitoneum (Fig. 28.1). The posterior peritoneum to the right of the aorta is incised. The duodenum is retracted to the right exposing the avascular plan under the pancreas. Careful dissection should be conducted as mesenteric vessels may be encountered at this level before the avascular plane is entered. The incision may need to be extended along the inferior border of the pancreas to obtain adequate posterior exposure. The

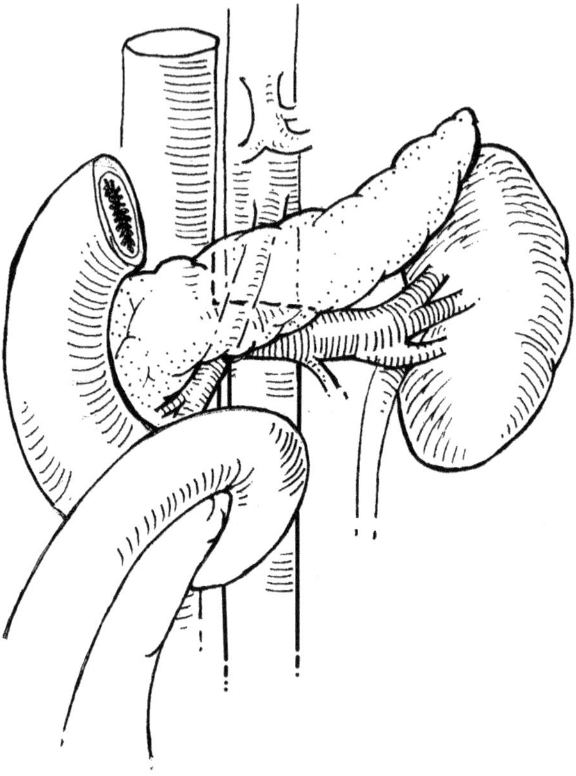

Fig. 28.1 Infra-mesocolic approach with the small bowel retracted to the right, and the colon retracted superiorly, allowing a midline exposure of the retroperitoneum

left renal vein is then mobilized, and the adrenal, gonadal, and lumbar veins ligated. The left renal vein can then be reflected superiorly (most commonly) or inferiorly, to aid in exposing the artery. (Fig. 28.2). The right renal artery at its origin can be exposed through the same approach, limited to the first 3–4 cm of the proximal right renal artery. The proximal portion of the right renal artery is exposed by retracting the left renal vein superiorly and the vena cava to the right (Fig. 28.2). The aorta which generally is used as the origin for both the right and left renal bypass is exposed for 5–8 cm below the renal artery origin down to or just below the origin of the inferior mesenteric artery. If a vein graft is being used, perioperative vein mapping is undertaken to identify the best available segment of greater saphenous vein. The author favors a distal end-to-end anastomosis with the distal anastomosis spatulated (Fig. 28.3). The aortic anastomosis to limit arterial ischemia to the kidney is performed first. The aorta is cross-clamped, both proximally and distally (or alternately, in a non-diseased aorta or with an aortic graft, a side-biting clamp may be utilized), and an aortotomy is made on the anterolateral aspect of the aorta with the aortotomy length extending 2.5× the vein caliber. The vein is slightly spatulated and the anastomosis carried out with 5-proline suture with the initial suture at the apex of the spatulated graft and the superior segment of the aortotomy (Fig. 28.4).

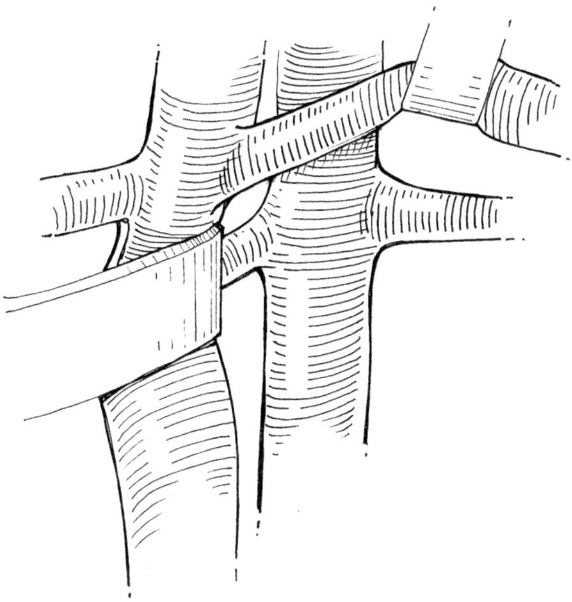

Fig. 28.2 Retraction of the inferior vena cava to the right and the left renal vein superiorly allowing exposure of the origins of both the right and left renal arteries

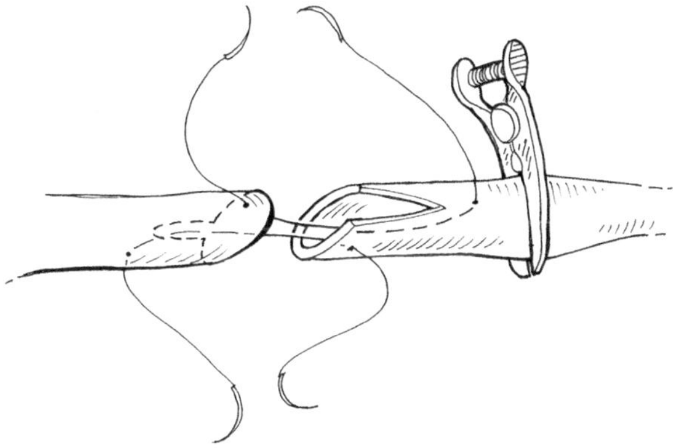

Fig. 28.3 Performance of an end-to-end spatulated renal artery anastomosis

Following the anastomosis, the flow in the aorta is restored, the vein graft is distended, and the conduit is assessed for orientation and length. Additionally, a side-biting clamp may be useful to avoid a pressured vein graft and allow for technically easier distal anastomosis. The diseased renal artery stump will need to be suture ligated. The distal anastomosis is accomplished via a spatulated technique (Fig. 28.3) with the spatulation of the renal artery on the anterior aspect and spatulation of the vein (or graft) on the posterior aspect (Fig. 28.4). The conduct of the bypass is similar whether vein graft or PTFE graft is utilized. In combined procedures, the author favors the use of PTFE graft with the only additional caveat that the proximal bypass anastomosis to the main body of the graft has been completed prior to the

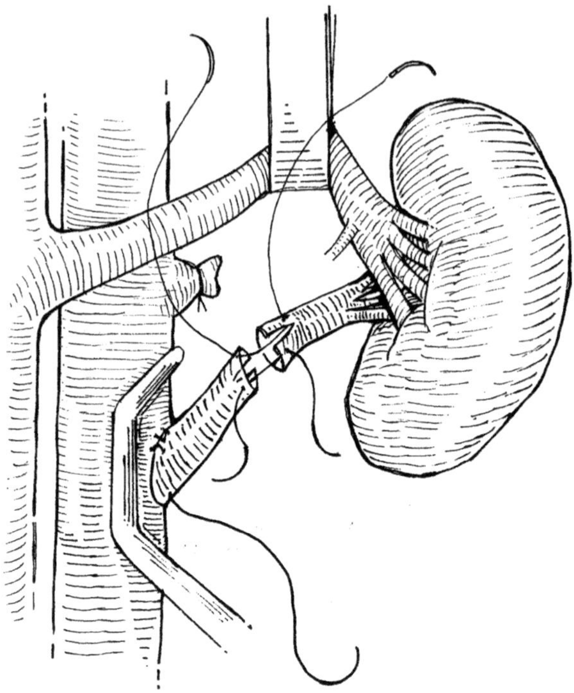

Fig. 28.4 Performance of the proximal anastomosis of a left aorto-renal bypass off the aorta (side-biting aortic clamp utilized) with spatulation of the distal anastomosis

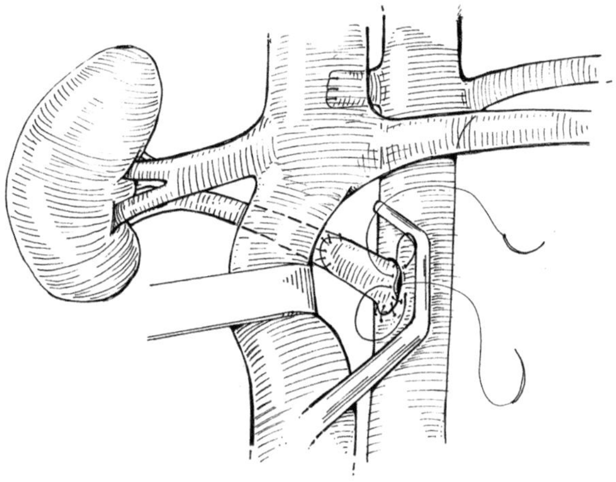

Fig. 28.5 Performance of the proximal anastomosis of a right aorto-renal bypass off the aorta (side-biting aortic clamp utilized) with a completed distal spatulated anastomosis posterior to the inferior vena cava

performance of the proximal aortic anastomosis. The operation on the right can be performed through the same exposure, accomplished with careful retraction of the left renal vein superiorly and the vena cava to the patient's right (Fig. 28.5). This approach should be for disease confined to the very proximal orifice of the right renal artery. The bypass is tunneled inferior to the IVC (Fig. 28.5).

Medial Visceral Rotation (Right Renal Artery Bypass and Distal Exposure of the Left Renal Artery)

The MVR allows for increased proximal aortic exposure along with improved exposure of the distal renal artery and its branches. Medial visceral rotation is accomplished through a midline abdominal incision. During the right MVR, the peritoneal reflection of the ascending colon at the white line of Toldt is excised, and the colon reflected anteromedially. The duodenum and pancreatic head are Kocherized and reflected medially, exposing the right kidney and Inferior vein cava (IVC) (Fig. 28.6). The right renal vein, which overlies the artery, must then be circumferentially cleared from the inferior vena cava junction. Any small branches should be ligated, including lumbar veins, which will aid in retraction of the IVC. The right renal vein can then be retracted superiorly to expose the artery (Fig. 28.6).

The left MVR requires the peritoneal reflection of the descending colon at the white line of Toldt to be excised, and the colon reflected anteromedially, exposing the left kidney. The left renal vein, lying anterior to the artery, can then be further

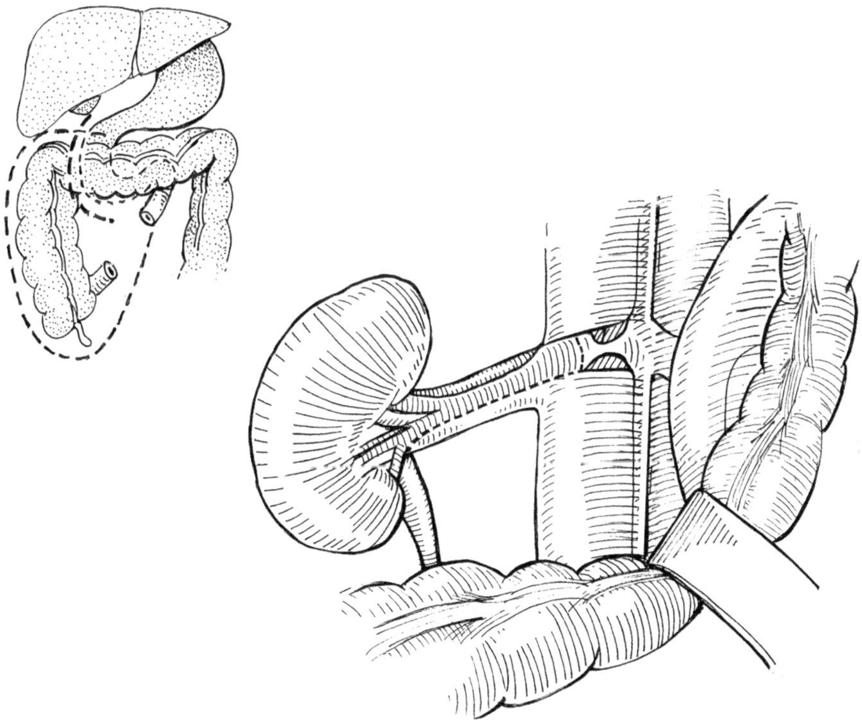

Fig. 28.6 Right medial visceral rotation with the location of the incision (insert) and mobilization of the right colon and duodenum to the left with exposure of the inferior vena cava and the distal right renal vessels (main diagram)

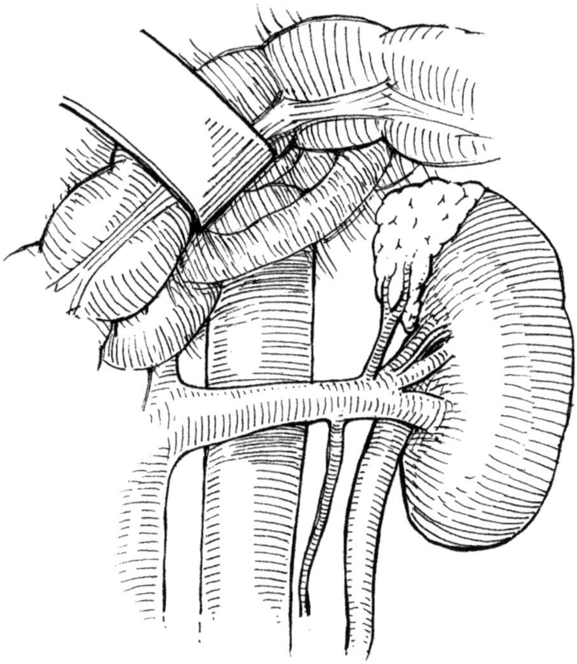

Fig. 28.7 Left medial visceral rotation with mobilization of the left colon anteromedially with exposure of the left renal vessels (the artery, not shown, lies just posterior to the vein)

mobilized by ligating the adrenal, gonadal, and lumbar branches and reflecting it either superiorly or inferiorly (Fig. 28.7). In practice, when an abdominal aortic aneurysm is being performed concomitantly with the left renal artery reconstruction, the authors prefer the left flank retroperitoneal approach (see chapter on AAA), and the renal artery bypass, typically performed with PTFE graft, is kept very short (<1 cm). There is a tendency for the bypass graft to be long, which once the retroperitoneal contents are returned to their anatomic position, the graft may prove to be redundant and prone to kinking. Whether the exposure is accomplished via the MVR approach or via the infra-mesocolic approach, the concepts and the technical exercise of the renal artery bypass remain the same.

Complications

The most common complications after renal artery bypass are early renal dysfunction, bypass graft occlusion or thrombosis (1%), unchanged or worsening hypertension, and recurrent stenosis. Early bypass graft occlusion is most often technical in nature. The mortality rate of renal artery bypass when combined with aortic reconstruction varies between 4.7% and 8.3%. Advanced age, female gender, chronic renal failure, bilateral procedures, congestive heart failure, and chronic lung disease were all independent risk factors of in-hospital mortality. Patency, while difficult to accurately assess due to the absence of routine surveillance, has been reported to be 95% at 3–5 years post bypass. Patency rates appear to be equivalent between saphenous vein bypass and prosthetic bypass.

Take-Home Points

1. Renal artery open reconstructions are less commonly performed, restricted now to specific indications owing to randomized trials failing to show an advantage or benefit to revascularization interventions. As such, isolated renal artery reconstructions are less commonly performed and are typically carried out now in the setting of concomitant aortic reconstruction.
2. Open renal revascularization is still utilized in instances of recurrent disease not amenable to repeat intervention, failure of attempted endovascular intervention, and anatomic pattern of disease which does not render itself to endovascular intervention. Specific disease states including renal artery aneurysm and mid-aortic syndrome may require open bypass or revascularization.
3. Key concepts of renal revascularization include (1) the aorta (or the aortic graft) primarily serves as the inflow (although alternate inflow sources can be used); (2) bypass can be performed with vein or PTFE with the caveat of a spatulated anastomosis; and (3) the exposure of the majority of renal artery bypasses is accomplished via a infra-mesocolic approach with the medial visceral rotation reserved for specific indications or considerations.

References

1. Cooper CJ, Murphy TP, Cutlip DE, Jamerson K, Henrich W, Reid DM, Cohen DJ, Matsumoto AH, Steffes M, Jaff MR, Prince MR, Lewis EF, Tuttle KR, Shapiro JI, Rundback JH, Massaro JM, D'Agostino RB Sr, Dworkin LD, Investigators CORAL. Stenting and medical therapy for atherosclerotic renal-artery stenosis. N Engl J Med. 2014;370(1):13–22.
2. Wheatley K, Ives N, Gray R, Kalra PA, Moss JG, Baigent C, Carr S, Chalmers N, Eadington D, Hamilton G, Lipkin G, Nicholson A, Scoble J, Investigators ASTRAL. Revascularization versus medical therapy for renal-artery stenosis. N Engl J Med. 2009;361(20):1953–62.

Chapter 29
Crossover Femoral-Femoral Bypass Graft and Iliofemoral Bypass Graft

Alice Lee

Femoral-Femoral Bypass

Anatomy

The inguinal ligament is located between the anterior superior iliac spine and the pubic symphysis. Above the ligament is the external iliac artery and below is the common femoral artery. Medial to the common femoral artery is the vein and the nerve is lateral. This area is called the femoral triangle. The medial border is formed by the medial aspect of the adductor longus and the lateral border is the medial aspect of the sartorius muscle. The branches of the common femoral artery include the superficial external pudendal artery, deep external pudendal artery, superficial circumflex iliac artery, and superficial epigastric artery. The superficial external pudendal artery, deep external pudendal artery, and superficial epigastric artery run medially. The superficial circumflex iliac artery runs lateral toward the anterior superior iliac spine. Branches of the external iliac artery include deep circumflex iliac artery and inferior epigastric artery. The profunda artery is the largest branch of the common femoral artery and runs laterally compared to the superficial femoral artery.

Indications

1. Active intra-abdominal infection. For example, mycotic abdominal aortic aneurysm, infected aortic prothesis, aorta-enteric fistula.

A. Lee (✉)
Henry Ford Hospital, Detroit, MI, USA
e-mail: alee18@hfhs.org

S. S. Hans et al. (eds.), *Primary and Repeat Arterial Reconstructions*,
https://doi.org/10.1007/978-3-031-13897-3_29

2. Hostile abdomen.
3. Adjunct to aorto-uni-iliac (AUI) stent graft for repair of abdominal aortic aneurysm.
4. Absence of endovascular options for iliac occlusive disease.

Procedure

Groin incisions are made in longitudinal fashion. It is helpful to use an ultrasound to mark the bifurcation prior to prepping. Dissect out and obtain control of the common femoral, superficial femoral, and profunda arteries. An endarterectomy may be needed depending on plaque burden/disease. A suprapubic subcutaneous tunnel anterior to the abdominal fascia is made in reverse C shape. This can be created with blunt dissection using fingers, a tunneling device, or a curved aortic clamp. Pass the graft (usually 8 mm PTFE with rings) using a tunneling device or a long aortic clamp. Heparinize for an ACT >250. If intervention is needed of the donor iliac, this should be completed. Donor anastomosis will be made in end-to-side fashion using 5-0 prolene. Prior to completion of anastomosis, artery should be forward and back-bled. The distal anastomosis is also completed in end-to-side fashion using 5-0 prolene, and prior to completion of anastomosis, the artery and graft should be flushed. Close the groins in multiple layers and take care to avoid compression/kinking of the graft. Pay particular attention to not leave a dead space which can lead to seroma formation and possible infection.

Diagrams of the Procedure

"Course/tunneling of femoral-femoral bypass with anastomosis over the origin of the profunda artery and origin of the superficial femoral artery" (see Fig. 29.1).

Pearls and Complications

1. Donor iliac needs to be free of disease and may need endovascular intervention.
2. When creating the tunnel, the "turn" of the graft should be several centimeters superior to the planned arteriotomy site to reduce kinking. Kinking commonly occurs at the heel if the "turn" is too steep or shallow.
3. A small amount of redundancy in the graft can decrease kinking of the graft at the heel.

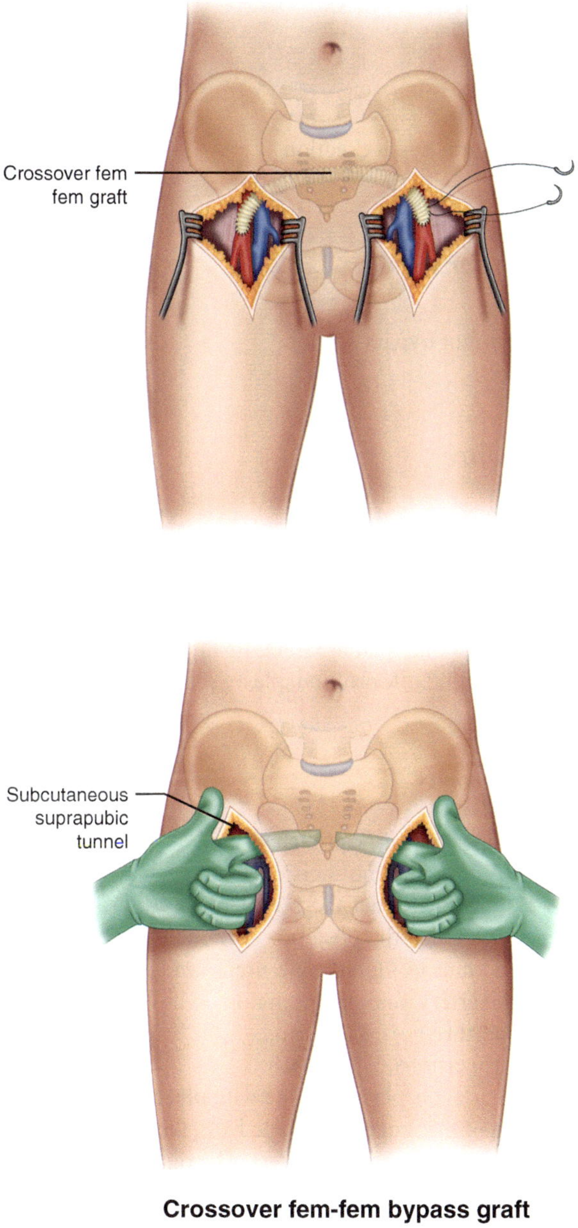

Fig. 29.1 Anastomosis of crossover femoral-femoral graft to the femoral artery is performed via subcutaneous suprapubic tunnel

4. If patient is high risk for general anesthesia, local anesthesia or epidural is an option.
5. If a subcutaneous tunnel is contraindicated, a tunnel can be made in the preperitoneal position but be wary of a bowel or bladder injury with tunneling.

Iliofemoral Bypass

Anatomy

See fem-fem bypass section.

Indications

See fem-fem bypass section.

Procedure

Groin Exposure

Groin incision can be made in longitudinal or transverse fashion. Obtain control of the common femoral, superficial femoral, and profunda arteries. If the profunda artery is the only patent target, ligate venous branches to ensure adequate exposure of the profunda. A profundaplasty may also be needed if there is heavy disease.

Iliac Exposure

A. Intraperitoneal Approach

A low midline incision is made. Place a self-retracting system to improve exposure. Retract the bowel to the right side. This will expose the aorta/iliac artery. Open the posterior peritoneum over the aorta and extend caudally. Very important to identify the ureter and retract lateral. Obtain control of common iliac artery and take care to avoid injury to the iliac vein that is located posteriorly.

B. Retroperitoneal Approach

Patient is placed supine with placement of a roll under the ipsilateral hip. The start of the incision is made from the midaxillary line halfway between the subcostal margin and iliac crest. The distal end of the incision should be 3 cm above the inguinal ligament at the lateral border of the rectus. The incision is oblique and there can be a slight curve. Divide external oblique aponeurosis in the direction of its fibers. Then the internal oblique and transversus abdominal muscles are divided in the line of the incision. Enter the retroperitoneum. Open the retroperitoneal space and retract the peritoneal sac and ureter medially. The common iliac artery will be just medial to the iliopsoas muscle.

Procedure

Create a tunnel using blunt dissection in the plane anterior to the iliac artery so that the ureter will be posterior to the graft. Be sure to tunnel underneath the inguinal ligament. Use an umbilical tape to mark the tunnel, then pass a Dacron or ringed PTFE graft (usually 8 mm) through the tunnel. Heparinize to achieve an ACT >250. Clamp the iliac artery and then create a longitudinal arteriotomy about 1.5 cm. Sew an end to side anastomosis using 5-0 prolene. Prior to completing the anastomosis, the artery and graft are flushed. Repeat for the distal anastomosis, end-to-side with 5-0 prolene. Close each muscle layer in the flank separately (generally interrupted sutures for transversus/internal oblique and continuous suture for external oblique aponeurosis) using 0 Vicryl. Close the groin in multiple layers.

Diagrams of the Procedure

"Course of ileofemoral bypass" (see Fig. 29.2).

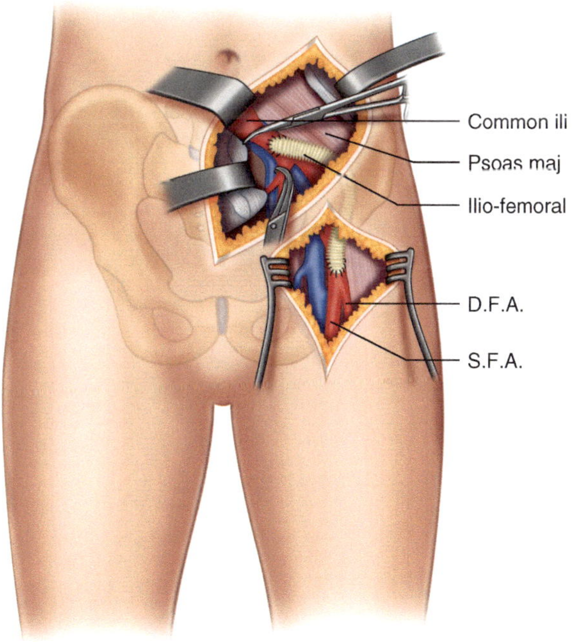

Fig. 29.2 Ileofemoral bypass course and anatomy

Pearls and Complications

1. Minimize dissection of left common iliac artery to preserve the autonomic nerve fibers (postoperative sexual dysfunction in male patients).
2. If the external iliac artery is needed for the bypass, an incision 2 cm above and parallel to the inguinal ligament is made.

Chapter 30
Axillo-Femoral Bypass

Alice Lee

Anatomy

The axillary artery consists of three parts. The first portion is distal to the lateral border of the first rib to the medial edge of the pectoralis minor. The superior thoracic artery arises in this section. The second portion is under the pectoralis minor. The first branch is the thoracoacromial trunk which divides into the acromial artery, pectoral artery, clavicular artery, and deltoid artery. The second branch is the lateral thoracic artery. The third portion of the artery is from the lateral edge of the pectoralis minor to the lateral border of teres minor. There are three branches which are the subscapular artery, anterior humeral circumflex artery, and posterior humeral circumflex artery. The vein lays medial to the artery.

Indications

1. Hostile abdomen
2. Abdominal infection
3. Poor surgical candidate due to comorbidities

A. Lee (✉)
Henry Ford Hospital, Detroit, MI, USA
e-mail: alee18@hfhs.org

S. S. Hans et al. (eds.), *Primary and Repeat Arterial Reconstructions*,
https://doi.org/10.1007/978-3-031-13897-3_30

Procedure

The donor arm is abducted 90 degrees and a towel roll is placed under the patient. A 10–12 cm transverse incision about one finger breath below the middle third of the clavicle is made (from the costosternal junction to the deltopectoral groove). Incise the pectoralis major fascia along the direction of its fibers. Usually the medial portion of the pectoralis minor muscle is divided to help mobilize the axillary artery or the muscle is retracted laterally. The axillary vein is anterior and caudal to the artery and may need to be isolated to improve exposure of the artery. Avoid injury to the cords of the brachial plexus that lay superior and posterior to the artery. Dissect out 4–5 cm of the axillary artery. Next an incision is made in the groin, and the common femoral, profunda, and superficial femoral artery is mobilized. The proximal graft is generally under the pectoralis minor muscle but can be placed on the anterior surface. A subpectoral muscle is created parallel to the axillary artery and continued in a subcutaneous plane in the axilla. The tunnel continues distally along the anterior axillary line and will gently curve at the level of the anterior superior iliac spine towards the groin. A counter incision made below the costal margin will help with tunneling. Next, an 8 mm-ringed PTFE is passed through the tunnel. If a femoral-femoral crossover graft is planned, the tunnel should be created next. A prefabricated graft for an axillobifemoral bypass can be used for this. Be sure to allow slight redundancy to the axillary tunnel to avoid avulsion with extreme arm abduction. Anticoagulate with heparin to achieve an ACT >250. An arteriotomy is made on the anterior inferior surface of the axillary artery, and an end-to-side anastomosis is sewn using 5-0 prolene. The bevel can be made in the traditional 30-degree angle or in cobrahead fashion. Prior to completion of the anastomosis, the artery is forward and back bled. Next create an arteriotomy on the common femoral artery which should be extended onto the profunda or superficial femoral artery. An end-to-side anastomosis is then sewn using 5-0 prolene. Prior to completion of the anastomosis, the artery is forward and back bled as well as the graft. See Chap. 29 for more information regarding femoral-femoral bypass.

Diagrams of the Procedure

Image showing "Proximal anastomosis of axillo-femoral bypass with two types of configuration" Fig. 30.1.

Figure 30.1a: 30° bevel

Figure 30.1b: Cobrahead bevel

Image showing "Course of tunnel for an axillobifemoral bypass," (see Fig. 30.2a).

Image showing "Details of femoral anastomosis," (see Fig. 30.2b).

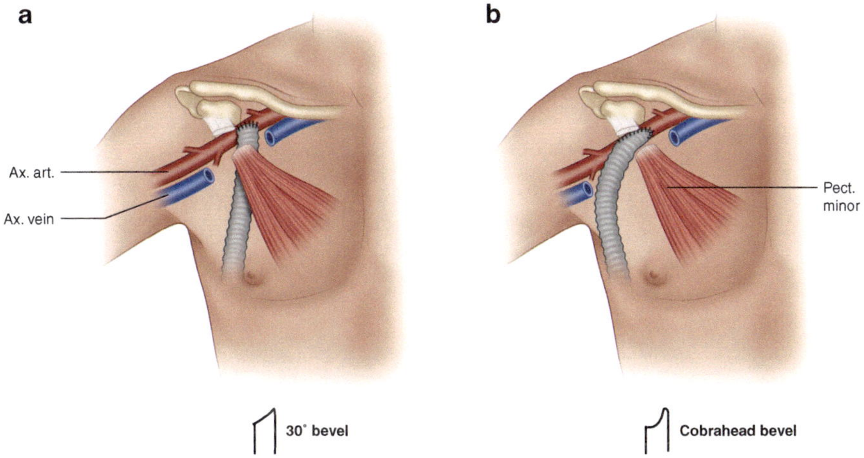

Fig. 30.1 Proximal anastomosis of axillo-femoral bypass graft – two types of configurations

Fig. 30.2 (**a**) Course of tunnel for axillobefemoral graft. (**b**) Details of femoral anastomosis

a

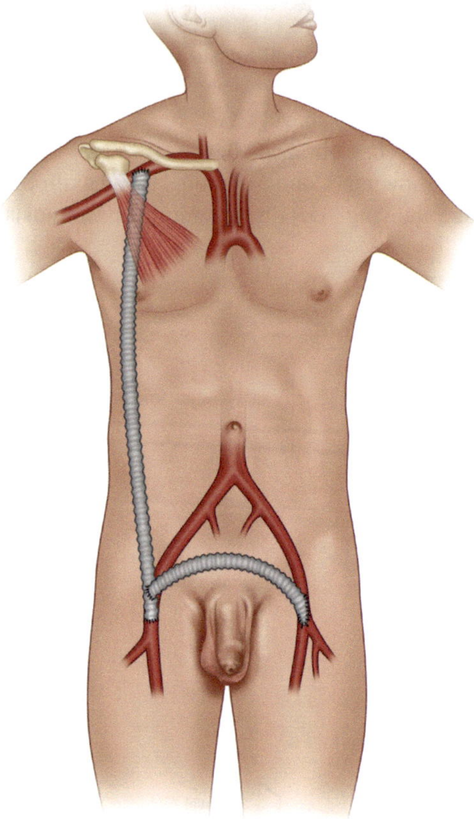

b

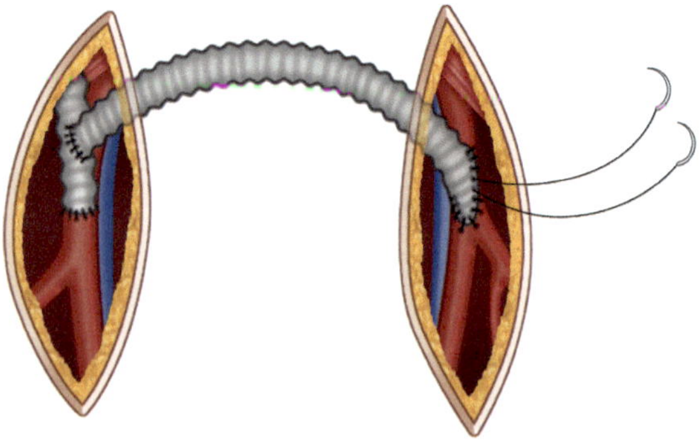

Pearls and Complications

1. To avoid avulsion or excessive tension with extreme arm abduction, be sure to leave a small amount of redundancy in the graft.
2. Either axillary artery can be used if there is no disease in the subclavian/axillary artery, but the right side is preferred if a left flank incision will be utilized in a future procedure.
3. If both axillary arteries are equal, inflow is usually the same side as the worst leg.
4. If there is a systolic pressure difference in the arms that is greater than 10 mmHg, choose the arm with the higher pressure.
5. The axillary artery is fragile – avoid excess tension when sewing the anastomosis.

Chapter 31
Iliac and Femoral Artery Endarterectomy

Farah Hanif Ali Mohammad

Surgical Anatomy

Common and External Iliac Artery

The aorta bifurcates into common iliac arteries at the level of L4–L5. They descend down into the pelvis further dividing into external and internal iliac arteries. The internal dives into the true pelvis, while the external runs medial to the psoas, going behind the inguinal ligament. It gives off deep circumflex and inferior epigastric branches near the ligament.

Operative Steps to Iliac Endarterectomy

The common iliac artery can be exposed via transperitoneal or retroperitoneal exposure (Fig. 31.1a). For transperitoneal exposure, the patient is placed supine, and the entire abdomen and pelvis are prepped. A longitudinal midline incision is made, and the peritoneum is entered (Fig. 31.1b). The omentum and transverse colon are reflected superiorly, and the small bowel is eviscerated to the right. The posterior peritoneum is then incised over the aorta lateral to the fourth portion of duodenum. This is following inferiorly over the iliac bifurcation. The iliac artery is then dissected out and encircled carefully to avoid injury to the iliac vein that runs posterolateral to it. One should be careful in dissecting the peri-adventitial tissue over the aortic bifurcation and left common iliac artery in males as the sympathetic nerves for ejaculatory function anatomically located in this region. As you dissect further

F. H. A. Mohammad (✉)
Henry Ford Hospital, Detroit, MI, USA

S. S. Hans et al. (eds.), *Primary and Repeat Arterial Reconstructions*,
https://doi.org/10.1007/978-3-031-13897-3_31

distally, the ureter runs adjacent to the iliac bifurcation and should be carefully retracted laterally. The external and internal iliac veins run posteromedial to their corresponding arteries. Depending on the extent and location of disease, the vessels are mobilized in anticipation of an endarterectomy.

If retroperitoneal exposure is planned, then the patient is positioned supine position but with ipsilateral hip elevated to 10° with a rolled sheet bump. An oblique incision is made extending from lateral border of the rectus muscle to approximately halfway between the subcostal margin and iliac crest in the direction of the midaxillary line (Fig. 31.2). The external and internal oblique muscles are divided parallel to their axis. The transversus abdominis and transversalis fascia are opened at the lateral half of the wound. The peritoneum is stripped off the lateral pelvic wall, and retroperitoneum is entered. The psoas muscle and the iliac vessels that lie medial to it are exposed. The ureter is left attached to the posterior peritoneum and retracted medially. Depending on the extent and level of exposure needed, the incision and dissection are carried out accordingly.

a

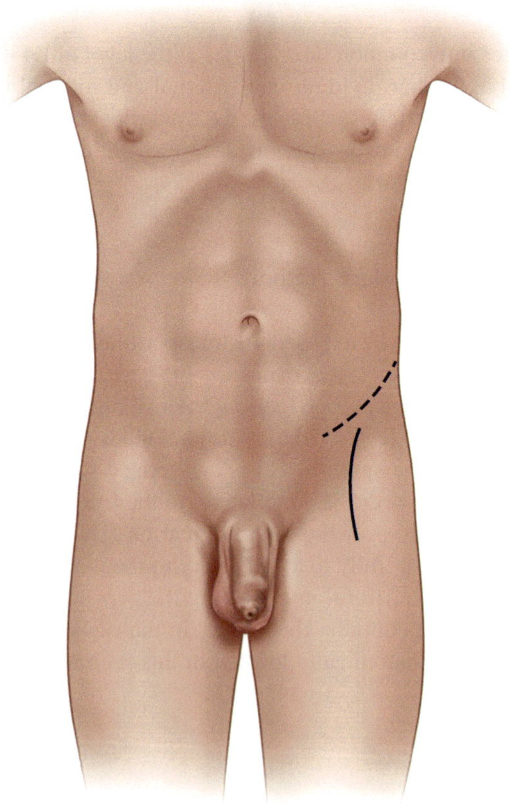

Fig. 31.1 (**a, b**) Midline transperitoneal exposure

b

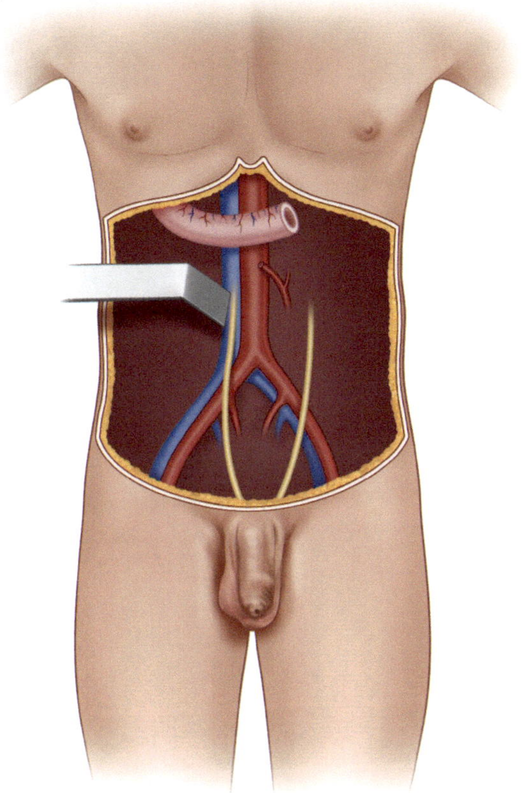

Fig. 31.1 (continued)

Complications

– Venous and ureteral injury: Careful dissection and orientation to corresponding veins and course of the ureter in relation to the artery are essential to avoid injury.

Common Femoral Artery

The femoral artery serves as the principal vessel supplying blood to the lower extremity. Inguinal ligament serves as a transition point between the external iliac and femoral artery. It lies approximately midway between the anterior superior iliac spine and the symphysis pubis. Common femoral artery along with the vein which lies medial to it is enclosed in the femoral sheath. Femoral nerve lies lateral to the artery. The vessels lie within the femoral triangle which is bounded laterally by the

Fig. 31.2 Retroperitoneal exposure of bifurcation of left common iliac artery

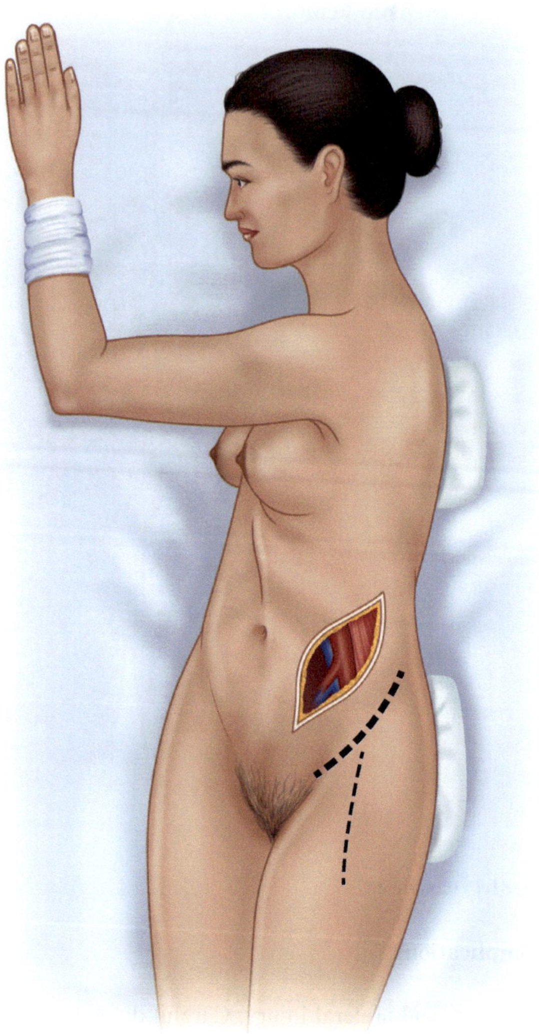

sartorius muscle, medially by the adductor longus muscle, and superiorly by the inguinal ligament. Femoral artery gives rise to three superficial branches which include superficial external pudendal, superficial epigastric, and superficial circumflex arteries. These branches may serve as essential collaterals in cases of significant iliac occlusive disease. The common femoral then continues onto to become superficial femoral artery after giving off the profunda femoris artery laterally approximately 4 cm distal to the inguinal ligament. There are two groups of superficial subinguinal lymph nodes that lie in the anterior groin incision and contribute to the rich plexus of lymphatic channels around the artery. Interruption of these channels can lead to a lymphocele formation.

Operative Steps to Femoral Endarterectomy

Patient is placed supine, and the lower abdomen up to the level of the umbilicus and mid-thigh is prepped. Bedside ultrasound to identify the femoral bifurcation allows accurate planning of the incision. Wide exposure of the femoral artery is best achieved by a vertical incision. The incision is made midway between the anterior superior iliac spine and the symphysis pubis. In morbidly obese patients with focal and short segment disease, a horizontal incision may be used to decrease the risk of wound complications (Fig. 31.3). Horizontal incision is made parallel along the inguinal ligament. As the incision is deepened, time should be taken to ligate the lymphatics to reduce the risk of lymphocele. The fascia forming the femoral sheath is opened along the medial border of the sartorius. Dissection should then be carried close the artery to avoid injury to the surrounding nerve and venous structures. Common femoral artery is dissected proximally usually up to the level of inferior epigastric artery or until a healthy segment of the common femoral is palpated. Occasionally, the disease extends into the external iliac artery in which partial division of the inguinal ligament assists in exposure. In case of significant proximal disease, hybrid approach can be taken with iliac artery stenting or angioplasty. The dissection distally extends to expose the femoral bifurcation. Depending on the extent of the disease, the proximal segments of SFA and profunda femoris may be dissected. Once adequate proximal and distal control is obtained, patient is heparinized, and clamps are placed. Artery is then opened, and endarterectomy is performed and patched with autogenous vein or bovine pericardium. The wound should be closed in multiple layers to close the dead space.

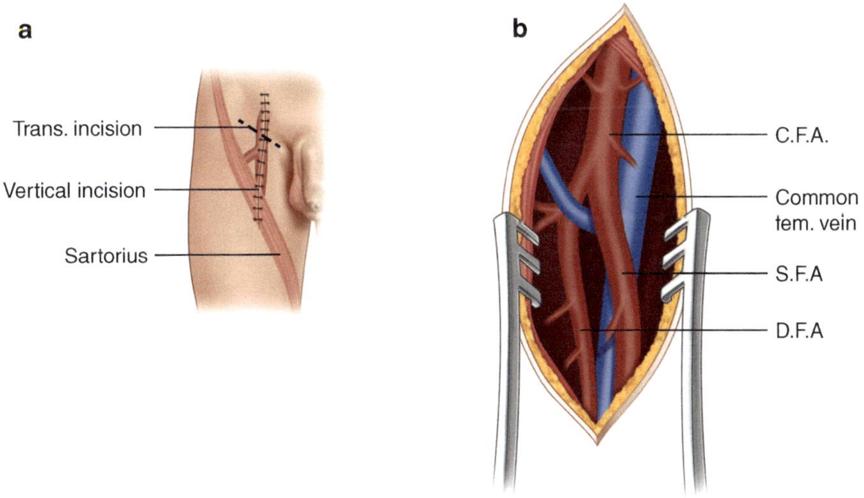

Fig. 31.3 (**a**, **b**) Exposure of common femoral artery and its bifurcation

Complications

- Wound complications: Groin wound complications including dehiscence, infection, lymphocele, and hematoma can be devastating. Gentle tissue handling and aggressive ligation of lymphatics are key to avoid wound problems.

Chapter 32
Femoral-Popliteal Bypass Graft

Abdul Kader Natour and Loay Kabbani

Introduction

It's estimated that 30 million North Americans are affected by peripheral artery disease (PAD), with a prevalence of almost 30% in people older than 70 years [1–2]. PAD significantly affects the quality of life and constitutes a major burden for healthcare-related expenditures [3–4]. Femoral-popliteal (FP) PAD symptoms can range from asymptomatic to claudication and to critical limb ischemia (CLI) [5]. The optimal approach to treating FP atherosclerotic disease remains controversial [6]. Although the use of endovascular treatment has been increasing over the past decades, there remain a significant number of patients best treated with open surgery. The indications for infrainguinal bypass include the presence of CLI manifested by tissue loss, rest pain, or gangrene. Persistent lifestyle-limiting claudication after medical therapy is also a relative indication.

A. K. Natour
Henry Ford Hospital, Detroit, MI, USA
e-mail: anatour1@hfhs.org

L. Kabbani (✉)
Department of Surgery, Henry Ford Hospital, Detroit, MI, USA

Wayne State University, Detroit, MI, USA

Michigan State University, Detroit, MI, USA

Henry Ford Hospital, Heart and Vascular Institute, Detroit, MI, USA
e-mail: lkabban1@hfhs.org

S. S. Hans et al. (eds.), *Primary and Repeat Arterial Reconstructions*,
https://doi.org/10.1007/978-3-031-13897-3_32

Surgical Anatomy

Common Femoral Artery

The common femoral artery (CFA) is the continuation of the external iliac artery at the level of the inguinal ligament. It's located in the femoral triangle, a wedge-shaped area situated within the superomedial aspect of the anterior thigh. The femoral triangle is bounded superiorly by the inguinal ligament, medially by the adductor longus muscle, and laterally by the sartorius muscle (Fig. 32.1). Within the femoral triangle, the anatomical relationship from medial to lateral is femoral vein, CFA, and femoral nerve (Fig. 32.1). The vein and artery are contained within a fascial covering called a fascial sheath while the nerve is not. The CFA branches in the femoral triangle into the profunda femoris and superficial femoral artery (SFA). The latter exits at the adductor hiatus to continue as the popliteal artery.

Popliteal Artery

The popliteal fossa is located at the back of the knee joint defined anteriorly by the upper tibia, femur, and popliteus muscle; laterally by biceps femoris and gastrocnemius muscles; and medially by semitendinosus and semimembranosus muscles.

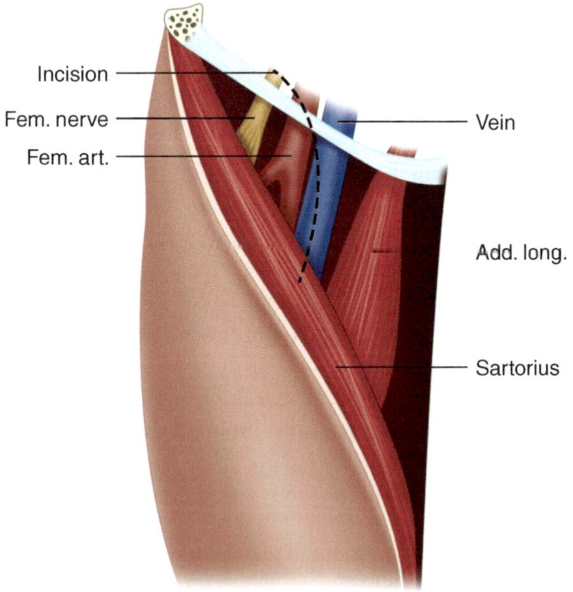

Fig. 32.1 Groin incision in the femoral triangle

The SFA artery exits the adductor hiatus at the apex of the popliteal fossa where it becomes the popliteal artery. The popliteal artery ends at the lower border of the popliteus muscle, where it branches into the anterior tibial artery and the tibioperoneal trunk.

Preoperative Planning

Traditionally, angiography has been the gold standard imaging modality. However, computed tomographic angiography has been used more frequently to assess the thigh vessels.

Proximal Anastomotic Site Assessment and Selection

Traditionally, the CFA is the inflow vessel of choice. If the CFA exhibits significant atherosclerotic disease, consideration of CFA endarterectomy is prudent. The profunda femoris or SFA provide effective sites when appropriately selected and have the added benefit of shortening the conduit length used. In reoperative procedures, access to the CFA may be limited, and the SFA or profunda femoris could serve as alternate inflow site (Figs. 32.2, 32.3, and 32.4).

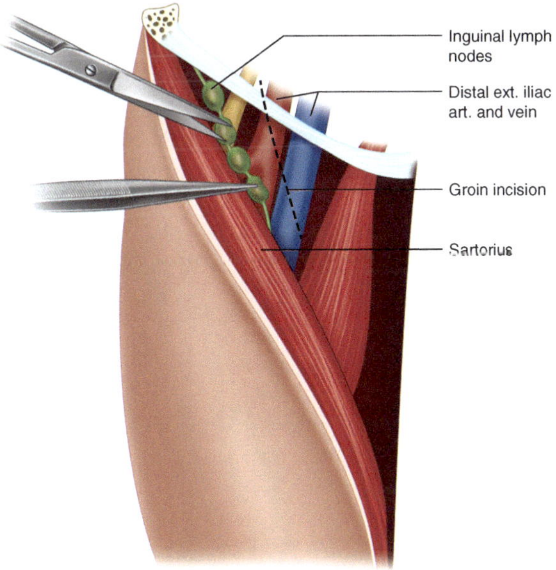

Fig. 32.2 Opening of the deep fascia over the femoral vessels

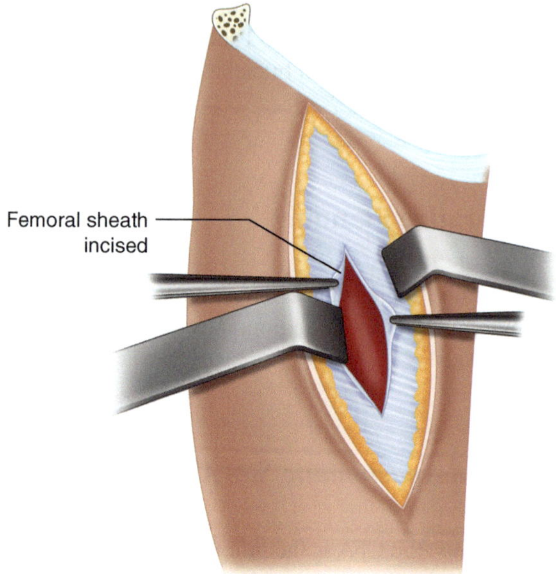

Fig. 32.3 Opening of the femoral sheath

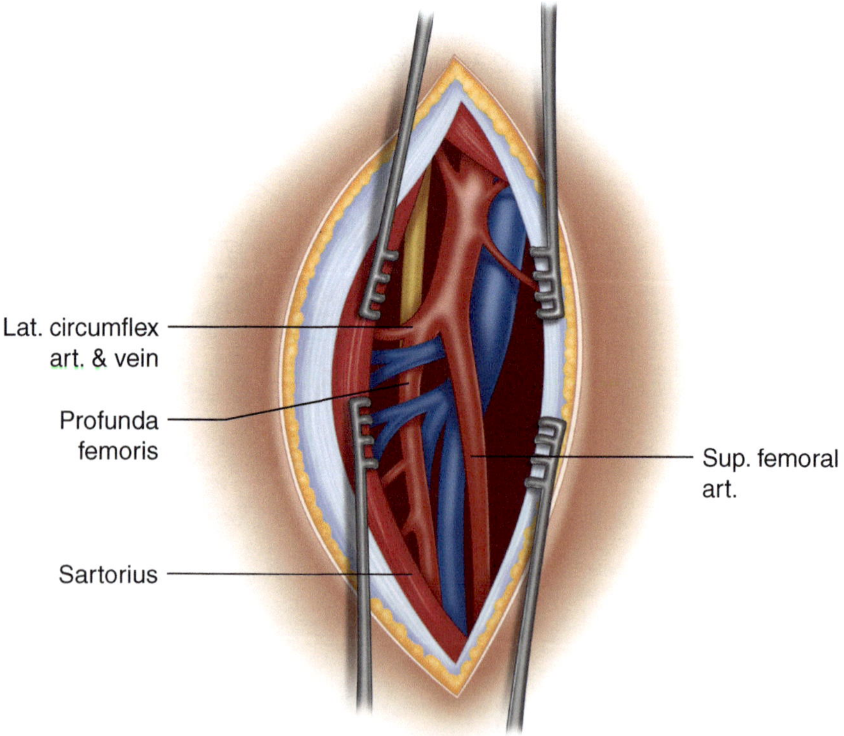

Fig. 32.4 Exposure of the femoral artery, its branches, and accompanying veins

Distal Anastomotic Site Assessment and Selection

The distal anastomotic site should be stenotic free and has at least one runoff artery to the foot. In addition, arteries distal to the outflow vessel should be free of hemodynamically significant atherosclerotic disease.

Conduit Selection

The two primary types of conduit available for bypass are autogenous and prosthetic. Autogenous conduits include the aforementioned veins, whereas prosthetic conduits include Dacron, polytetrafluoroethylene (PTFE), expanded PTFE, and polyester.

Autogenous Conduit

In general, autogenous veins are preferred due to their higher patency and limb salvage rates in infrainguinal bypass procedures [7–10]. The GSV is the most used and best-performing autogenous conduit, providing 70% for above the knee and 50–70% below the knee patency at 5 and 3 years postoperatively, respectively [7, 8, 11, 12]. The GSV could be used in either reversed or in situ configurations, with equal effectiveness [13, 14]. In the absence of appropriate GSV, alternative sources of veins could be used, including harvesting the cephalic or basilic veins, or connecting spliced short segments of veins with venovenostomies to achieve appropriate graft length. These alternative veins may also be used in reversed or in situ configurations; however, due to their smaller size and thinner walls, they are more prone to injury and hence are more commonly used as reversed grafts.

Preoperative Vein Assessment

Preoperative vein mapping is done via duplex imaging to determine the quality of the vein conduit. Namely, the vein diameter, flow, compressibility, and wall thickness are evaluated. For optimal patency, the diameter of the vein should be at least 3 mm.

Prosthetic Conduit

For patients with no suitable autogenous conduits, prosthetic grafts are used. The expanded PTFE is (ePTFE) is the most used prosthetic graft for lower extremity bypasses. It provides slightly lower patency than autogenous graft in above-knee

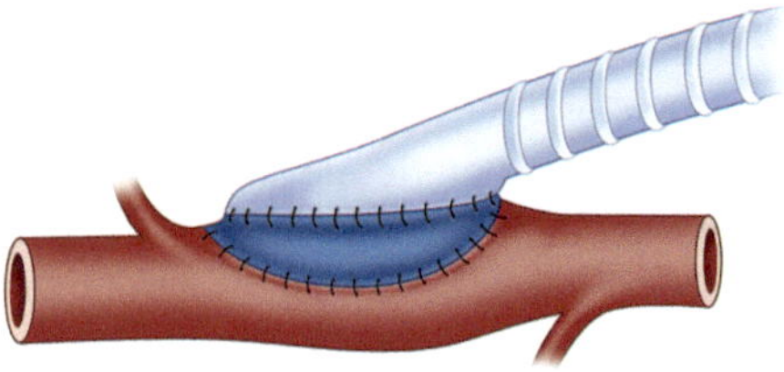

Fig. 32.5 Miller vein cuff

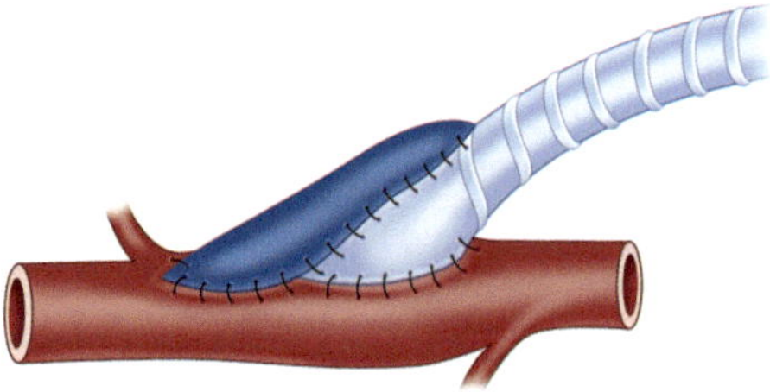

Fig. 32.6 Taylor vein patch

popliteal bypasses [8, 15]. In below-the-knee popliteal bypasses, prosthetic bypasses have uniformly poor patencies [12]. Adjunctive Miller vein cuff (Fig. 32.5) or Taylor vein patch (Fig. 32.6) could be used to further improve the patency of below-the-knee prosthetic bypasses [16]. Prosthetic grafts do have some advantages, including decreased operative time, spare vein harvesting with its associated potential wound complications, and provide better size match to the inflow and outflow arteries.

Operative Technique

Vein Harvesting

The GSV is found on the medial aspect on the femoral triangle. Preoperative vein mapping can be used to delineate the GSV pathway.

Incision

1. Using a #10 blade, an oblique incision directly overlying the GSV is made to prevent subcutaneous skin flaps. The GSV can be identified in the fossa ovalis as it enters the common femoral vein.
2. Once the GSV is identified, distal circumferential dissection directly over the vein is made. To avoid direct grasping of the vein with forceps, silicone elastomer loops can be used.

3. Skip incisions are preferred over continuous incision to minimize wound complications. Typically, three incisions are made each extended for 8 to 10 cm with two intervening skin bridges of around 4 cm. The proximal incision is used for exposure of the femoral vessels and to harvest the proximal great saphenous vein. If performing a below-the-knee bypass, a fourth incision is made below the knee.
4. 3-0 silk sutures are used to ligate small vein tributaries. It's advisable to leave a short stump when tying next to the vein to prevent graft stenosis.
5. Dissection is continued distally until adequate vein length is achieved.
6. A small clamp is placed flush with the common femoral vein. The GSV is then ligated proximally, and two layers of monofilaments are used to oversaw the stump.
7. A bulldog clamp is used to clamp the proximal aspect of the graft, and heparinized blood with papaverine is flushed under gentle pressure from the distal end to identify untied branches or tears. Avoid overdistention of the vein.
8. 6-0 propylene sutures can be used to repair any leak due to tears or small, untied branches. Any focal areas with stenosis are resected.
9. Graft is then temporarily stored in a chilled, heparinized blood until creation of the tunnel.

Femoral to Above-Knee Popliteal Bypass

CFA Exposure

Incision

1. A vertical incision is made 1 to 2 cm proximal to the inguinal crease directly over the femoral pulse and continued 3 to 4 cm distally (Fig. 32.1). If the pulse is absent, the common femoral artery can be located two fingerbreadths lateral to the pubic tubercle.
2. Electrocautery is used to deepen the dissection and expose the femoral artery in a longitudinal fashion to avoid lymphatic disruption (Figs. 32.2 and 32.3). Lymphoadipose tissue (inguinal lymph nodes) is mobilized medially. The deep fascia is incised, and the femoral sheath can be adequately exposed using self-retraining retractors (Fig. 32.4). Any bleeding or lymphatic disruption is controlled with ligation.
3. The dissection is carried proximally to the level of the inguinal ligament and distally to the level of the SFA and profunda femoris on the anterior surface of the CFA. Dissection of the profunda femoris at its origin should be done carefully to avoid disrupting collateral branches and the one or two satellite vein branches crossing at its initial anterior segment.
4. Silastic vessel loops are placed around each vessel using a right-angled clamp to establish vessel control.

Above-Knee Popliteal Artery Exposure

Incision

1. With the knee flexed at 30° and leg externally rotated, an incision is made anterior to the sartorius muscle in the lower third of the thigh and extended to the medial aspect of the knee (Fig. 32.7).
2. Electrocautery is used to dissect the deeper tissue and fascia anterior to the sartorius muscle, and the sartorius is retracted posteriorly.
3. The popliteal fossa is entered, and the popliteal artery can be identified with palpation. The sheath of the artery is opened, and division of the adductor magnus tendon may be required to achieve adequate exposure.
4. Venous network on the surface of the artery is separated from the adventitia, and the branches are divided and ligated.
5. The artery is carefully mobilized from the popliteal vein. The popliteal artery is then freed for an appropriate healthy length, and vessel loops are placed around it proximally and distally (Fig. 32.8).

Conduit Tunneling

A tunneling device is passed from the femoral incision to the popliteal fossa below the sartorius muscle. A red rubber catheter attached to an aortic clamp can be used as a tunneling device as well.

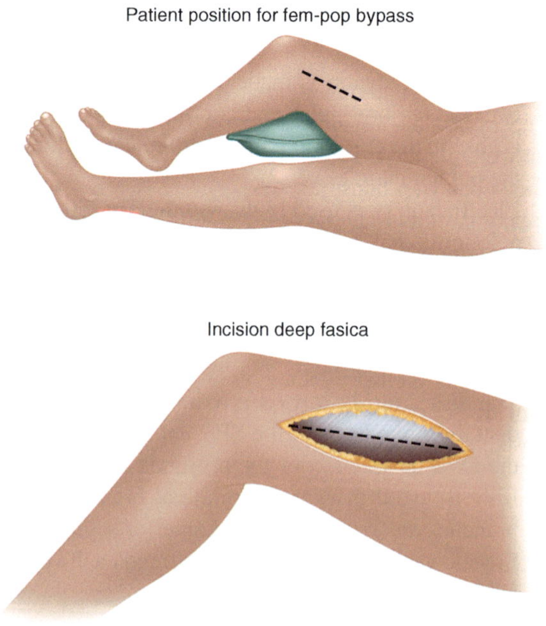

Fig. 32.7 Patient positioning and distal incision with opening of deep fascia for AK femoral-popliteal bypass

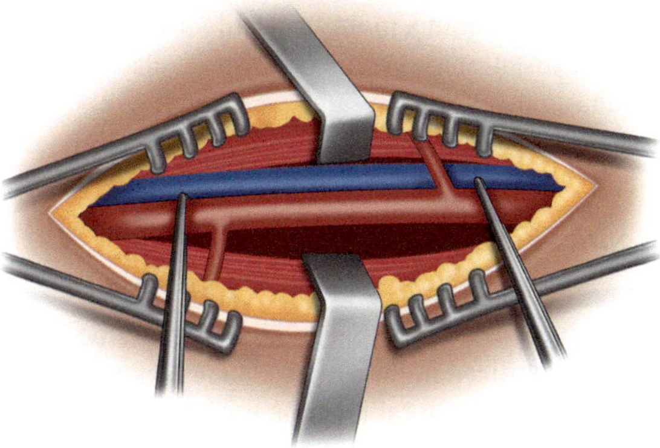

Fig. 32.8 Exposure of the popliteal artery above the knee

Proximal and Distal Anastomosis

Heparin is administered at least 5 min before arterial clamping. Usually 100 U of heparin are given for each kg of body weight. Activated clotting times are monitored, and the anticoagulation is adjusted appropriately. Proximal anastomosis is typically performed first after the clamps are applied to the inflow vessels.

Incision

1. A #11 knife blade is used to perform a longitudinal arteriotomy on the anterior wall of the CFA. Arteriotomy is then enlarged with a scalpel or Potts angled scissors to achieve an opening length of approximately twice the vessel diameter.
2. A longitudinal incision over the end of the graft is made. If using a reversed GSV technique, the segment is reversed so that its proximal end becomes its distal end for anastomosis.
3. 5-0 polypropylene continuous suture starting at the heel of the graft and proceeding toward the toe is made in an end-to-side fashion.
4. The clamps are released after flushing, and if a vein graft is used, it is distended and checked for bleeding.
5. The graft is then tunneled. The graft is marked for orientation and then attached to the obturator of the tunneler and pulled into position.
6. The tunneler is removed, and graft orientation is checked and insured not to be twisted.
7. A soft clamp is placed on the proximal end of the graft until the distal anastomosis is complete.
8. Vessel clamps or loops are used to control the above-knee popliteal artery. After the arteriotomy is performed, any atheromatous or calcified edges are excised with scissors.

9. The orientation of the graft is rechecked, and the bulldog clamp is released and should result in a highly pulsatile flow through the graft.
10. The distal anastomosis is sewn in place using 6-0 prolene in an end-to-side anastomosis.

In Situ Vein Grafts

1. The proximal GSV is identified as described previously. The distal segment is then mobilized in the projected anastomotic location.
2. The saphenofemoral junction is divided, and the first venous valves are removed with Potts scissors under direct visualization.
3. The proximal anastomosis is performed next in an end-to-side fashion. Valvulotomies are then created starting from the distal GSV and advanced proximally. Blood flow through the vein is then analyzed and should be pulsatile.
4. Distal anastomosis is performed, and the graft is evaluated with Doppler ultrasound to exclude any continuous flow indicating an arteriovenous fistula (AV). Ligation of any AV fistula identified should be done before closure.

Femoral to Below-Knee Popliteal Bypass

If the upper and middle portion of the popliteal artery exhibit significant atherosclerosis, the lower portion is used instead.

Below-Knee Popliteal Artery Exposure

Incision

1. With the knee flexed at 30° and leg externally rotated, a vertical incision is made 1–2 cm behind the posteromedial surface of the tibia and extended one third of the way down the calf (Fig. 32.9). Care must be taken to avoid injury to the GSV. If a GSV is to be used, the same incision can be made for artery exposure and vein harvesting.
2. The crural fascia is exposed and opened along its fibers. The sartorius, gracilis, and semitendinosus tendons are mobilized and divided if more proximal exposure is needed (Fig. 32.10).
3. The medial head of the gastrocnemius muscle is mobilized and retracted posteriorly, exposing the neurovascular structures within the popliteal fossa (Fig. 32.11).

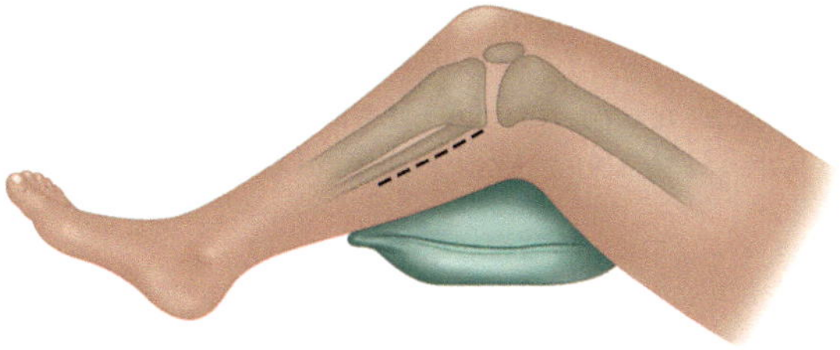

Fig. 32.9 Patient position and incision line for below-the-knee femoral-popliteal bypass

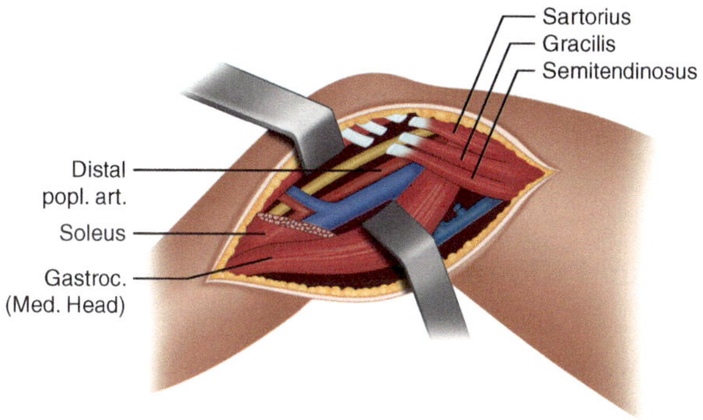

Fig. 32.10 Exposure of the distal popliteal artery

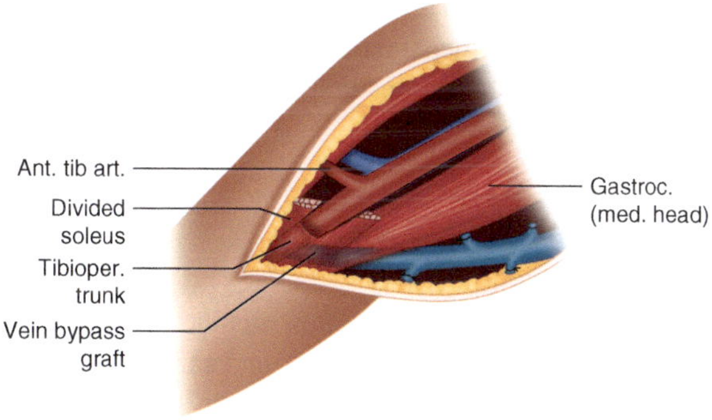

Fig. 32.11 Exposure of the popliteal artery bifurcation with a partial takedown of the soleus from the soleal line

4. Metzenbaum or tenotomy scissors are used to enter the fascial sheath. The popliteal veins are carefully dissected from the artery, and associated bridging veins are divided with 3-0 silk sutures.
5. Vessel loops are used to obtain proximal and distal control.

Tunneling

The tunneling device is passed through the two heads of the gastrocnemius muscle in the popliteal fossa, advanced posterior to the knee between the femoral condyles, and then through the subsartorial space to the groin incision. The graft is passed through the tunnel while maintaining proper orientation.

Proximal and Distal Anastomosis

Same steps are performed for the proximal and distal anastomosis as described in the femoral to above-knee popliteal bypass section.

Intraoperative Assessment of Femoral-Popliteal Bypass

A Doppler probe can be used to check for the presence and quality of blood flow to the foot. Duplex imaging of the graft is used to assess any stenosis, outflow obstruction, or other potential conduit defects. Similarly, intraoperative angiogram can be performed.

Wound Closure

The wound can be closed once the bypass is determined to be successful. Hemostasis is then achieved with reversal of heparin. Absorbable sutures are used to approximate the fascia, taking care not to close the deep fascia of the popliteal fossa. Subcutaneous tissue is then closed in layers, and the skin is finally closed subcuticularly. Skin closure in an interrupted fashion using running nylon sutures is done for patients with significant edema or diabetes. If there are any concerns for lymphatic leak, closed suction drains may be placed in the groin incision.

Complications

1. Possible early complications include postoperative bleeding, wound infection and dehiscence, lymphedema, and early graft thrombosis (<30 days).
2. Possible late complications include late graft thrombosis, arterial aneurysms, infection, and persistent lymphedema.

References

1. Henry TD, Schwartz RS, Hirsch AT. "POBA plus": will the balloon regain its luster? Circulation. 2008;118(13):1309–11.
2. Norgren L, Hiatt WR, Dormandy JA, et al. Inter-society consensus for the management of peripheral arterial disease (TASC II). J Vasc Surg. 2007;45(Suppl S):S5–S67.
3. Regensteiner JG, Hiatt WR, Coll JR, et al. The impact of peripheral arterial disease on healthrelated quality of life in the peripheral arterial disease awareness, risk, and treatment: new resources for survival (PARTNERS) program. Vasc Med. 2008;13(1):15–24.

4. Hirsch AT, Hartman L, Town RJ, et al. National health care costs of peripheral arterial disease in the Medicare population. Vasc Med. 2008;13(3):209–15.
5. Femoral Endarterectomy and Femoral Popliteal Bypass Christopher J. Smolock Y Keith Glover Netter's Surgical Anatomy and Approaches second eddition, Elsevier, Inc. 2021;479–486.
6. Erwin PA, Shishehbor MH. Contemporary management of femoral popliteal revascularization.
7. Klinkert P, Schepers A, Burger DHC, et al. Vein versus polytetrafluoroethylene in above-knee femoropopliteal bypass grafting: five-year results of a randomized controlled trial. J Vasc Surg. 2003;37:149–55.
8. Pereira CE, Albers M, Romiti M, et al. Meta-analysis of femoropopliteal bypass grafts for lower extremity arterial insufficiency. J Vasc Surg. 2006;44:510–7.
9. Conte MS, Pomposelli FB, Clair DG, Geraghty PJ, JF MK, Mills JL, Moneta GL, Murad MH, Powell RJ, Reed AB, Schanzer A, Sidawy AN, Society for Vascular Surgery; Society for Vascular Surgery Lower Extremity Guidelines Writing Group. Society for Vascular Surgery practice guidelines for atherosclerotic occlusive disease of the lower extremities: management of asymptomatic disease and claudication. J Vasc Surg. 2015;61(3 Suppl):2S–41S.
10. Ambler GK, Twine CP. Graft type for femoro-popliteal bypass surgery. Cochrane Database Syst Rev. 2018;2:CD001487.
11. Johnson WC, Lee KK. A comparative evaluation of polytetrafluoroethylene, umbilical vein, and saphenous vein bypass grafts for femoral-popliteal aboveknee revascularization: a prospective randomized Department of Veterans Affairs cooperative study. J Vasc Surg. 2000;32:268–77.
12. Veith FJ, Gupta SK, Ascer E, et al. Six-year prospective multicenter randomized comparison of autologous saphenous vein and expanded polytetrafluoroethylene grafts in infrainguinal arterial reconstructions. J Vasc Surg. 1986;3:104–14.
13. Harris PL, Veith FJ, Shanik GD, et al. Prospective randomized comparison of in situ and reversed infrapopliteal vein grafts. Br J Surg. 1993;80:173–6.
14. Watelet J, Soury P, Menard JF, et al. Femoropopliteal bypass: in situ or reversed vein grafts? Ten-year results of a randomized prospective study. Ann Vasc Surg. 1999;18:149–57.
15. Mills JL Sr. P values may lack power: the choice of conduit for above-knee femoropopliteal bypass graft. J Vasc Surg. 2000;32:402–5.
16. Stonebridge PA, Prescott RJ, Ruckley CV. Randomized trial comparing infrainguinal polytetrafluoroethylene bypass grafting with and without vein interposition cuff at the distal anastomosis. The Joint Vascular Research Group. J Vasc Surg. 1997;26:543–50.

Chapter 33
Femoral-Infrapopliteal (Crural and Paramalleolar) Bypass Graft

Sachinder Singh Hans

Femoral-infrapopliteal bypass remains one of the most common open vascular reconstructions performed to treat patients with critical limb ischemia (ischemic rest pain, ischemic ulceration, and toe gangrene). In general, bypass to infrapopliteal arteries is not offered to patients for treatment of intermittent claudication.

Preoperative Planning

Preoperative planning is pivotal for infrapopliteal bypass reconstruction. Detailed anatomic characterization is necessary to define adequate inflow vessel free of proximal hemodynamic significant stenosis, as well as distal outflow arterial target. The ideal distal target must be of adequate size, axially patent to the foot, and sufficiently free of calcium that performing an anastomosis is feasible. Advances in computed tomographic arteriography (CTA) and magnetic resonance angiography (MRA) have led to increasing number of patients undergoing noninvasive imaging studies for this assessment [1]. However, both CTA and MRA may overestimate the degree of stenosis/occlusion, especially in cases of significant calcification and thus fail to identify possible targets for distal bypass. If a target for distal bypass is not well identified with CTA or MRA, high-quality catheter-directed, digital angiography should be performed prior to determining a patient not anatomically a candidate for bypass.

S. S. Hans (✉)
Vascular and Endovascular Services, Henry Ford Macomb Hospital,
Clinton Twp, MI, USA

S. S. Hans et al. (eds.), *Primary and Repeat Arterial Reconstructions*,
https://doi.org/10.1007/978-3-031-13897-3_33

Proximal Anastomotic Site

See discussion in Chap. 32.

Distal Anastomotic Site

The selected distal target vessel should be free of significant atherosclerotic disease from the planned site of anastomosis and distal to that site. However, the presence or absence of plantar arch should not be a sole consideration for recommendation of distal arterial bypass graft. In selecting a target artery for patients undergoing distal bypass with advanced ischemia of the foot (gangrene of the toes), posterior tibial and anterior tibial artery of suitable diameter and free of significant disease should be preferred over the peroneal artery, though later has proven satisfactory target artery for distal bypass in patients with occlusion of both posterior and anterior tibial artery. If all the crural arteries are patent (uncommon findings in patients with critical limb ischemia), the author's preference is the posterior tibial artery, then anterior tibial, followed by peroneal artery.

Conduit Selection

The most satisfactory conduit for infrapopliteal bypass is autologous vein. Options include ipsilateral and contralateral greater saphenous vein, lesser saphenous vein, cephalic/basilic vein, and occasionally superficial femoral vein. Because of the better size matching, author prefers in situ configuration to reversed vein as a conduit for femoral crural and paramalleolar bypasses. Preoperative vein mapping with duplex imaging should be performed to evaluate the diameter, compressibility, and wall thickness of the conduit. For optimal patency, the vein diameter should be at least 3 mm, although satisfactory results have been reported with compressible veins between 2 and 3 mm used for tibial/peroneal artery bypasses. If adequate length of greater saphenous vein is not available, a variety or combination of veins can be used. Upper extremity veins (cephalic or basilic) can provide adequate length, but due to their thin wall harvesting, the veins can be challenging. Lesser saphenous vein (patient prone) has also provided suitable conduits for femoral popliteal/infrapopliteal bypasses. Short segments of veins can be connected to one another with venovenostomies to obtain adequate length. The ends of each vein are spatulated when performing spliced vein bypasses to aide in creation of wide anastomosis. As a last resort for limb salvage, a prosthetic graft may occasionally be considered with the use of a distal vein patch or cuff.

Vessel Control

Small arteries in the calf and distally are controlled with nontraumatic clamps such as Yasergill (cerebral aneurysm clamp, Aesculap Tuttlingen Germany) or a micro bulldog clamp. However, clamping a small diameter calcified artery can result in dissection with resulting occlusion. Tourniquet occlusion in the thigh prior to the performance of distal anastomosis aids in "bloodless" visualization of the operative field with minimal dissection of target vessels in the calf is a significant advance in performance of small vessel anastomosis for lower extremity arterial reconstruction. Since clamp application to the calcified and friable artery is avoided, early failure may be improved [2, 3]. Uncommonly in patients with severe arterial calcification, tourniquet occlusion may not be successful as arteries may be incompressible.

Special Considerations

Skip incisions in the thigh and calf decrease the incidence of surgical site infection. Meticulous medial mobilization of the groin lymph nodes and ligation of the lymphatics decrease the incidence of postoperative lymph leak.

In Situ Bypass

1. In some instances, greater saphenous veins may not be able to reach the common femoral artery for proximal anastomosis. Therefore, common femoral endarterectomy with patch graft is a useful adjunct.
2. Valvulotome – Several commercially available valvulotome LeMaiter, WL Gore, and leather modification of Mills valvulotome are available, and operator should be familiar with their use.
3. Arteriovenous fistula – Careful ligation of significant size branches of greater saphenous vein is necessary to avoid residual arterial venous fistula that may threaten the patency of the graft. Visual inspection of the side branches, Doppler insolation, and in some instances completion arteriography will aide in the detection of medium to large size arteriovenous fistulas. In general, if the fistula's communication does not outline the deep venous system, it may not require ligation.

Distal Anastomosis to Posterior Tibial Artery

Exposure of Posterior Tibial Artery

A proximal one-third of the posterior tibial artery – the proximal segment of posterior tibial artery can be exposed via the popliteal fossa. Tendons of the pes anserinus (sartorius), gracilis, and semitendinosus may need to be divided at their insertion into the tibia. The medial head of the gastrocnemius is retracted posteriorly, and the soleus muscle is taken down from the soleal line (Figs. 33.1, 33.2, and 33.3), taking care to protect the underlying vessels. It is not necessary to divide the origin of the anterior tibial vein for exposure of the proximal posterior tibial artery. For exposure of the distal popliteal artery and its bifurcation for femoral popliteal bypass below the knee the origin of anterior tibial vein as it crosses transversely at the popliteal artery bifurcation. Distal portion of the tibial-peroneal trunk and its division into posterior tibial and peroneal artery can be visualized, and anastomosis carried out with 7-0 CV polypropylene continuous suture usually starting in a parachute manner and then as a continuous suture at the apex of the anastomosis to be tied on the lateral wall of the arteriotomy in the proximal posterior tibial artery. This should be carried out as the arteriotomy with Potts scissors is from the 1 o'clock to the 7 o'clock position so that autogenous vein is in satisfactory alignment with the plane of posterior tibial artery thus avoiding any kink at the distal anastomosis.

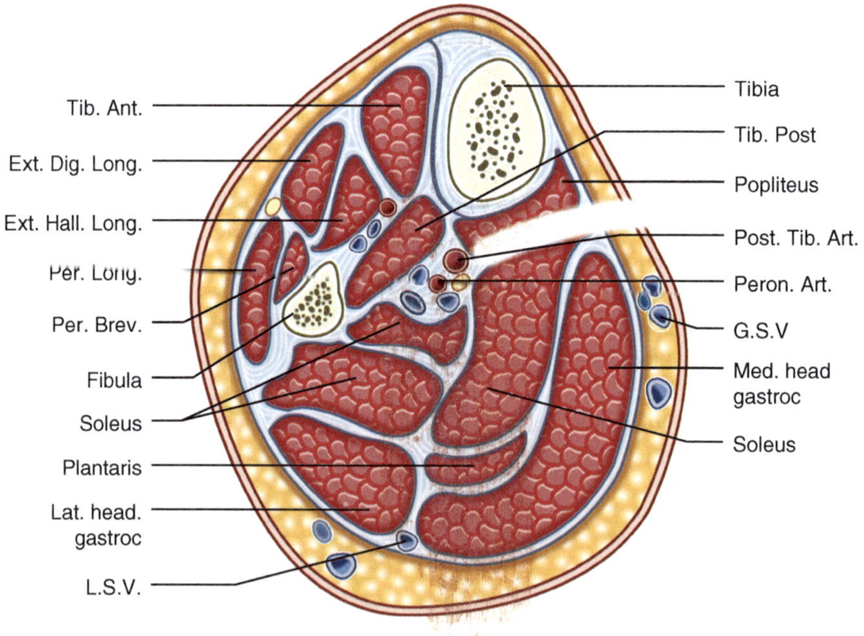

Fig. 33.1 Transverse section of upper leg 10 cm below the knee joint for exposure of proximal post. Tibial artery

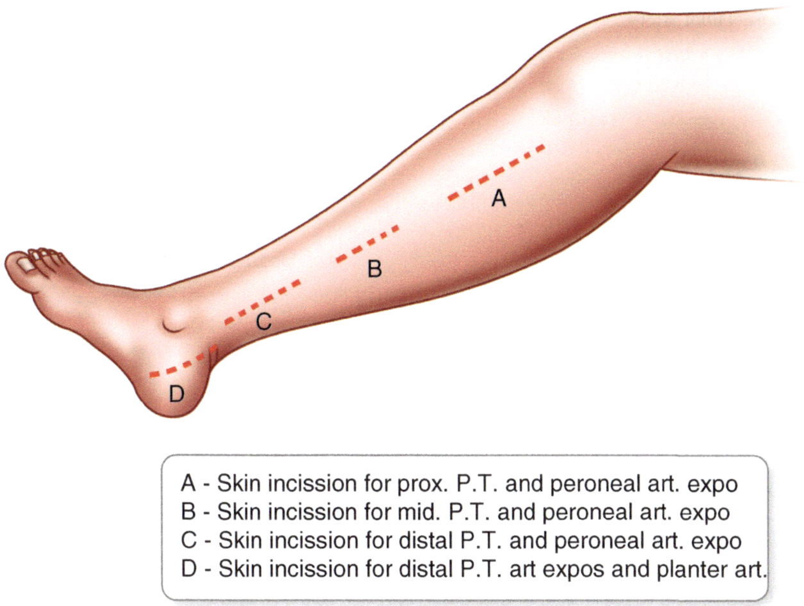

Fig. 33.2 Skin incision sites for exposure of post. Tibial and peroneal artery

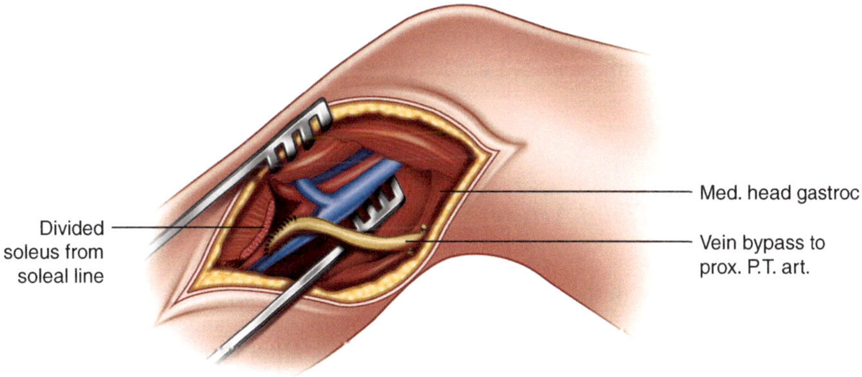

Fig. 33.3 Exposure of proximal post. Tibial and peroneal artery with takedown of soleus from the soleal line

Mid-Segment Posterior Tibial Artery

The exposure of the mid-posterior tibial artery in the mid-calf is obtained by an incision, approximately 8–10 cm in length performed 2 cm posterior and parallel to the medial border of the tibia (Fig. 33.2). The medial head of gastrocnemius is retracted

Fig. 33.4 (**a**, **b**) Exposure of mid-post. Tibial artery

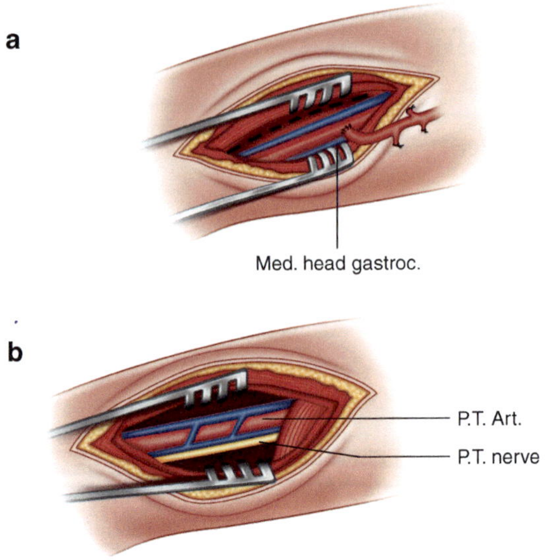

posteriorly along with the soleus. The neurovascular bundle lies in the groove between the flexor digital longus medially and tibialis posterior laterally (Fig. 33.4a, b). Posterior retraction of the soleus and gastrocnemius may result in tear of small arterial and venous branches. Posterior tibial artery at this site is accompanied by vena comitans with crossing veins. The crossing veins should be carefully ligated and divided with 4-0 silk, and 2–3 cm length of posterior tibial artery is carefully exposed.

Distal Posterior Tibial Artery

Posterior tibial artery in the distal one-third of the leg is exposed via longitudinal incision between the post promedial border of the tibia and tendons achilles (Fig. 33.2). The deep fascia anterior to the tendons achilles is incised, and the neurovascular bundle is exposed between the flexor digital longus and flexor hallucis longus. In situ bypass can be easily routed for distal anastomosis at this site. Reversed vein bypass (prosthetic graft-uncommonly) is tunneled from the groin to the popliteal fossa deep to the sartorius and then brought down distally in the subcutaneous position. At the ankle, longitudinal incision is made in the middle of the tip of the medial malleolus and the calcaneus, and the fascial sheath is incised exposing the posterior tibial artery with accompanying veins (Fig. 33.5). Distal anastomosis should be carried out to one of the plantar arteries if necessary, plantar arteries exposing the bifurcation of posterior tibial artery toward the heel. Lateral

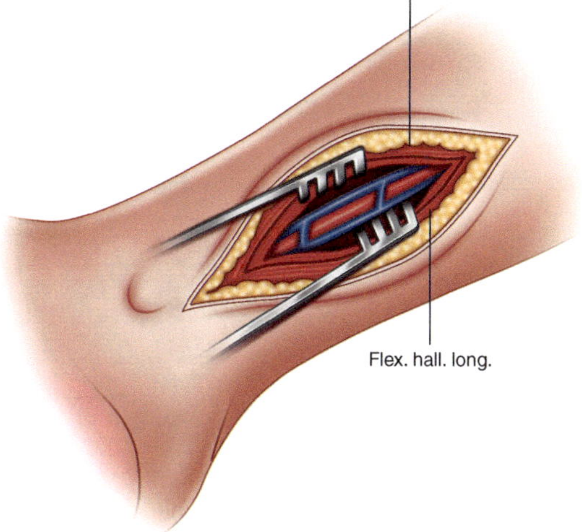

Fig. 33.5 Exposure of distal post. Tibial artery

plantar artery is usually larger than the medial plantar artery. Anastomosis to plantar arteries can be formed in the first 2 cm and may require partial division of the origin of plantar muscles (Fig. 33.6).

Bypass to the Anterior Tibial Artery

Distal anastomosis to the anterior tibial artery in the upper and middle third of the leg is best accomplished via anterior approach (Fig. 33.7). The limb is positioned with 60°–90° knee flexion with a knee "bump" associated with dorsi flexion of the foot, and the operating table slightly tilted to the contralateral side (if right femoral anterior tibial artery is planned, the right side of the table is tilted upward and the left side of the table is tilted downward about 15°–20°). A longitudinal incision about 8–10 cm length is made over the patent anterior tibial artery just lateral to the tibial crest (Fig. 33.8). The fascia is incised longitudinally, and the dissection is done over the palpable groove between the tibialis anterior and the extensor digitorum longus muscle (Fig. 33.9). The neurovascular bundle is exposed, and the Weitlaner retractor is applied for exposure. The artery is carefully separated from the vena comitans, and bridging veins are ligated and divided. Anterior tibial artery is carefully mobilized with a double-loop silastic loop if tourniquet occlusion technique is not used. An adequate tunnel from the medial aspect of upper calf to the anterior tibial artery via interosseous membrane is constructed for the passage of vein graft (Fig. 33.10). In patients with tourniquet occlusion, complete mobilization of the anterior tibial artery is not necessary.

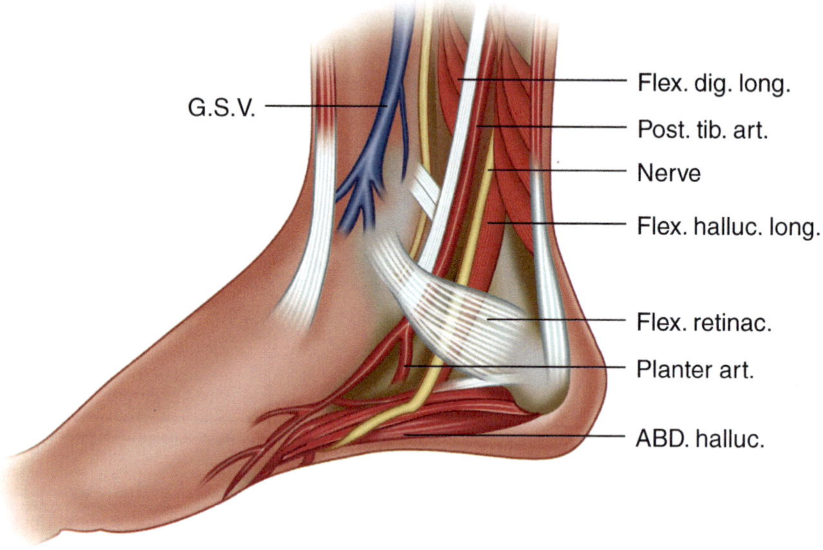

Fig. 33.6 Exposure of distal post. Tibial artery and prox. Planter arteries

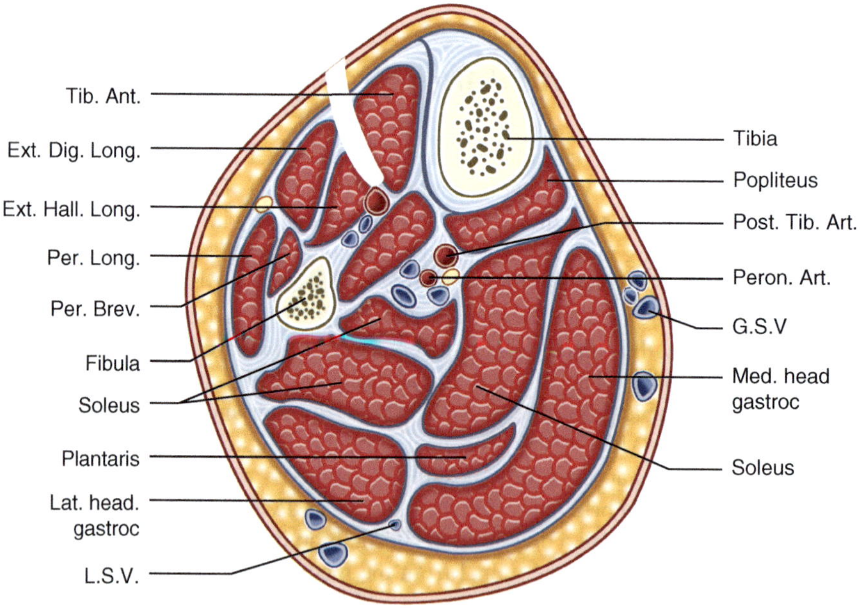

Fig. 33.7 Transverse section of upper leg for exposure of proximal ant. Tibial artery

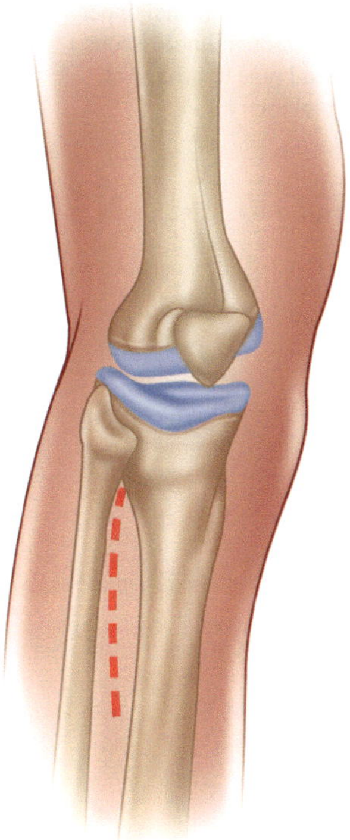

Fig. 33.8 Skin incision for exposure of prox. Ant. tibial artery

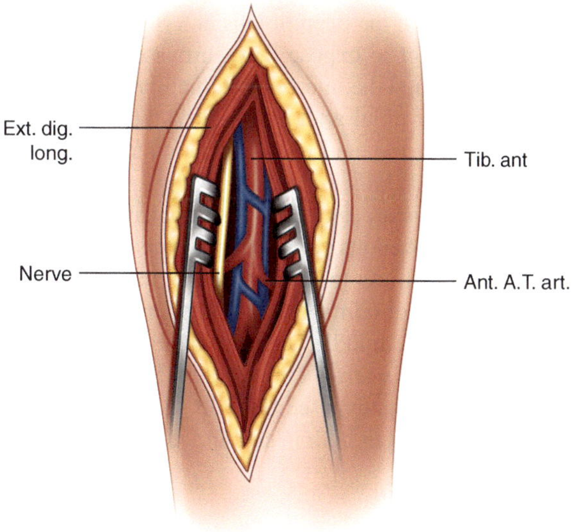

Fig. 33.9 Ant. tibial artery exposure proximally between tib. Ant. and ext. dig. long

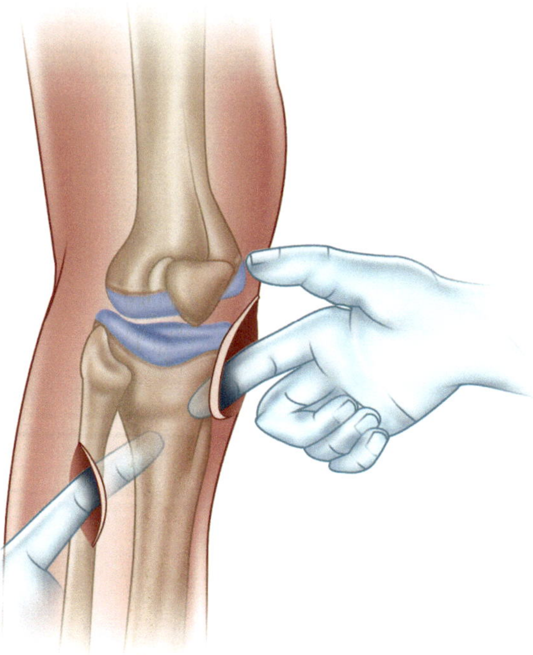

Fig. 33.10 Creation of tunnel from medial upper calf through interosseous membrane to prox. Ant. tibial artery

In exposure of the anterior tibial artery in middle third of the leg following a longitudinal skin incision about 8–10 cm long in the anterior compartment about 2 cm lateral to the lateral border of tibia, the fascia is incised, and dissection is performed between the deep tibialis anterior muscle, and the extensor hallucis longus muscle in order to expose the neurovascular bundle, and the vein bypass graft is tunneled through the interosseous membrane for performance of distal anastomosis to the anterior tibial artery. Similarly, the dorsalis pedis artery is identified proximally between the tendons of extensor hallucis longus and extensor digitorum longus and more distally between the extensor hallucis brevis and the digitorum longus. In situ vein bypass can be easily tunneled at this level because of the proximity of the greater saphenous vein to the dorsalis pedis artery.

The anastomosis to distal anterior tibial and dorsalis pedis artery is performed following a longitudinal or a slightly curved incision made just above the ankle and continued in the middle between the medial and lateral malleolus for exposure of the dorsalis pedis artery (Fig. 33.11). Extensor retinaculum is divided, and neurovascular bundle is exposed (Fig. 33.12). The subcutaneous plane is suitable for the tunnel to be used in both in situ and reversed vein bypasses at this level.

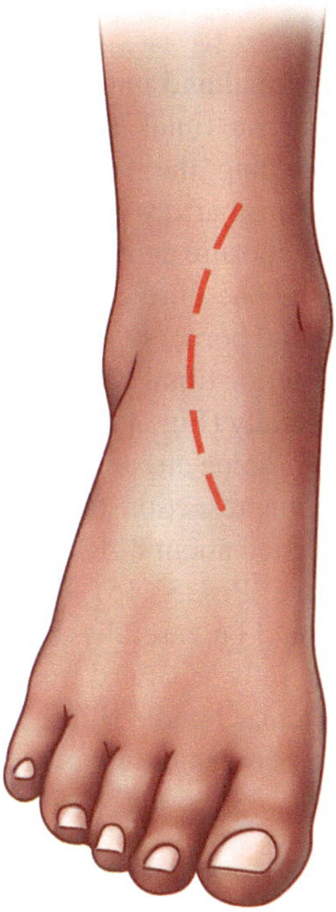

Fig. 33.11 Skin incision for exposure of distal ant. Tibial artery and dorsalis pedis artery

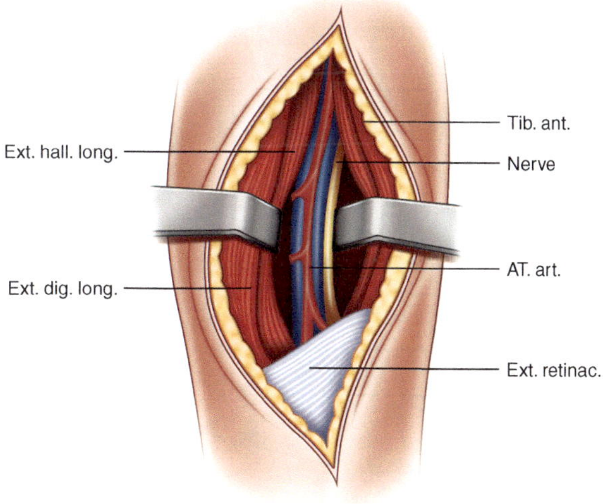

Fig. 33.12 Exposure of distal ant. Tibial artery and dorsalis pedis artery

Anastomosis to Peroneal Artery

Proximal and middle third of the peroneal artery can be exposed like exposure of posterior tibial artery with takedown of soleus muscle from the soleal line and unroofing the fascia covering the flexor hallucis longus muscle (Fig. 33.13). Peroneal artery is the deepest artery and runs along the medial border of the fibula. Its exposure can be difficult in patients with "heavy" legs. The peroneal artery in the distal one-third can also be performed via medial incision 1.5–2 cm posterior to the medial border of the tibia and dissection carried out similarly to the exposure of the posterior tibial artery between flexor hallucis longus and tibialis posterior antero-medially (Fig. 33.14).

In some circumstances, particularly in patients with obesity, lateral approach following resection of the distal fibula with a podiatric oscillating saw following a skin incision about 8–10 cm long on the skin covering the fibula at this lower end can be made (Fig. 33.15). As the fibula is divided, the neurovascular bundle underneath should be carefully protected with periosteal elevators, and periosteum should be carefully separated from the bone circumferentially to prevent damage to the neurovascular bundle (Figs. 33.16 and 33.17). More commonly, the medial approach to the peroneal artery is preferable in its distal one-third segment.

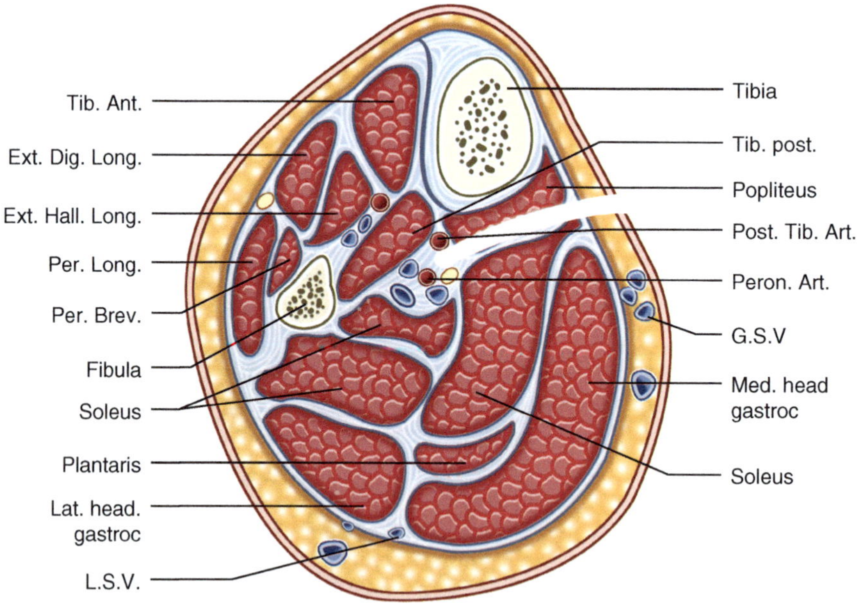

Fig. 33.13 Transverse section of upper right leg for exposure of proximal peroneal artery

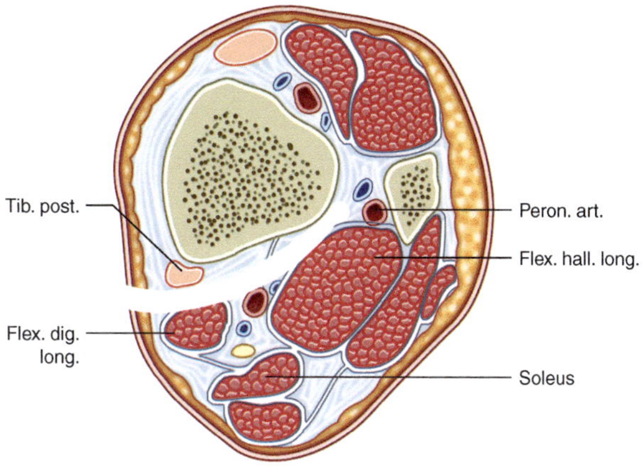

Fig. 33.14 Transverse section of lower left leg for exposure of distal peroneal artery

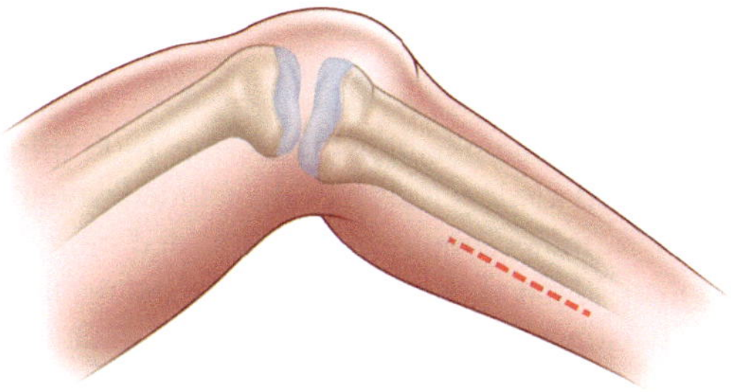

Fig. 33.15 Skin incision of exposure of distal peroneal artery via lateral approach

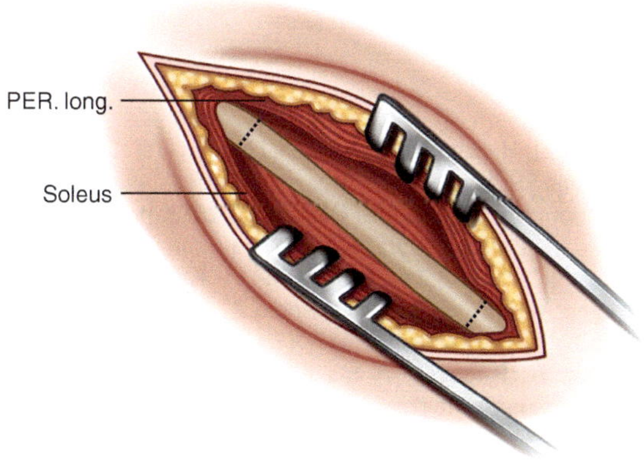

Fig. 33.16 Exposed fibula

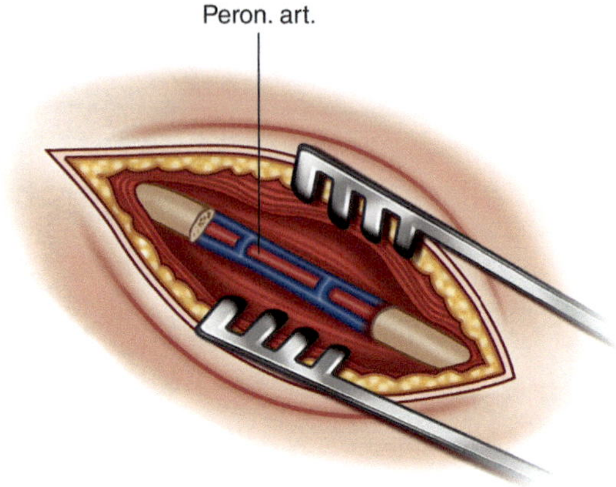

Fig. 33.17 Partial fibulectomy

Complications

Postoperative complications following 1400 infra-inguinal grafts for chronic limb ischemia reported by Kalish et al. included wound complications of 4%, graft occlusion 5.2%, major amputations 1.8%, and mortality of 2.7% [4]. Early thrombosis (less than 30 days) is most commonly the result of inadequate conduit (vein) kinking or twisting of the graft, poor outflow. Patient should be taken back to the operating room for thrombectomy and arteriography. Late complications include persistent lymphedema, aneurysmal changes vein bypass conduits, graft stenosis, and infection.

References

1. Davis FM, Henke PK. Infrainguinal bypass graft for lower extremity arterial occlusive disease. In: Hans SS, Shepard AD, Weaver MR, et al., editors. Endovascular and open vascular reconstruction. Boca Raton, FL: CRC Press; 2018. p. 319–27.
2. Ciervo A, Dardik H, Qin F, et al. The tourniquet revisited as an attempt to lower limb revascularization. J Vasc Surg. 2000;31(3):436–42.
3. Wagner WH, Treiman DV, Cossman JL, et al. Tourniquet occlusion for tibial artery reconstruction. J Vasc Surg. 1993;18:637–47.
4. Kalish JA, Farber A, Homa K, et al. Factors associated with surgical site infection after lower extremity bypass in the society for vascular surgery, quality initiative. J Vasc Surg. 2014;16(5):1238–46.

Chapter 34
Upper Extremity Artery Bypass

Farah Hanif Ali Mohammad

Surgical Anatomy

Axillary Artery

The axillary artery has three parts based on pectoralis minor. The first part is superior and medial to the pectoralis minor and begins as continuation of the subclavian artery at the lateral edge of the first rib. Here it gives off its first branch named the superior thoracic artery. The second portion lies underneath the pectoralis minor and gives off thoracoacromial and lateral thoracic artery. Third portion lies lateral to the pectoralis minor and gives off subscapular, anterior, and posterior humeral circumflex artery. It continues on to become brachial artery at the lower margin of teres major. The axillary vein runs along its entire course medially. The brachial plexus runs posterior to the first and then interlaces the second and third part (Fig. 34.1).

Brachial Artery

The axillary artery continues on to become the brachial artery past the inferior border of teres major. The brachial artery passes between the biceps and triceps muscles. In the antecubital fossa, it divides into the radial, interosseous, and ulnar

F. H. A. Mohammad (✉)
Henry Ford Hospital, Detroit, MI, USA

S. S. Hans et al. (eds.), *Primary and Repeat Arterial Reconstructions*,
https://doi.org/10.1007/978-3-031-13897-3_34

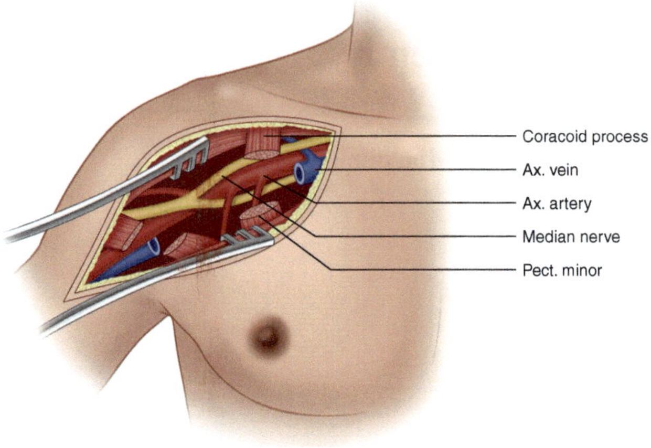

Fig. 34.1 Exposure of axillary artery

arteries to supply the soft tissues of the forearm. The median nerve runs along the artery crossing from relatively lateral to medial position as it goes distally. Its first major branch called the deep brachial artery runs posteriorly and serves as a major collateral in the setting of brachial injury. Two brachial veins closely run along the artery in the brachial sheath. The brachial artery divides into radial and ulnar arteries at the level of the radial tuberosity (Fig. 34.2).

Radial Artery

Radial artery arises in the antecubital fossa and runs distally along the anterolateral border of the forearm underneath the brachioradialis muscle. It continues on to pass through the anatomical snuff box and becomes part of the deep palmar arch. Along its course, it's accompanied by paired radial veins and gives off multiple collateral branches (Fig. 34.2).

Ulnar Artery

After its origin at the level just below the antecubital fossa, it passes obliquely distally, underneath the superficial flexor muscles along the anteromedial portion of the forearm. It passes over the ulnar border of the wrist over the pisiform bone, terminating in the superficial palmar arch (Fig. 34.2).

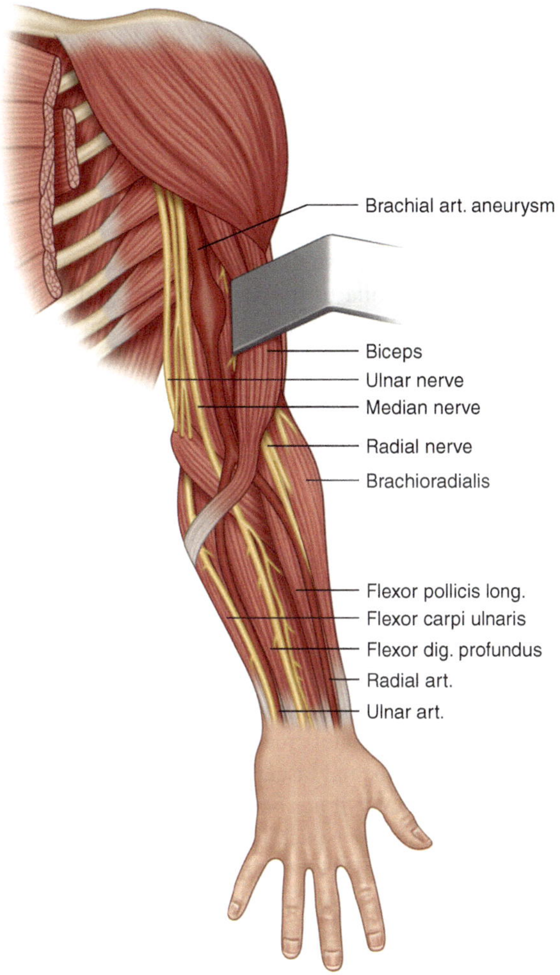

Fig. 34.2 Exposure of brachial, radial and ulnar artery (Left)

Surgical Exposure

Once the extent of disease has been determined, the bypass can be planned accordingly. The proximal and distal vessel is exposed, and chosen conduit is tunneled.

Axillary Artery

The patient is positioned supine with the ipsilateral arm abducted to 90°. The first and second portions of the axillary artery are best exposed with an infraclavicular incision approximately 2 cm below the clavicle. The incision is made from mid-clavicle to anterior surface of deltoid, approximately 7–8 cm in length. If more lateral or if the third portion needs exposure, the incision would have to be extended on to the deltopectoral groove. (Details in Chap. 31).

Brachial Artery

The patient is placed supine with the arm abducted to 90° over an arm board. Entire arm from the axilla to the hand are prepped and draped. To expose the brachial artery in the arm, an axial incision is made on the medial aspect of the arm between the biceps and triceps muscles. At the antecubital fossa, usually a transverse incision just inferior to the antecubital crease may be sufficient. However, if the aneurysm is large or more extensive exposure is needed, then an S-shaped incision is more suitable. (Details in Chap. 31).

Radial Artery

Proximal radial artery can be exposed in via a transverse incision in inferior to the antecubital fossa. In the forearm depending on the level, the radial artery is exposed via a longitudinal incision over the volar forearm (Fig. 34.1). Landmarks include midpoint of antecubital crease to styloid process of radius. After ligating superficial veins, the antebrachial fascia is incised along the medial border of the brachioradialis muscle. Distally, it lies between tendons of brachioradialis and flexor carpi radialis muscles. At this aspect, the superficial radial nerve runs along its lateral aspect and should be preserved during dissection. The accompanying paired veins should be carefully mobilized off the artery.

Ulnar Artery

Proximal ulnar artery can be exposed in via a transverse incision in inferior to the antecubital fossa. It then dives deep underneath the superficial flexor muscle group. In the forearm, it can be exposed via a longitudinal incision along the medial border extending from the medial condyle of the humerus to the pisiform (Fig. 34.1). After incising the antebrachial fascia, the ulnar artery can be isolated by laterally retracting the flexor digitorum superficialis muscle in the proximal forearm. As it progresses distally, the best way to expose would be to medially retract the flexor carpi ulnaris. The ulnar nerve runs medially along the artery in the mid- to distal forearm.

Bypass and Conduit

Autogenous vein grafts are conduits of choice. Lower extremity veins especially great saphenous veins are preferred. Cephalic vein can be used however is usually very thin walled and may not be a good size match. Ultrasound should be used to map the desired length of the vein. Prosthetic reconstruction may be utilized if there are no adequate vein conduits for axillary and brachial bypasses.

Once the vein is harvested, based on size match, it may be used in a reverse or non-reversed fashion. If non-reversed orientation is chosen, then the vein should be distended with heparinized saline. Mills or Lemaitre valvulotome can be used to perform valvulolysis. For axillary artery bypasses, the conduit can be tunneled anatomically. For more distal bypasses, a subcutaneous tunnel is usually created.

Complications

Nerve Injury: Understanding the relation to the artery to the surrounding structures is key to avoiding technical complications. Injury to the brachial plexus during proximal axillary dissection can lead to significant morbidity. Median and ulnar nerve injury can lead to hand numbness and tingling. Radial nerve injuries can lead to radial nerve palsy, which can cause pain and a loss of function in the wrist, hands, and fingers.

Chapter 35
Arterial Reconstructions in Patients with Hostile Groin

Sachinder Singh Hans

Surgical Anatomy

The common femoral artery is a continuation of the external iliac artery as the latter ends at the inguinal ligament midway between the anterior superior iliac spine and symphysis pubis. The common femoral artery bifurcates into the profunda femoral artery which supplies blood flow to the thigh and the superficial femoral artery. The superficial femoral artery runs longitudinally and at the middle and distal third of the thigh as it passes through an opening in the adductor magnus tendon to become the popliteal artery.

Common Femoral Artery

The common femoral artery (CFA) is the continuation of the external iliac artery as it crosses under the inguinal ligament. Coursing in the femoral triangle and not passing through the femoral triangle whose borders include the inguinal ligament superiorly, the medial border of the sartorius muscle laterally, and the medial border of the adductor longus muscle medially. Here it is surrounded by the femoral sheath

S. S. Hans (✉)
Vascular and Endovascular Services, Henry Ford Macomb Hospital,
Clinton Twp, MI, USA

S. S. Hans et al. (eds.), *Primary and Repeat Arterial Reconstructions*,
https://doi.org/10.1007/978-3-031-13897-3_35

with the femoral vein running just medial to the artery. Common femoral artery gives off small branches which may include superficial epigastric artery, superficial circumflex iliac artery, and superficial and deep external pudendal artery. The artery ends when it gives off its largest branch the profunda or deep femoral artery which arises approximately 3.5 cm below the inguinal ligament. The deep femoral artery runs posteriorly and continues downward between the pectineus and adductor longus muscle. After the profunda femoral artery branch point, the common femoral artery continues distally in the extremity as the superficial femoral artery. The superficial femoral artery extends beneath the sartorius muscle in the thigh eventually passing through the adductor canal and continues as the popliteal artery.

Deep Femoral Artery

Deep femoral artery near its origin is crossed anteriorly by lateral circumflex femoral vein, and it gives three branches:

1. Lateral circumflex femoral artery which divides into ascending branch, transverse branch, and descending branch.
2. Medial circumflex femoral-transverse and ascending branch.
3. Perforating arteries.

Adductor Canal (Hunter or Subsartorial Canal)

Adductor canal is a tunnel in the middle third of the thigh in which femoral vessels and saphenous nerve are enclosed. Femoral vessels continue from the subsartorial canal into the popliteal fossa. The sartorius muscle lies anteriorly in the subsartorial canal.

Anatomic Variations

Common and superficial femoral artery (SFA) may be absent and replaced by the inferior gluteal artery which accompanies sciatic nerve into the popliteal fossa. The deep femoral artery may arise from the medial or posterior aspect of CFA. The origin of deep femoral artery is usually 2.5–5 cm below the inguinal ligament.

Hostile Groin

In patients with previous multiple arterial reconstructions in the groin, prior history of graft infection, femoral artery infections in patients with intravenous drug abuse, and those with history of groin radiation pose technical challenges for arterial reconstruction in the groin. Management options in such cases include arterial reconstruction with axillo-popliteal bypass with prosthetic graft or autologous bypasses such as the use of femoral and popliteal veins. In such situations, an alternative approach is to perform distal anastomosis to the mid- or distal SFA via lateral approach, or consideration of obturator bypass for arterial reconstruction.

Obturator Bypass

Obturator bypass is considered in patients with unilateral graft limb infection secondary to a previous aortobifemoral graft (ABF) reconstruction. Evaluation of CT imaging should confirm the absence of infection in the main body of the graft or involvement of the contralateral limb by the absence of perifluid/gas collection to consider reconstruction using obturator bypass as an alternate to standard arterial reconstruction. At the time of intra-abdominal or retroperitoneal exploration, the main body of the graft should be well incorporated. The affected limb is transected, and opening is made in the anteromedial aspect of the obturator membrane by palpation of the pubis, and moving the finger laterally till the edge of the firm obturator membrane can be palpated (Figs. 35.1 and 35.2). Metzenbaum scissors is used to incise the obturator membrane over the guidance of the finger. A blunt-tipped tunneler such as Gore or Garrett tunneler is passed from the obturator fossa into the medial thigh anterior to the adductor longus muscle. Superficial femoral artery is exposed under the sartorius muscle in the midthigh, and distal anastomosis of an 8 mm PTFE graft (interring) is performed to the mid- or distal superficial femoral artery. The distal anastomosis to the popliteal artery may need to be performed in patients with occlusion of SFA. The proximal graft anastomosis is performed prior to passage of the graft through the obturator tunnel in an end-to-end fashion with the previously placed limb which is divided flush at the body of the graft with 4-0 CV polypropylene suture [1]. After both anastomoses are completed, the patient is redraped, and retroperitoneal incision and the incision on the middle thigh are isolated, and groin incision is opened; all the prosthetic materials are removed, as well as excisional debridement of the tissues is performed. Common femoral artery is oversewn by a monofilament suture such as 4-0 CV polypropylene.

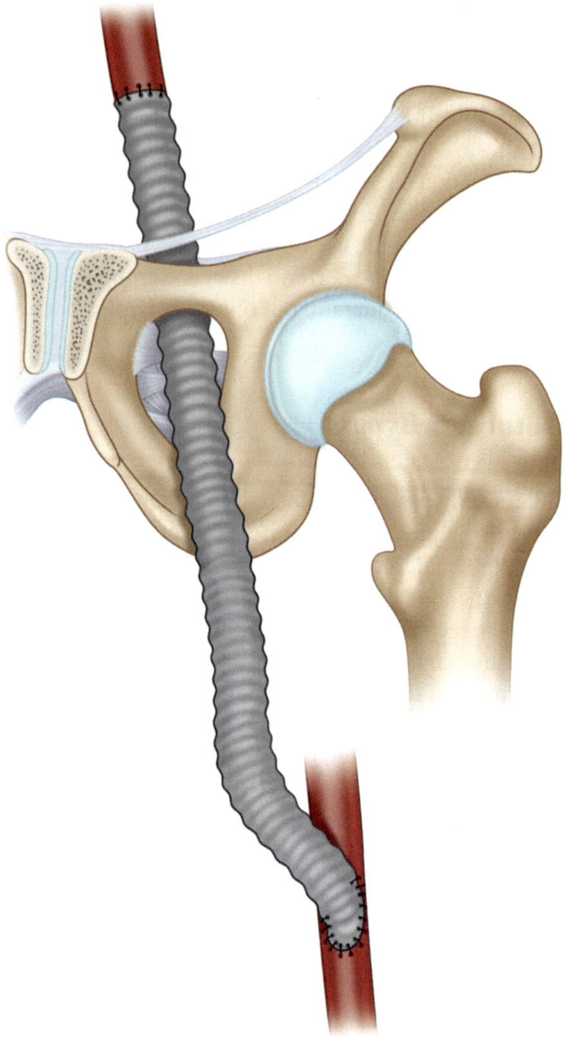

Fig. 35.1 Obturator bypass with prosthetic graft anastomosed to the left limb of the aortic bifurcation graft brought through the obturator foramen with distal anastomosis at the mid-SFA level

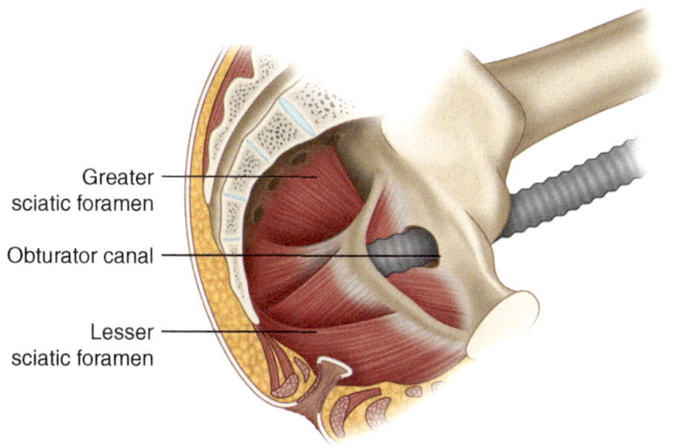

Fig. 35.2 Inside view of the pelvis showing prosthetic graft tunneled through the obturator foramen and extending to the mid-thigh

Lateral Approach for Exposure of SFA

Lateral approach for exposure of SFA can be used for both proximal and distal anastomosis in patients with hostile groin. The groin is isolated by placing a 4 × 4 and an Ioban drape (3M Antimicrobial). Patients are placed in the operating table with the leg externally rotated and the ipsilateral knee flexed to 25–30° by a "knee bump."

Exposure of the SFA in its Proximal Portion

The sartorius is mobilized medially by incising the fascia along its lateral border following a skin incision parallel to the lateral border of the sartorius (Fig. 35.3). The dissection is done under the sartorius muscle, and the muscle is retracted. The dissection plane is established between the vastus medialis and the adductor longus muscle. The femoral vein and the SFA are dissected carefully. Sharp dissection is done to separate the femoral vein as it is formerly adherent to the artery, and its branches may be crossing the artery anteriorly. Silastic vessel loop is passed proximally and distally as 3–4 cm length of the SFA near the apex of the femoral triangle is exposed (Fig. 35.4).

Exposure of the SFA in the Middle Thigh

An incision is made in the middle of the thigh along the lateral border of sartorius muscle. Dissection is performed under the subsartorial canal between the vastus medialis and the adductor longus muscle (Fig. 35.5). If the SFA is the site of distal

Fig. 35.3 Lateral exposure of the proximal one-third of the SFA and DFA through an incision along the lateral border of the sartorius and upper thigh. Lateral exposure of the middle third of the SFA with an incision along the lateral border of the sartorius. The dissection is done between the plane between vastus medialis and adductor longus

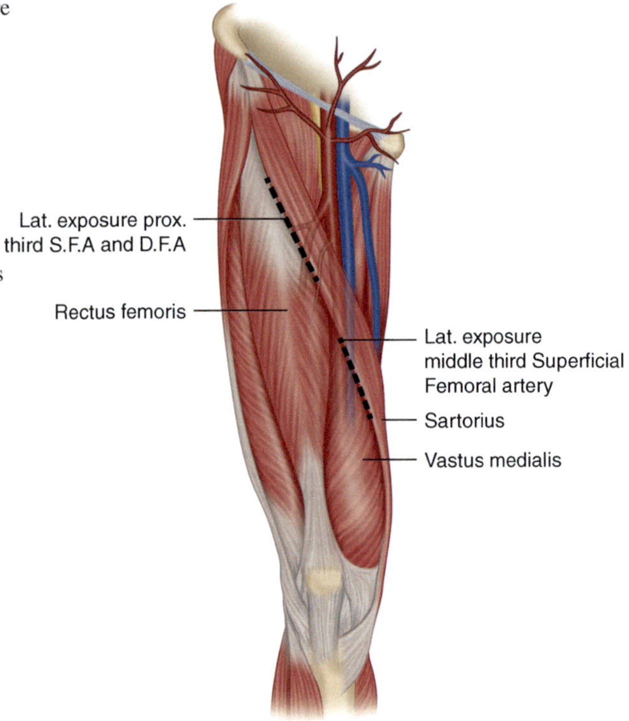

Fig. 35.4 Prox deep femoral artery exposure

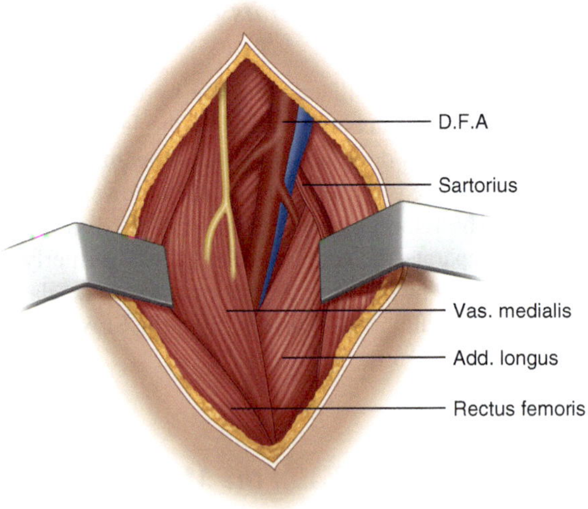

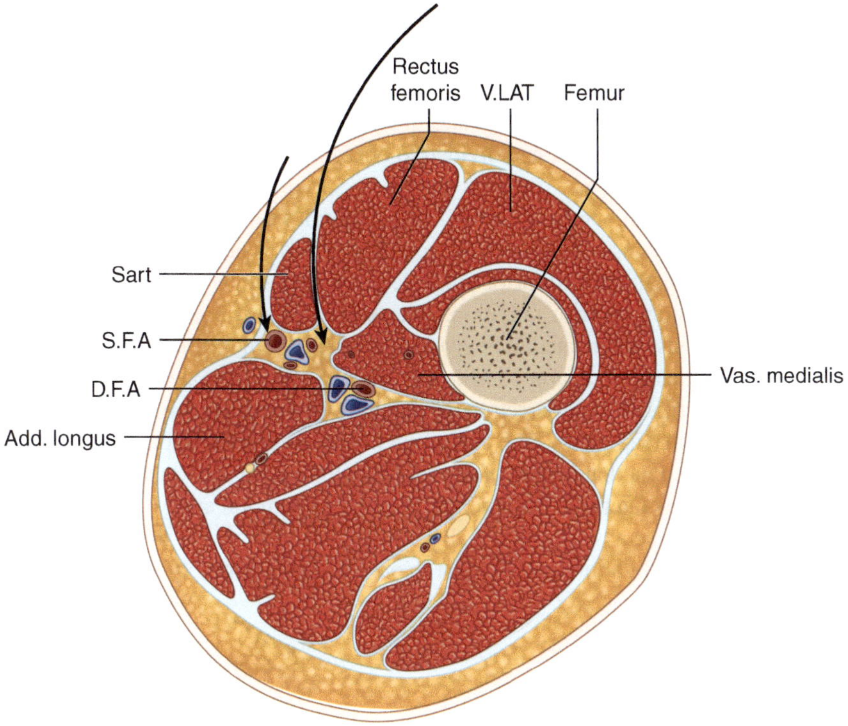

Fig. 35.5 Right thigh at the apex of the femoral triangle. Both SFA and DFA are seen with dissection done along the lateral border of the sartorius between vastus medialis and adductor longus

anastomosis in a patient with hostile groin, the proximal anastomosis is performed to the external iliac artery or iliac limb of the graft as the need may be via a supra-inguinal incision. The external oblique fascia is incised, and retroperitoneal space is entered. The graft is brought over the iliac crest in a lateral route after proximal anastomosis is performed. Following completion of the distal anastomosis, and closure of the incisions, sterile dressings are applied. The groin is opened under the Ioban dressing and excisional debridement with removal of the soft tissues and graft if necessary is performed.

Exposure of Profunda Femoral Artery (Deep Femoral Artery)

Proximal exposure of the profunda femoris (deep femoral artery) is via a longitudinal incision in the upper anterior thigh. The incision can be extended proximally or distally for additional exposure. In obese patients, proximal incision is extended in a "hockey stick" manner just above and parallel to the inguinal ligament to avoid wound complications. For exposure of the proximal deep femoral artery, CFA and SFA are looped with a silastic vessel loop and are retracted medially. Sharp dissection is done at the origin of deep femoral artery which usually has a small branch arising superiorly and laterally. The lateral circumflex vein crosses the artery anteriorly and needs to be ligated and divided to obtain an additional length of exposure of the deep femoral artery.

Exposure of distal segment of the deep femoral artery is useful regardless of whether the artery is used as an outflow vessel or serves as inflow source. This exposure is useful in patients with prior multiple groin exposures, groin infection, or in patients with history of prior radiation. The skin incision is made along the medial border of sartorius (anteromedial approach) or lateral border of the sartorius which is preferable (anterolateral approach); once the dissection is done along the deeper plane, the sartorius muscle is retracted medially or laterally depending upon the selected approach (Fig. 35.6). The dissection is done lateral to SFA and accompanying nerve between medial border of the adductor longus muscle (medially) and into the vastus medialis laterally. Profunda femoris (deep femoral artery) and its accompanying vein can be visualized. Small vein tributaries crossing the deep femoral artery may require ligation and division to obtain satisfactory exposure of the deep femoral artery.

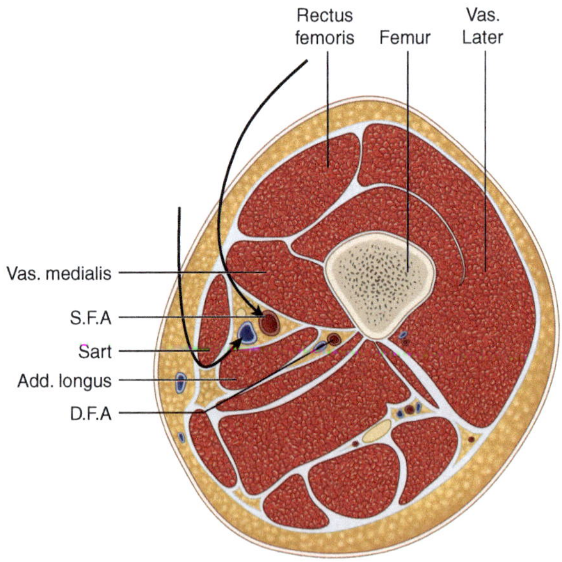

Fig. 35.6 Right middle thigh showing the exposure of mid-SFA as well as deep location of the DFA

Reference

1. Bath J, Rahimi H, Long B, et al. Clinical outcomes of Obturator canal bypass. J Vasc Surg. 2017;66(1):160–6.

Part III
Amputations

Chapter 36
Lower Extremity Major Amputations

Chinmayee Potti and Andi Peshkepija

Introduction

As recently as the 1970s, up to 70% of patients who underwent minor amputations progressed to limb loss within 3 years. However, better understanding of the disease process, modification of risk factors, and the ability to perform femoral-to-popliteal and more distal arterial bypass grafts, and, more recently, catheter-based interventions have led to contemporary limb salvage rates approximating 80% at 5 years [1]. A properly timed and executed minor amputation can avoid the metabolic, quality of life, cost, and ambulatory adversities associated with a major amputation. This chapter describes pertinent surgical anatomy and techniques for commonly performed major amputations and further delves into possible complications, how to avoid and tackle them. This chapter primarily describes below-knee, above-knee, and hip disarticulation. However, toe, transmetatarsal, hind quarter amputations, as well as through-knee disarticulation are excluded from this chapter.

C. Potti (✉)
Henry Ford Hospital, Detroit, MI, USA
e-mail: cpotti1@hfhs.org

A. Peshkepija
Henry Ford Hospital, Detroit, MI, USA

Wayne State University, Detroit, MI, USA

S. S. Hans et al. (eds.), *Primary and Repeat Arterial Reconstructions*,
https://doi.org/10.1007/978-3-031-13897-3_36

Below-Knee Amputations (BKA)

Indications

The healing potential of the skin at the amputation level is dependent on the vascularity at the level of amputation. Less than 25% of BKAs healed when a femoral pulse was absent [2]. Furthermore, significantly more energy is required to ambulate with an above-knee prosthesis (50–70%) compared to below knee (10–40%) [1]. Considering these factors, on occasion, endovascular or even open arterial reconstruction might be necessary to ensure that the planned BKA will have adequate perfusion. Evolving from the earliest forms of amputations which were done predominantly for wounded warriors, trauma is less often an indication for amputation except in unsalvageable limbs. The most common of indications for below-knee amputation are critical limb ischemia and diabetes with infectious gangrene. A large portion of amputations, 82% [1], are done due to ischemia, despite aggressive thrombectomies or repeated arterial reconstructions. In cases of severe infection, active cellulitis first needs to be controlled prior to amputation. If infection and necrosis are severe, a guillotine amputation is performed 2–3 cm above the ankle for source control followed by a more definitive below-knee amputation. The level of amputation should be decided after assessing the level of pathology, potential for rehabilitation, and the presence of adequate perfusion [3].

Pertinent Surgical Anatomy

There are four fascial compartments in the lower leg (Fig. 36.1). Anterior compartment, laying anteromedial to the tibiofibular interosseous membrane, contains the tibialis anterior, extensor halluces longus, extensor digitorum longus, peroneus tertius, anterior tibial artery and vein, as well as deep peroneal nerve running alongside the vessels. The anterior tibial artery is the main blood supply to the anterior compartment, aided by perforating branch of peroneal artery. The lateral compartment, laying posterior to the anterior compartment and lateral to the fibula, contains peroneus longus, peroneus brevis, and the superficial peroneal nerve. The posterior superficial contains the soleus, gastrocnemius, and plantaris muscles. The deep posterior compartment contains tibialis posterior, plantar flexors of the foot and toes, the tibial nerve, and the posterior tibial artery which supplies this compartment.

***Guillotine amputation*:** While several techniques can be adopted to perform the guillotine amputation, the goal is to ensure source control. The initial step is simply making a circumferential incision just proximal to the malleoli. Any patent named vessels are suture ligated. The ligamentous attachments of the ankle are incised, exposing the periosteum of the tibia and fibula. The periosteum is elevated, and a saw is used to divide the bones. Electrocautery can be used to ensure hemostasis. Cultures can be sent and dressings applied. Definitive revision can take place in 5–7 days.

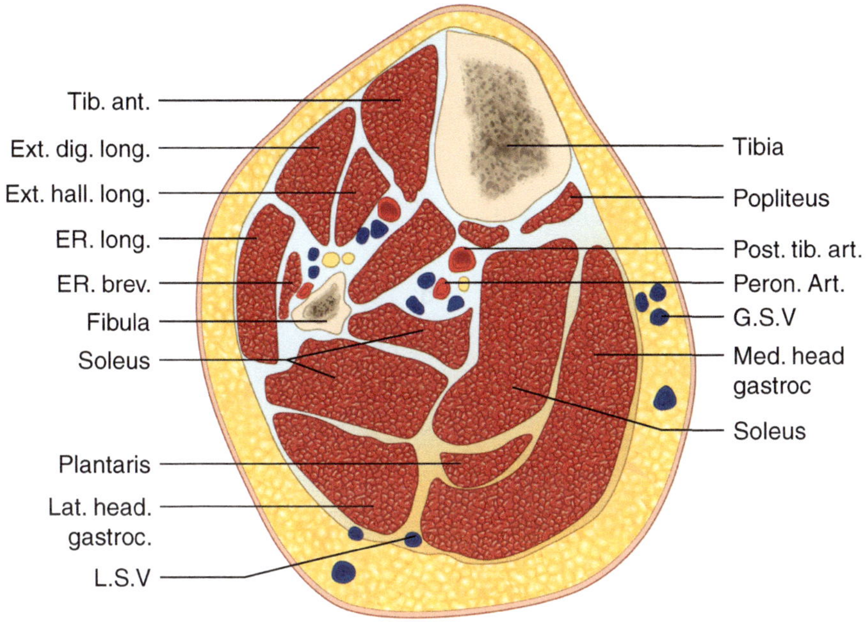

Fig. 36.1 Cross-sectional anatomy of below-knee lower extremity

Preoperative Preparation

- Nutritional optimization to ensure healing.
- Cardiopulmonary risk stratification and optimization when feasible.
- General or regional anesthesia.
- Prophylactic antibiotics to reduce wound infection rates.
- Venous thromboembolism prophylaxis. There is an estimated 12.5% risk of venous thromboembolism in the perioperative period.

Operative Technique

- **Skin incision** (Fig. 36.2): The skin at the planned site of incision must be healthy without infection, breakdown, or ischemia. Most common technique is the long posterior flap. The anterior skin incision typically extends two-thirds of the circumference of the leg. This is made at least 10–12 cm or four fingerbreadths distal to the tibial tuberosity, which is the level at which the tibia is transected. Although a longer stump may aid functionally, functional stumps are achieved with as little as 5 cm of residual tibia. A thicker posterior flap aids in vascularity although can have cosmetic hitches while approximating the incision. Although various alternative flaps are described, the posterior flap is easy to construct and

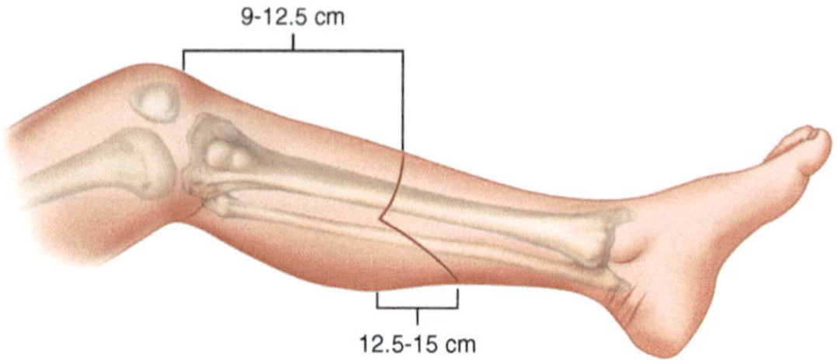

Fig. 36.2 BKA skin incision

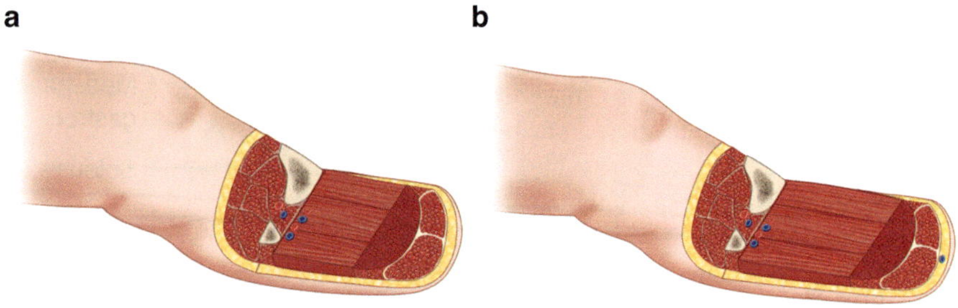

Fig. 36.3 (**a**) BKA – At the end of neurovascular ligation. (**b**) BKA – At the end of division of tibia and fibula

offers adequate coverage and padding of the stump. The length of the posterior flap should be 5–6 in or longer to ensure tension-free closure of the stump.

- **Neurovascular ligation** (Fig. 36.3a): Understanding anatomy is of utmost importance in order to anticipate and ligate structures appropriately. Major vessels are suture ligated, including anterior tibial, posterior tibial, and peroneal arteries. Large nerves are grasped, advanced, tied, and transected and allowed to retract into the depths of the wound to avoid neuroma formation.
- **Division of tibia and fibula** (Fig. 36.3b): The periosteum of the tibia is elevated circumferentially proximally for 2 cm using a periosteal elevator and divided using a powered oscillating saw or a Gigli saw perpendicular to the axis of the tibia. The anterior edge of the tibia is then bevelled to eliminate sharp edges that can protrude through the skin. The fibula is transected using a saw or bone cutter 1–2 cm proximal to the tibia. Excessively short fibula can result in a conical stump that is difficult to fit with a prosthesis. However, excessively long fibula will be functionally inept.
- **Stump closure** (Fig. 36.4a, b): Hemostasis should be ensured. Stump closure is in two layers, an interrupted layer of absorbable suture for fascia and interrupted loose nylon sutures for skin approximation to avoid skin ischemia. The stump is placed in padded dressing.

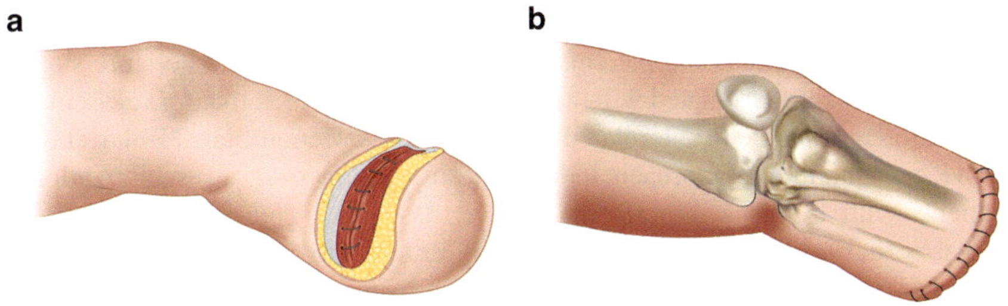

Figs. 36.4 (**a, b**) BKA – stump closure

Potential Complications

- Inappropriate stump length.
- **Flexion contracture of knee in BKAs** – This can be prevented with knee immobilization in neutral position in immediate postoperative period and early rehabilitation.
- **Hematoma**, if significant especially in early postoperative period, should be evacuated to avoid a nidus for infection.
- **Wound complications** can include breakdown secondary to ischemia and wound infection. Wound infections are more common when performed for infectious indications, and in patients with risk factors such as diabetes, malnutrition, malignancy, wound hematoma, and prior prosthetic grafts.
- **Stump ischemia** can manifest as pallor, persistent pain, coolness of the stump, and progress to skin blisters and eventual necrosis. This results from lack of adequate vascularity or constrictive dressings. Stump trauma can occur secondary to pressure-induced necrosis from underlying bone or tourniquet-type dressing or shear injury.
- Furthermore, about 10–20% of patients eventually undergo above-knee amputations. Up to 30% of amputations can have wound complications. The estimated mortality at 3 years after an amputation is up to 43%.

Above-Knee Amputation (AKA)

Indications

The most common indications for AKA include acute limb ischemia, chronic limb ischemia, and infection [4]. These are followed by trauma and malignancy. AKAs are performed in patients with irreversible acute limb ischemia, chronic limb ischemia after failed repeated revascularizations, patients with persistent severe chronic limb ischemia, and patients with BKA complications. Literature suggests that mortality rate associated with major amputation exceeds that for revascularization, although this could be related to an implicit selection bias. Nehler et al. [5] provide a qualitative approach indicating amputation over revascularization for patients with extensive severity in two of these three categories: comorbidities (notably diabetes, end stage renal disease), complexity of revascularization, and extent of tissue loss. Approximately 95% of AKAs heal compared to 80% of BKAs. An estimated 70% more energy is expended to walk on an AKA prosthesis compared to 40% on a BKA prosthesis. A palpable femoral pulse usually predicts AKA healing.

Pertinent Surgical Anatomy

The thigh is divided into anterior, posterior, and medial compartments (Fig. 36.5). The anterior compartment contains the vastus medius, vastus lateralis, vastus intermedius, rectus femoris, and genu articularis. Branches of the femoral nerve supply the anterior compartment. The sartorius runs anterior proximally to medial as it

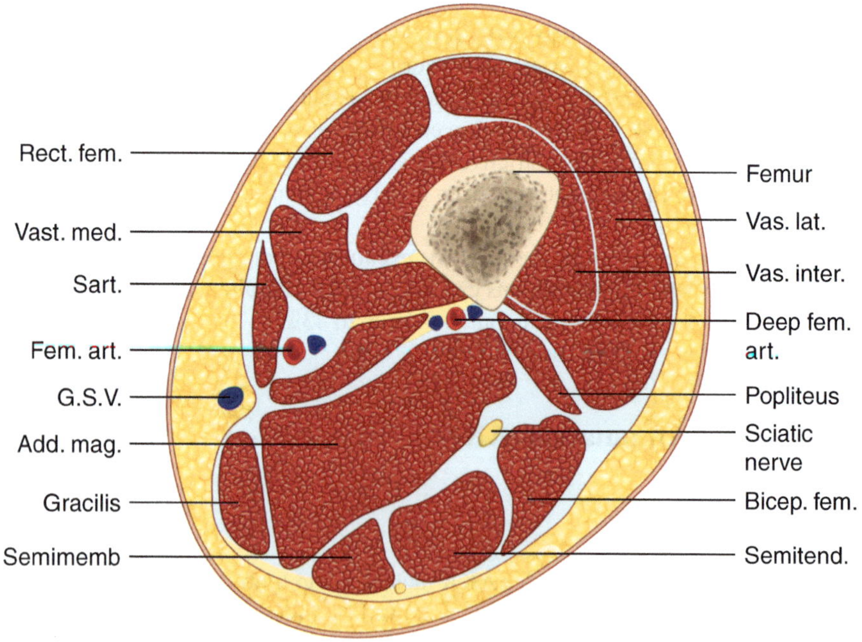

Fig. 36.5 AKA – surgical anatomy

inserts distally onto the proximal tibia as a part of the pes anserinus. Saphenous nerve, a cutaneous branch of the femoral nerve, supplies the medial skin of thigh and leg. The medial compartment contains the adductor magnus, adductor longus, adductor brevis, and gracilis. While adductor magnus receive innervation from sciatic as well as obturator nerves, the rest of the medial compartment muscles are innervated by the obturator nerve. The medial compartment contains the femoral artery and vein which pass through the adductor hiatus to course posteriorly. The femoral artery provides blood flow to the muscles of the thigh and the femoral shaft through deep branches. The posterior compartment contains the long and short heads of biceps femoris, semitendinosus, semimembranosus, and the sciatic nerve which supplies this compartment. The great saphenous vein runs superficially along the medial aspect of the thigh.

Operative Technique

- **Skin incision** (Fig. 36.6): A tourniquet can be used when there is sufficient salvageable femur length. The junction of middle and distal thirds is the most common site of femur transection. Although many incisions are described, a transverse fishmouth incision with equal anterior and posterior flaps is commonly used. Alternatives include circular incision with progressive layer deepening to the bone or sagittal flaps.
- Superficial femoral artery and vein are identified and suture ligated.
- **Division of femur** (Fig. 36.6): The femur is transected proximal to the skin incision using an oscillating saw; the edges are shaped in order to reduce pressure necrosis of the skin. Bone wax can be used to control bleeding from the marrow.
- Sciatic nerve is identified, sharply divided under tension, ligated, and allowed to retract into the deeper tissue.
- **Wound closure**: Stabilization of adductors by myopexy in order to avoid abduction and flexion of the proximal femur may be beneficial, though not commonly done for vascular pathology. Myopexy is performed by sewing the muscles of the posterior and medial compartment to the periosteum anterolateral to the femur. Deep fascia is approximated using absorbable suture. Skin is closed using interrupted monofilament sutures or staples which are removed in 4–6 weeks.

Postoperative Care

- **Edema** of the stump is an expected outcome, with an underappreciated component of lymphatic edema. While some surgeons use vacuum-assisted dressings, some use rigid plaster dressings, and some use stump shrinkers to reduce this

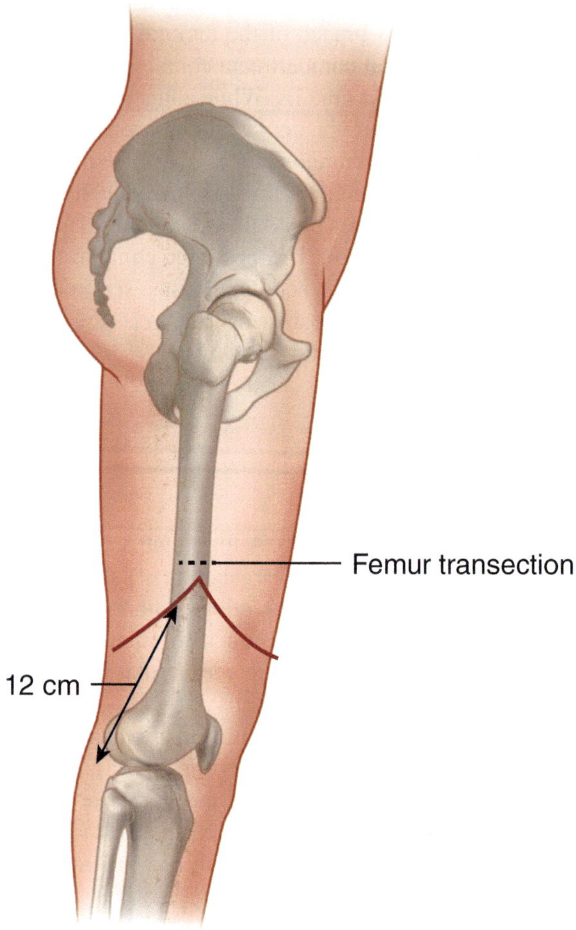

Fig. 36.6 AKA – skin incision and transection of femur

edema and wound complications that are associated with it. Elevation of the stump also reduces edema.

- Psychological support as well as targeted multimodal pain control are critical postoperatively. About 5% of these patients experience phantom pain.
- **Incision**: Skin sutures are not removed till at least 6 weeks. A nonadherent gauze followed by dry dressing is typically used. Regular monitoring for wound complications is essential. Constrictive dressings must be avoided.

Potential Complications

- **Hematoma**, if significant especially in early postoperative period, should be evacuated to avoid a nidus for infection.

- **Wound complications**, seen in up to 40% cases, can include breakdown secondary to ischemia and wound infection. Wound infections are more common when performed for infectious indications, and in patients with risk factors such as diabetes, malnutrition, malignancy, wound hematoma, and prior prosthetic grafts. An aggressive approach to wound care must be adopted including liberal debridement, systemic antibiotics when appropriate, and nutritional optimization. Vacuum-assisted dressings can be particularly useful. In rare situations where local wound care is ineffective secondary to ischemia, aggressive attempts at revascularization should be perceived as more proximal amputations can result in the same outcome.
- **Stump ischemia** can manifest as pallor, persistent pain, coolness of the stump, and progress to skin blisters and eventual necrosis. This results from lack of adequate vascularity or constrictive dressings. Stump trauma can occur secondary to pressure-induced necrosis from underlying bone or tourniquet-type dressing or shear injury.
- **Deep vein thrombosis and pulmonary embolism** are seen in up to 50% patients after major lower extremity amputations. All patients should be on venous thromboembolic prophylaxis.
- **Postoperative pain** can be debilitating – could arise from the incision, ischemia, neuropathy, phantom pain or infection. Multimodal therapy including regional anesthesia can prove beneficial. Physical and mental rehabilitation are key to recovery.
- **Mortality** perioperatively after an AKA ranges from 11% to 18%, most commonly secondary to sepsis, pneumonia, and cardiac complications. Survival rate at 1 year is approximately 50%, and less than 10% of elderly can walk on a prosthesis.

Hip Disarticulation

Indications

Hip disarticulation refers to the removal of the entire lower extremity through the hip joint. Hip disarticulation, when performed, is most often performed for treatment of high-grade diaphyseal tumors distal to the lesser trochanter, sometimes after massive trauma, for arterial insufficiency, for severe infections, for massive decubitus ulcers, or for certain congenital limb deficiencies [6]. Although prostheses are available, few patients are able to utilize them, and energy requirements to use a prosthesis have been estimated to be 200% of normal ambulation. Mortality rates vary between 0% and 44%.

Operative Procedure

1. **Incision** (Fig. 36.7): Equal anterior and posterior flaps are utilized. With the patient in the lateral decubitus position, an anterior racquet-shaped incision is made beginning one fingerbreadth medial to the anterior superior iliac spine and curving it distally and medially almost parallel with the inguinal ligament to the pubic tubercle, pubic bone, and a point on the medial aspect of the thigh 5 cm distal to the origin of the adductor muscles (two fingerbreadths distal to the ischial tuberosity). The posterior incision continues around the posterior thigh along the lateral aspect of the thigh about two fingerbreadths anterior to the greater trochanter.

   If the buttock flap is extremely thick, the anterior incision can be moved laterally. The distance distal to the gluteal crease is directly proportional to the anterior-posterior diameter of the pelvis to allow for appropriate approximation of the flaps.
2. **Femoral triangle exposure** (Fig. 36.8): The skin, subcutaneous tissue, and Scarpa's fascia are dissected till the external oblique aponeurosis is identified. Superficial epigastric artery, branches of external pudendal artery, and branches of saphenous vein are divided and ligated. While the superficial inguinal lymph nodes are included in the specimen, the spermatic cord and round ligament are not.

Fig. 36.7 Disarticulation hip – skin incision

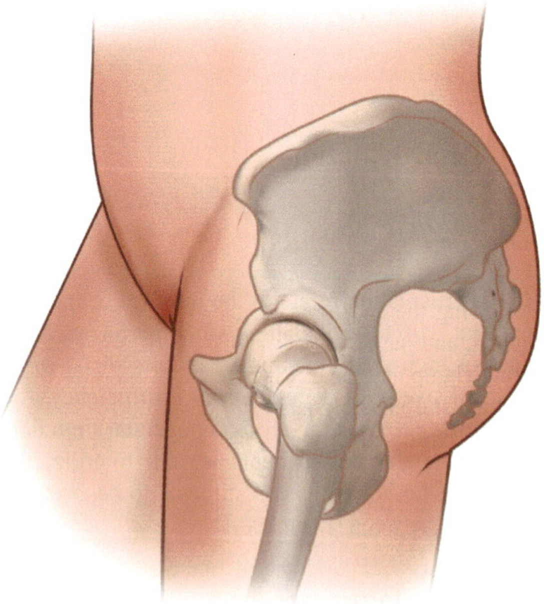

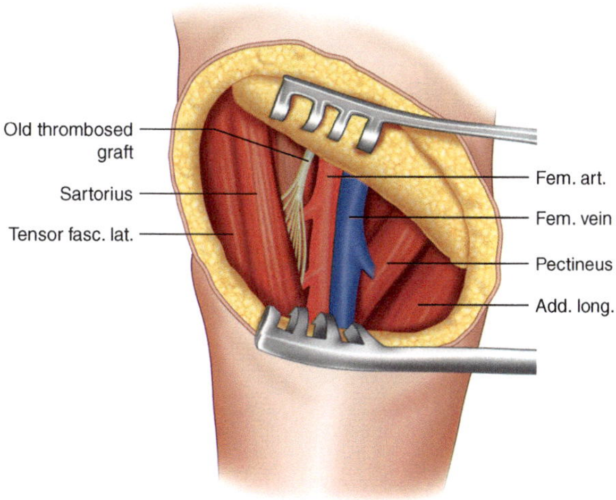

Fig. 36.8 Femoral triangle exposure

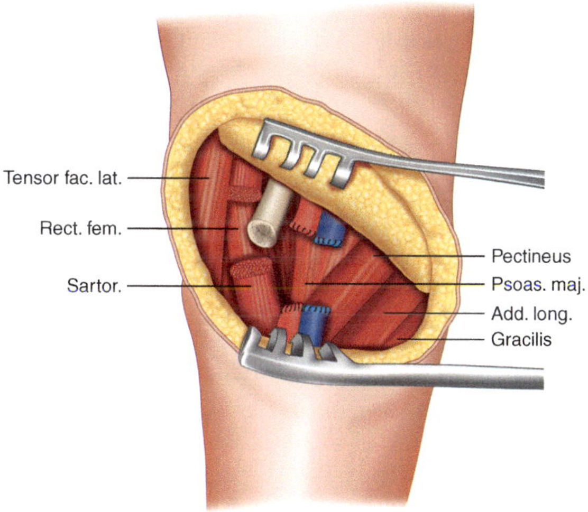

Fig. 36.9 Division of femoral vessels

3. **Division of femoral vessels** (Fig. 36.9): The femoral vessels are double ligated and transected. The femoral nerve is placed on gentle traction, ligated so that when divided, it retracts beneath the external oblique aponeurosis, so that if a neuroma forms, it will not be in a weight-bearing portion of the stump.
4. **Division of muscles** (Figs. 36.10 and 36.11): The **sartorius** is detached from the anterior superior iliac spine and **rectus femoris** from the anterior inferior iliac spine. The femoral sheath posterior to the femoral vessels is also incised using electrocautery to expose the hip joint capsule.

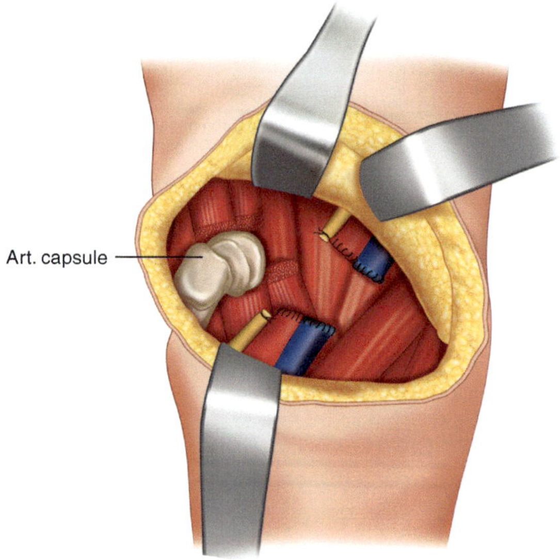

Fig. 36.10 Division of muscles (sartorius, rectus femoris)

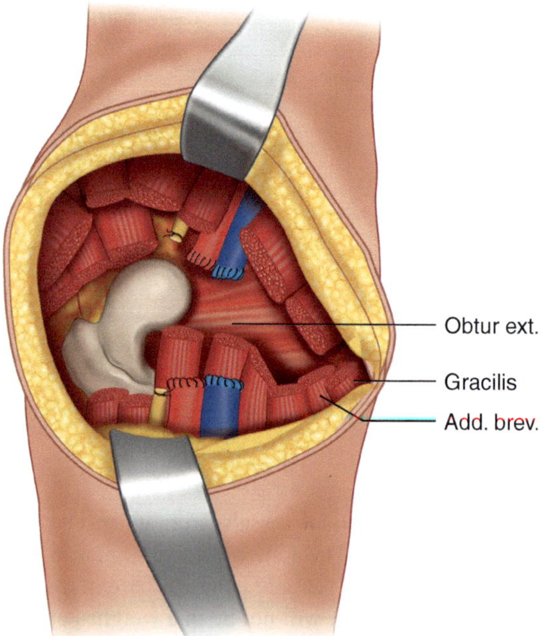

Fig. 36.11 Division of adductors, gracilis

The hip is flexed slightly to relax the **iliopsoas**; this allows for blunt finger dissection around the muscle in a mediolateral fashion. The entire muscle is dissected until the lesser trochanter is clearly identified while taking care to secure vessels that pass anterior to this muscle. The iliopsoas is divided at its insertion into the lesser trochanter.

- The **adductors** are then released from their origin on the pelvis. To preserve the **obturator externus** over the pelvis, its tendon arising from the lesser trochanter is identified to develop the plane between pectineus and obturator externus. A finger is passed beneath the **pectineus**, and it is released at its origin from the pubis using electrocautery. Beneath this, branches of the obturator artery, vein, and nerve are visualized.
- The adductor and **gracilis** muscles are detached from the pubis, and the part of the adductor magnus that arises from the ischium is divided at its origin. **Obturator vessels and nerves** are divided at this time. These bifurcate around the adductor brevis. *The branches of the obturator artery should be carefully secured during dissection to prevent accidental rupture, retraction into the pelvis, and hemorrhage that is difficult to control.* The **abductor muscles** are transected at their origin at the pubic symphysis.
- *The obturator externus muscle is divided at its insertion on the femur instead of at its origin on the pelvis because otherwise the obturator artery may be severed and might retract into the pelvis, leading to hemorrhage that could be difficult to control.*

5. **Identification of the sciatic nerve** (Fig. 36.12): The extremity is hyperabducted to help locate the ischial tuberosity. Cut ends of the abductor are retracted to find the tuberosity. **Quadratus femoris, flexors, and sciatic nerve** are identified. The quadratus femoris and the sciatic nerve are preserved. The **semimembranous, semitendinosus, and the long head of the biceps** are transected at their origin from the ischial tuberosity. *Care should be taken to avoid the circumflex femoral vessels.*

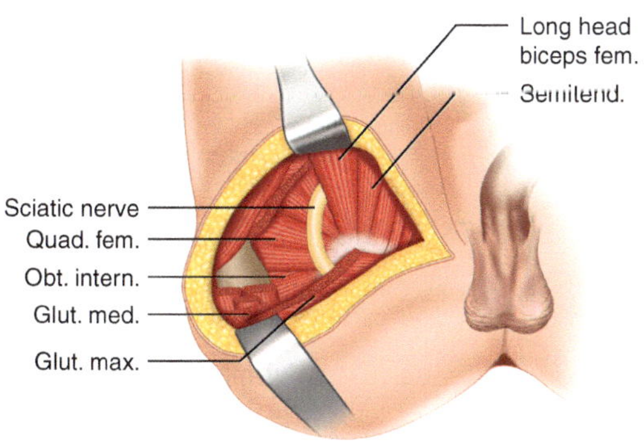

Fig. 36.12 Identification of the sciatic nerve

At this point, all anterior and posterior muscle groups have been divided. The joint capsule overlying the head of the femur is incised, and ligamentum teres transected.

6. **Posterior skin incision, transection of tensor fascia lata, gluteus maximus**: The patient's torso is tilted posterolateral to anterolateral position. The skin incision posteriorly is taken down through the gluteal fascia. The tensor fascia lata and gluteus maximus are divided (neither at the origin not at the insertion).

   Once the gluteus maximus is divided (Fig. 36.13), the common tendon containing multiple muscles – gluteus medius, gluteus minimus, piriformis, superior gemellus, obturator internus, inferior gemellus, and quadratus femoris – inserting into the greater trochanter is exposed. These muscles are divided close to their insertion into the greater trochanter.
7. **Release of the specimen**: The posterior portion of the joint capsule is incised. The **sciatic nerve** is dissected free, transected high near the sciatic notch, and allowed to retract beneath the piriformis.
8. Closure (Fig. 36.14) must consist of **tenodesing the remaining muscles** over the acetabulum.

   The **obturator externus and gluteus medius** are approximated over the joint capsule of the acetabulum to provide soft tissue coverage of bony prominences. The **gluteal fascia** is then elevated and approximated to the inguinal ligament and the pubic ramus. Sutures are placed bisecting the fascial edge uniformly prior to being tied as the posterior myocutaneous flap is much longer than the anterior fascia. Subfascial drains are placed prior to closure. The skin is closed over this. Subcutaneous drains can also be used prior to skin closure.

Fig. 36.13 Division of gluteus maximus

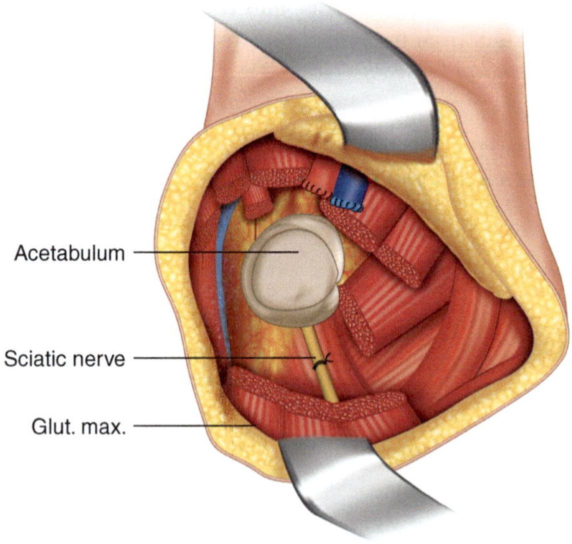

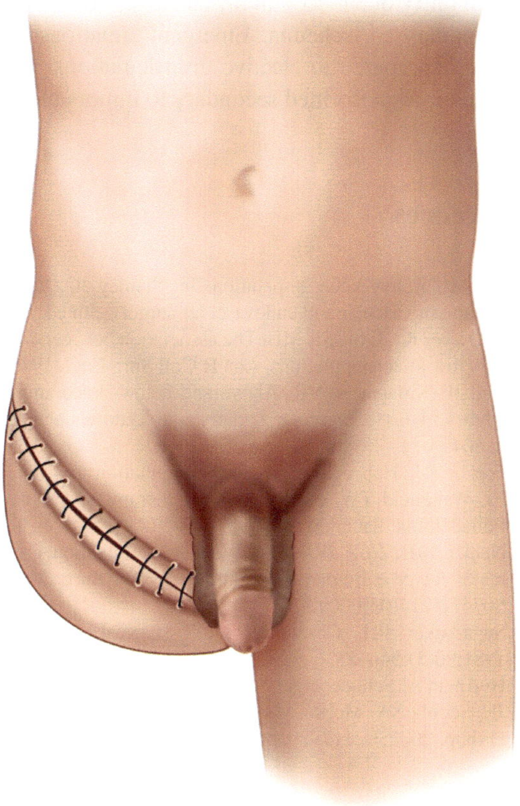

Fig. 36.14 Closure

Complications

Hip disarticulations are extremely invasive and mutilating procedures. Optimizing nutritional status and preparing for transfusions are vital to reduce morbidity. In addition to thromboembolism, debilitating pain seen in other major lower limb amputations, the morbidity and mortality seen with hip disarticulations are higher.

- **Phantom limb:** It is reported that patients who undergo hip disarticulations are 1.53 times more likely to experience Phantom limb pain than patients undergoing below-knee amputations [7].
- **Wound complications:** Complication rates for hip disarticulation, including events such as infection, wound healing, and hematoma formation, have been reported to be as high as 60% [7]. Wound complications were more frequently noted in disarticulations performed for ischemic or infectious indications. Flap necrosis and wound sloughs are also common complications. Patients with a posterior flap, who had ligation of the common iliac vessels, were 2.7 times more likely to have flap necrosis than those patients who had ligation of the external iliac vessels. Extent of gluteal or flap dissection is quoted to have some bearing on flap necrosis.

– **Mortality** of 37–55% in 5 years is reported when disarticulations are performed secondary to ischemia. Emergent situations have increased mortality as well when compared to elective disarticulations. Generally, patients with hip disarticulations performed secondary to tumors have better outcomes.

References

1. KE MI. Below knee amputation. In: Stanley JC, Veith FJ, Wakefield TW, editors. Current therapy in vascular and endovascular surgery. 5th ed. Philadelphia: Saunders; 2014. p. 647–8.
2. O'Dwyer KJ, Edwards MH. The association between lowest palpable pulse and wound healing in below knee amputations. Ann R Coll Surg Engl. 1985;67(4):232–4.
3. Eidt JF, Kalapatapu VR. Above and below- knee amputation. In: Chaikof EL, Cambria RP, editors. Atlas of vascular surgery and endovascular therapy. Philadelphia: Elsevier; 2014. p. 604–9.
4. Feezor RJ, Huber T. Above-knee amputation and hip disarticulation. In: Stanley JC, Veith FJ, Wakefield TW, editors. Current therapy in vascular and endovascular surgery. 5th ed. Philadelphia: Saunders; 2014. p. 649–51.
5. Nehler MR, Coll JR, Hiatt WR, et al. Functional outcome in a contemporary series of major lower extremity amputations. J Vasc Surg. 2003;38(1):7–14. https://doi.org/10.1016/S0741-5214(03)00092-2.
6. Sugarbaker PH, Chretien PB. A surgical technique for hip disarticulation. Surgery. 1981;90(3):546–53.
7. Huffman A, Schneeberger S, Goodyear E, West JM, O'Brien AL, Scharschmidt TJ, Mayerson JL, Schulz SA, Moore AM. Evaluating hip disarticulation outcomes in a 51-patient series. J Orthop. 2022;31:117–20. https://doi.org/10.1016/j.jor.2022.04.008.

Part IV
Misscelanous

Chapter 37
Carotid Body Tumor Resection

Mitchell R. Weaver

Preoperative Planning and Anatomy

The diagnostic finding of a carotid body tumor is a vascular mass displacing the internal and external carotid arteries at the carotid bifurcation. Several noninvasive imaging studies including color flow duplex ultrasound, computed tomography, and magnetic resonance imagining are available to confirm the diagnosis and inform surgical planning. Adequate preoperative imaging defines the extent of the tumor, the presence of any synchronous ipsilateral or contralateral tumors, as well as associated carotid arterial occlusive disease. These findings inform the surgical approach, allowing preparation for extended distal exposures and arterial reconstructions. Invasive catheter-directed angiography is typically limited to cases in which highly selective tumor embolization is considered with goal of reducing operative blood loss. When employed, preoperative embolization is usually reserved for larger tumors (greater than 5 cm) that appear to pose significant technical challenge to resection. Preoperative embolization does have risks of complications including stroke, and when performed, surgical resection is recommended within the next 48 h to avoid the post embolization inflammatory response in the surrounding tissue.

Pertinent surgical anatomy includes arterial structures: common, external, and internal carotid arteries, as well as nerves – hypoglossal, vagus, superior laryngeal, and glossopharyngeal nerves (Fig. 37.1). Due to risk of cranial nerve injury with carotid body tumor resection, it is important to perform and document a thorough cranial nerve exam.

M. R. Weaver (✉)
Henry Ford Hospital, Detroit, MI, USA

Wayne State University School of Medicine, Detroit, MI, USA
e-mail: mweaver1@hfhs.org

S. S. Hans et al. (eds.), *Primary and Repeat Arterial Reconstructions*,
https://doi.org/10.1007/978-3-031-13897-3_37

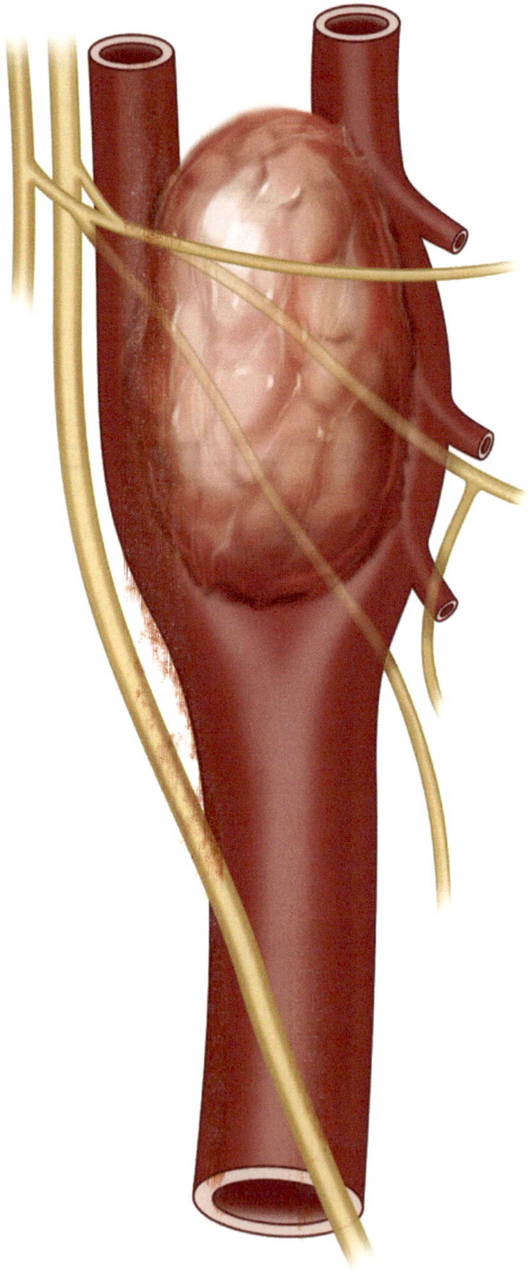

Fig. 37.1 Image demonstrating key anatomic structures including common, internal and external carotid arteries, vagus nerve, hypoglossal nerve, and ansa cervicalis

The extent of the tumor involvement with its surrounding anatomy and thus anticipated difficulty in resection has traditionally been based on the classification system described by Shamblin. This scheme classifies tumors in relation to their involvement with the carotid artery. According to this classification system, group 1 tumors can be resected without significant trauma to the vessel wall or to the tumor capsule. Tumors in group 2 are more adherent to the adventitia and partially surround the artery making their resection more difficult but still possible without sacrificing the vessel. Group 3 tumors completely encase and are best treated by resection of the involved artery with the tumor.

Additional operative preparations include ensured type, and crossed blood is available as well as considers the use of autotransfusion for larger tumors. Intraoperative cerebral monitoring with electroencephalography should be used in operations that may require carotid artery clamping or reconstruction. Additionally, when the need for arterial reconstruction is a possibility, duplex ultrasound vein mapping and preparation of a saphenous vein harvest site are performed. Bipolar cautery is also employed to avoid heat conduction injury to adjacent nerves. A harmonic scalpel is useful in facilitating the resection of carotid body tumors as well as a self-retaining retractor.

Nasal intubation and mandibular subluxation employed when the need for distal internal carotid artery exposure for tumors extending cranially are demonstrated by preoperative imaging. Mandibular subluxation is performed efficiently and safely by our head and neck surgery colleagues after induction of anesthesia but prior to prepping and draping for the tumor resection. Mandibular subluxation displaces the ramus of the mandible forward and alters the normally narrow triangular field into a rectangular field. This provides additional distal internal carotid artery exposure; however, anatomy becomes slightly distorted. The posterior belly of the digastric muscle and the hypoglossal nerve are displaced anteriorly and superiorly, while the carotid bifurcation and internal and external carotid arteries are rotated medially.

Surgical Management

The operation is performed under general anesthesia, and once induced, if mandibular subluxation is planned, it is performed at this time. The patient is placed in the Semi-Fowler's position and a roll are placed under the patient's shoulders. The neck is extended and rotated slightly to the contralateral side. A slightly oblique longitudinal incision is made along the anterior sternocleidomastoid, like that for a carotid endarterectomy (Fig. 37.2). The dissection continues through the subcutaneous tissue and the platysma muscle which are divided. The sternocleidomastoid muscle is encountered and mobilized laterally along with the internal jugular vein. Medial branches of the internal jugular that are not directly draining the tumor are ligated and divided. Lymphatic tissue is divided and ligated as well. If suspicious lymph nodes are encountered, biopsy should be performed, and if nodal metastasis identified, a modified neck dissection should be performed.

Once the tumor is visualized, assessment of the carotid artery is performed, and dissection is typically directed to achieve control of the common carotid artery proximally and then the external and internal carotid artery distally to the tumor. Typically the more proximal common carotid artery which is uninvolved is easily exposed, and then dissection can follow along the artery distally to the carotid bulb.

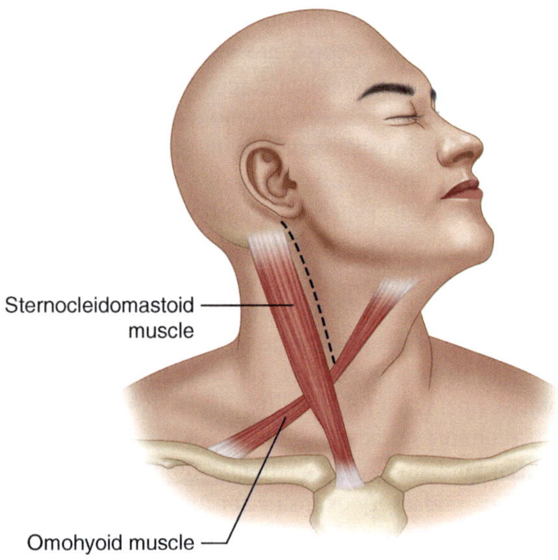

Fig. 37.2 Incision for exposure of carotid bifurcation along the upper two-thirds of the anterior border of the sternocleidomastoid muscle

During this dissection, the vagus nerve is also identified proximally along the common carotid artery and followed distally.

Distal exposure of the external and internal carotid arteries beyond the extent of the tumor is then performed (Fig. 37.3). During dissection of the external carotid artery, one needs to be aware of the hypoglossal nerve anteriorly and superior laryngeal nerve posteriorly. In exposing the internal carotid artery, one must be aware of several nerves including the mandibular branch of the facial nerve, the proximal hypoglossal nerve, the distal vagus nerve, the pharyngeal branch of the vagus nerve, the spinal accessory nerve, and the glossopharyngeal nerve. This dissection can be facilitated utilizing standard techniques such as division of the posterior belly of the digastric muscle taking care not to injure the glossopharyngeal nerve which is then mobilized. Ligation and division of the occipital artery will assist with this. The next maneuver is division of the stylohyoid muscle groups. At this point, if further exposure is required, styloidectomy and mastoidectomy are described but carry with them increased risk of morbidity with cranial nerve injury.

Having completed proximal and distal exposure of the arterial structures, further intervention is based on the extent of the tumor (Fig. 37.4). The vagus nerve as well as other adjacent noninvolved cranial nerves are separated from the tumor and protected by dissecting though the tumor pseudocapsule. Once the nerves are free, for less advanced tumors, attempt is made to create a periadvential dissection plane between the tumor and the artery and taking care not to violate the media, resecting the tumor in a caudal to cranial fashion leaving the arterial wall intact (Fig. 37.5). The blood supply for these tumors originates from the external carotid artery, and these multiple feeding artery branches are sequentially ligated and divided. However it is not unusual to find branches originating from the internal carotid artery as well. For larger, more advanced tumors, the external carotid artery may be ligated and

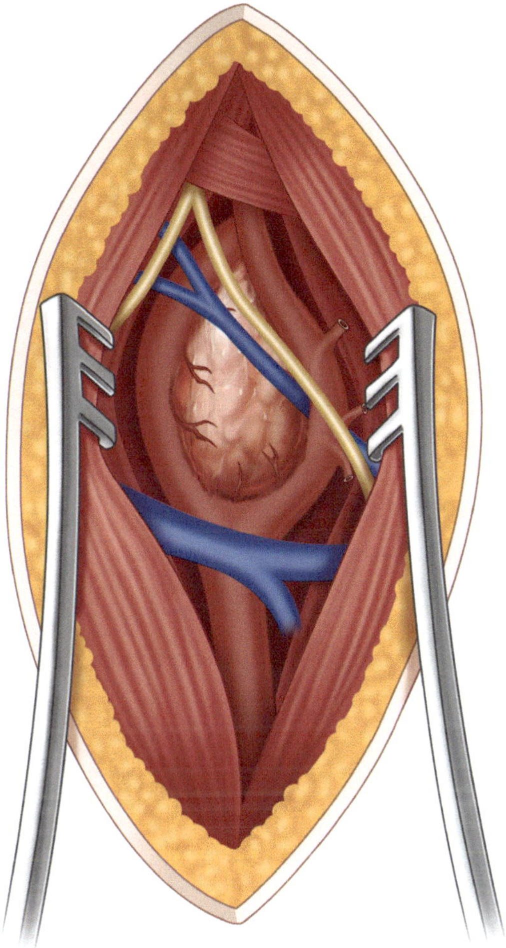

Fig. 37.3 Image demonstrating exposure of carotid bifurcation and carotid body tumor

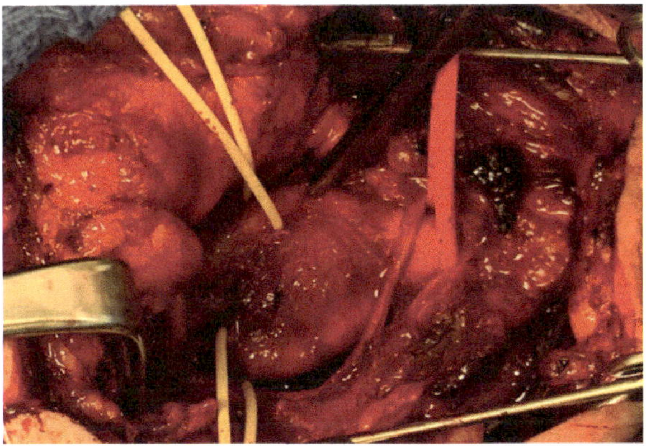

Fig. 37.4 Intraoperative photo demonstrating isolation of the common, internal, external carotid arteries and separation of the tumor from the adjacent nerves prior to resection of tumor

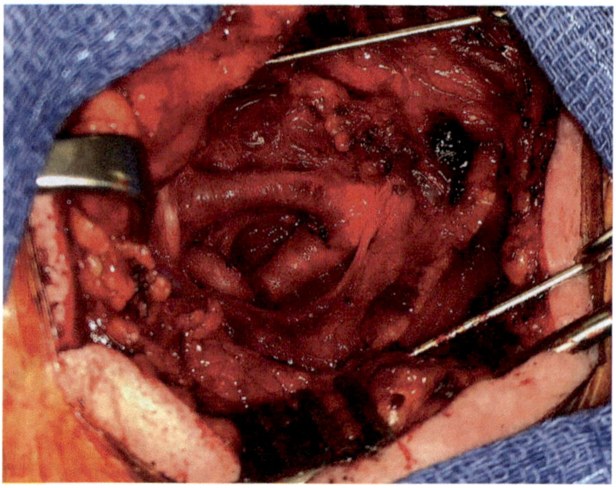

Fig. 37.5 Intraoperative photo following tumor resection with preservation of arterial structures

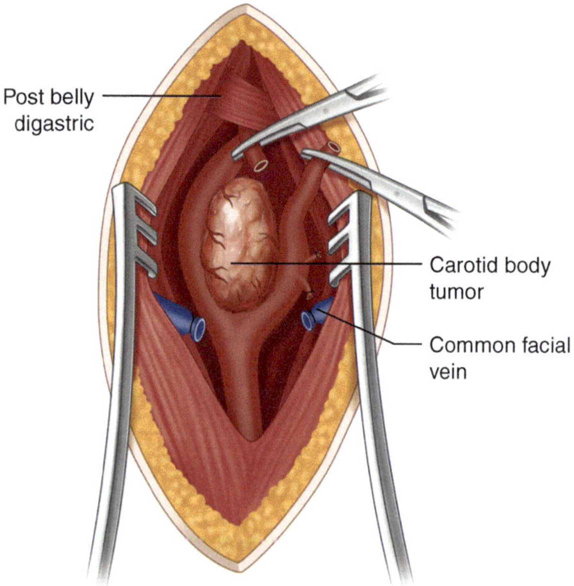

Fig. 37.6 Image illustrating ligation external carotid artery in case of complex carotid body tumor

divided to assist with mobilization and resection (Fig. 37.6). This maneuver also serves to devascularize the tumor.

More advanced tumors with greater involvement with the artery will require arterial resection of the carotid bulb, or internal carotid artery will require some type of arterial repair such as lateral arteriorrhaphy, patch angioplasty, or bypass (Fig. 37.7). In cases where the tumor completely encases the artery, the tumor and artery are resected en bloc, followed by arterial reconstruction usually with saphenous vein. When carotid artery clamping and/or reconstruction are required, monitored anticoagulation is instituted, along with selective shunting depending on the

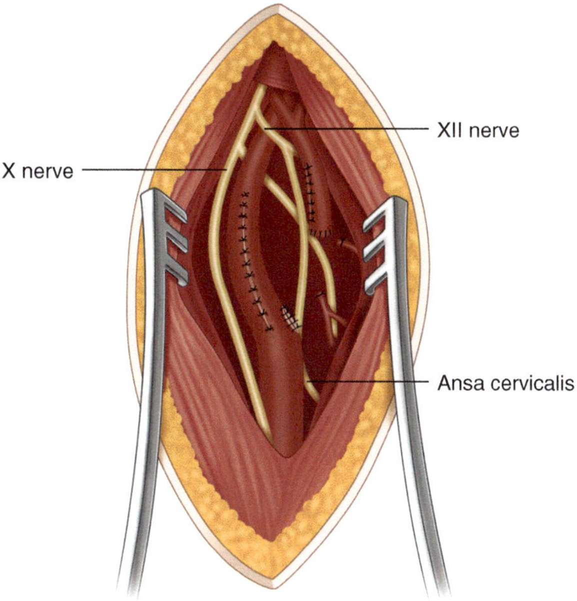

Fig. 37.7 Image illustrating external carotid artery excision and internal carotid artery repair in case of complex carotid body tumor excision

intraoperative electroencephalography findings. Attempt is made to remove all tumors as incomplete excision made lead to local recurrence.

Having completed resection of the tumor and any arterial reconstruction, hemostasis is ensured, and any heparin effect if present reversed with protamine. A closed suction drain is placed prior to closure to control residual blood or fluid in the resulting dead space and usually removed on post-op day 1 or 2. The platysma is closed over the drain with absorbable suture, and the skin is closed with a running subcuticular suture. Perioperative complications include nerve injury, stroke/transient ischemic attack, and bleeding. Most nerve injuries are secondary to stretch and resolve over time.

Chapter 38
Multiple-Choice Questions

Sachinder Singh Hans and Alexander D. Shepard

Chapter 1: Basic Techniques

Question 1

During arterial reconstructions under systemic heparin administration, ACT should be maintained at:

A. Less than 200 seconds
B. 200–250 seconds
C. 251–300 seconds
D. Greater than 300 seconds

Correct answer: C

Question 2

Interrupted closure of an arteriotomy is most commonly done for closure of the:

A. Femoral artery
B. Internal carotid artery
C. Brachial artery
D. External iliac artery

Correct answer: C

S. S. Hans (✉)
Vascular and Endovascular Services, Henry Ford Macomb Hospital, ClintonTwp, MI, USA

A. D. Shepard
Division of Vascular Surgery, Henry Ford Hospital, Detroit, MI, USA

S. S. Hans et al. (eds.), *Primary and Repeat Arterial Reconstructions*,
https://doi.org/10.1007/978-3-031-13897-3_38

Question 3
Eversion endarterectomy is most commonly performed in the:

A. External iliac artery
B. Femoral artery
C. Common carotid artery
D. Internal carotid artery

Correct answer: D

Question 4
During repair of a large femoral anastomotic aneurysm with obliteration of tissue planes, the control of deep femoral artery is best obtained by:

A. Control with a balloon angioplasty catheter via contralateral femoral approach
B. Ligation of deep femoral artery
C. Exposure of distal deep femoral artery in an undissected tissue plane
D. Intraluminal control

Correct answer: D

Chapter 2: Abdominal Aortic Aneurysm
Question 1
Just superior to the right renal artery, suprarenal aorta is separated from the IVC by the:

A. Right crus
B. Median arcuate ligament
C. Left crus
D. Cisterna chyli

Correct answer: A

Question 2
Patient with a retroaortic left renal vein is to undergo open AAA repair using left flank retroperitoneal approach.

A. Left kidney should be moved anteriorly.
B. Left kidney should be left in its bed.
C. Retroperitoneal approach is contraindicated.
D. Left renal vein can be ligated close to IVC as in transperitoneal approach.

Correct answer: B

Question 3
During repair of AAA without involvement of common and external iliac arteries, distal anastomosis to femoral artery should be avoided in order to prevent:

A. Surgical site infection and late development of an anastomotic aneurysm
B. Increased incidence of graft seroma
C. Increased incidence of graft limb occlusion
D. Increased incidence of sigmoid colon ischemia

Correct answer: A

Question 4
During left flank retroperitoneal repair of a large AAA, control of the right common iliac artery is most safely obtained by:

A. Direct clamping
B. Ligation of right common iliac artery and anastomosis to right external iliac artery using right extraperitoneal approach
C. Endoluminal control
D. Ligation of right common iliac artery and crossover femoral-femoral graft

Correct answer: C

Chapter 3: Open Repair of Juxtarenal and Infrarenal Abdominal Aortic Aneurysm

Question 1
A patient with 7.5 cm infrarenal AAA has a pelvic kidney with its arterial supply originating from the common iliac arteries on each side. The best management option is:

A. Open repair of AAA with renal autotransplantation
B. Axillobifemoral bypass graft during AAA repair to maintain retrograde arterial flow to the pelvic kidney
C. Nephrectomy of the pelvic kidney
D. Reimplantation of the renal arteries into the prosthetic graft during AAA repair

Correct answer: D

Question 2
A 70-year-old male has 7 cm juxtarenal AAA with significant COPD. CTA of the abdomen and pelvis shows a normal left renal vein. Preferred mode of repair is:

A. Transperitoneal midline repair
B. Transperitoneal transverse incision approach
C. Left flank retroperitoneal approach with kidney left in the anatomical position
D. Left retroperitoneal approach with plane of dissection behind the left kidney

Correct answer: D

Question 3
During repair of a large juxtarenal AAA and right common iliac artery aneurysm via a transperitoneal approach, proximal clamping of the aorta is facilitated by:

A. Ligation of left renal vein medial to the gonadal and adrenal vein
B. Ligation of left renal vein lateral to the gonadal vein and adrenal vein
C. Supraceliac control
D. Balloon occlusion of the supraceliac aorta via left brachial artery approach

Correct answer: A

Chapter 4: Paravisceral Abdominal Aortic Aneurysm Repair Questions
Question 1
During open repair of a suprarenal aortic aneurysm, the best exposure can be achieved using a:

A. Midline celiotomy with an infra-mesocolic approach
B. Thoracoabdominal incision through the eighth intercostal space
C. Midline celiotomy with right medial visceral rotation
D. Left flank retroperitoneal approach through the tenth intercostal space

Correct answer: D

Question 2
In a patient with an AAA extending to the level of the SMA, proximal control of the aorta is best obtained by:

A. Clamp placement at the supraceliac level
B. Clamp placement above the SMA but below the celiac
C. Intraluminal control by advancing and inflating an aortic balloon occlusion catheter in the supraceliac aorta
D. Balloon catheter occlusion of the supraceliac aorta using femoral artery access

Correct answer: A

Question 3
During open repair of a paravisceral AAA, renal ischemia time >30 min is anticipated. The best management strategy to reduce the risk of AKI consists of:

A. Mannitol infusion prior to aortic cross clamp
B. Infusion of sodium bicarbonate during the period of proximal aortic clamping
C. Perfusion of the renal arteries with a solution of cold Ringer's lactate + heparin, mannitol, and methylprednisolone during aortic occlusion
D. Maintaining the patient's temperature at 32–34 °C

Correct answer: C

Question 4
During open repair of a paravisceral AAA, the left renal artery can be reconstructed by:

A. Leaving it on an anterior tongue of aorta including the right renal, SM, and celiac arteries.
B. Bypassing it with a side-arm graft previously sewn on to the aortic prosthesis.
C. Reimplanting it directly on to the aortic prosthesis.
D. All are acceptable techniques depending on the local anatomy.

Correct answer: D

Chapter 5: Open Thoracoabdominal Aortic Aneurysm Repair
Question 1
Repair of a thoracoabdominal aortic aneurysm (TAAA) should be considered when the aneurysm reaches the maximum transverse/AP diameter:

A. 5 cm
B. 5.5 cm
C. 6 cm
D. 7 cm

Correct answer: C

Question 2
The best strategy for reducing the risk of spinal cord ischemia during repair of a TAAA is:

A. Epidural cooling
B. Distal aortic perfusion using a temporary axillary-femoral shunt
C. Distal aortic perfusion with intraoperative motor evoked potential monitoring
D. Quick clamp-and-sew technique without distal aortic perfusion

Correct answer: C

Question 3
During repair of a TAAA, left atrial femoral bypass is initiated. Mean distal perfusion pressure should be maintained as:

A. 35–39 mmHg
B. 40–50 mmHg
C. 51–59 mmHg
D. 60–70 mmHg

Correct answer: D

Question 4

Operative mortality for open TAAA repair 8–16%. Open repair of such aneurysm is contraindicated in chronic kidney disease patients with a GFR less than:

A. 30 cc
B. 40 cc
C. 50 cc
D. 60 cc

Correct answer: A

Chapter 6: Inflammatory Abdominal Aortic Aneurysm

Question 1

Inflammatory abdominal aortic aneurysm has a thickened aortic wall with dense adhesions to:

A. Jejunum
B. Duodenum and ureter
C. Sigmoid colon
D. Left renal vein

Correct answer: B

Question 2

During transperitoneal repair of an inflammatory AAA:

A. Third portion of duodenum should be left attached to aneurysmal wall.
B. Third portion of duodenum carefully separated from duodenal wall.
C. Ligament of Treitz should not be mobilized.
D. Left renal vein and inferior mesenteric vein always need ligation and division in order to obtain proximal control.

Correct answer: A

Question 3

Open repair of an inflammatory AAA:

A. It should always have placement of ureteral stent prior to open repair.
B. Transperitoneal repair is safer than retroperitoneal repair.
C. Inflammatory AAA has much lower incidence of rupture as compared to noninflammatory aneurysm of similar size.
D. Dense inflammatory reaction in the retroperitoneal tissues extends from below the origin of renal arteries to just above the common iliac artery bifurcation.

Correct answer: D

Question 4

During repair of an inflammatory AAA, there is an injury to right common iliac vein which is repaired by lateral venorrhaphy. On second post-op day, the patient develops mild discomfort in the right thigh. The patient should undergo:

A. Venogram right lower extremity
B. EMG right lower extremity
C. Duplex venous study of right lower extremity
D. Close observation

Correct answer: C

Chapter 7: Repair of Aortoenteric Fistula

Question 1

The repair of aortoenteric fistula is to be performed in a relatively stable patient who had undergone open repair of AAA previously. The best conduit for aortic reconstruction following removal of remotely placed prosthetic graft is:

A. Rifampin-soaked Dacron graft
B. Cryopreserved arterial allograft
C. Reconstruction with deep veins (femoral/popliteal)
D. Axillobifemoral graft

Correct answer: B

Question 2

During repair of aortoenteric fistula, the best method of proximal control of aorta is:

A. Supraceliac aorta via a laparotomy
B. Suprarenal aorta via laparotomy
C. Balloon occlusion of aorta via femoral artery access
D. Balloon occlusion of supraceliac aorta via left brachial artery access

Correct answer: A

Question 3

Following repair of an aortoenteric fistula with a direct inline aortic reconstruction, antibiotics should be administered for:

A. 2 weeks
B. 6 weeks
C. 3 months
D. 6 months–possible lifetime

Correct answer: D

Chapter 8: Ruptured AAA

Question 1

A 72-year-old female presents to ER with profound hypotension secondary to a ruptured AAA. The patient should undergo:

A. Thoracic aortic balloon occlusion via femoral approach in ER
B. Thoracic aortic balloon occlusion via left brachial approach in OR
C. Supraceliac aortic control in OR
D. Retrograde passage of a large Foley balloon catheter through the aortic neck in OR

Correct answer: C

Question 2

During open repair of a ruptured AAA, there is injury to the left renal vein close to IVC with a 40% loss of circumference. Mean BP is 70 mmHg. Optimal management consists of:

A. Lateral repair of left renal vein
B. Ligation of left renal vein
C. Splenic vein to left renal vein bypass
D. Vascular clamps on either side of injured left renal vein and repair of injury following completion of Proximal anastomosis

Correct answer: A

Question 3

During exposure of the supraceliac artery, which portion of the diaphragm is dissected?

A. Right crus
B. Left crus
C. Median arcuate ligament
D. Right dome of diaphragm

Correct answer: A

Question 4

During completion of distal anastomosis following open repair of a ruptured AAA, the patient has diffuse oozing from the exposed surfaces. Hgb = 9.2 Gm, Hct= 26, PTT = 54 s (normal 25–35), pro time = 16.8 s with INR = 1.8, fibrin split products are normal. The most common cause of this abnormality is:

A. Disseminated intravascular coagulopathy
B. Secondary fibrinolysis from hepatic ischemia with supraceliac clamping
C. Dilutional coagulopathy
D. Primary fibrinolysis

Correct answer: C

Chapter 9: Explant of Abdominal Aortic Endograft

Question 1

The incidence of late open conversion after EVAR is:

A. Less than 1%
B. 1–5%
C. 6–10%
D. Greater than 10%

Correct answer: B

Question 2

When complete excision of EVAR graft with suprarenal stent is required, the best strategy to facilitate complete removal of suprarenal struts is:

A. Release of barbs from the main body with a wire cutter circumferentially
B. Use of a 20 cc syringe as a sheath to encircle and collapse the suprarenal component
C. Iced saline on nitinol elements to help collapse the metal
D. All of the above

Correct answer: D

Question 3

The mortality rate for elective explant of an EVAR graft should be

A. Less than 5%
B. 5–10%
C. 11–20%
D. Greater than 20%

Correct answer: A

Chapter 10: Splanchnic Aneurysms

Question 1

Asymptomatic splenic artery aneurysm in a 56-year-old female should be repaired once the aneurysm measures:

A. 1.5 cm in AP/transverse diameter
B. 1.6–1.9 cm
C. 2.0–2.4 cm
D. Should be repaired regardless of its size

Correct answer: C

Question 2

Hepatic artery aneurysms constitute what percentage of splanchnic artery aneurysms?

A. Less than 12%
B. 13–20%
C. 21–24%
D. 25% or greater

Correct answer: B

Question 3
Celiac artery aneurysm is considered for repair once aneurysm measures:

A. 1.5 cm in AP/Tr diameter
B. 1.6–2.0 cm
C. 2.1–2.4 cm
D. 2.5 cm or greater

Correct answer: D

Question 4
Rupture rate of SMA aneurysms is:

A. Less than 20%
B. 20–25%
C. 26–34%
D. 35% or greater

Correct answer: D

Question 5
SMA aneurysms are most commonly located at:

A. Origin of SMA
B. About 4 cm from the origin of SMA
C. Near the origin of the middle colic artery
D. Near the origin of the right colic artery

Correct answer: B

Chapter 11: Renal Artery Aneurysm
Question 1
The major risk factor for a ruptured renal artery aneurysm is:

A. Size greater than 2 cm with pregnancy
B. Size between 1.5 and 2 cm
C. Size between 1 and 1.4 cm
D. Aneurysms associated with FMD

Correct answer: A

Question 2

During repair of a renal artery aneurysm, the renal ischemia time is greater than 30 min. The most practical strategy to prevent kidney injury is:

A. Optimal volume status prior to renal artery clamping and cooling the mobilized kidney with the ice
B. Repair using autotransplantation technique
C. Endovascular therapy, which is preferable
D. Optimal volume status and renal perfusion with cold RL at 4 °C with added heparin and methylprednisolone

Correct answer: D

Question 3

The incidence of bilateral renal artery aneurysms is:

A. 10–12%
B. 13–15%
C. 16–20%
D. 25%

Correct answer: B

Chapter 12: Femoral and Femoral Anastomotic Aneurysm

Question 1

The guideline for repair of asymptomatic femoral aneurysms based on size alone is:

A. 2–2.5 cm
B. 2.6–3.0 cm
C. 3.1–3.4 cm
D. Greater than 3.5 cm

Correct answer: D

Question 2

An 80-year-old man presents with a leaking 10 cm femoral anastomotic aneurysm. Proximal control is most safely obtained by:

A. Exposing the proximal graft through a groin incision (old scar)
B. Suprainguinal transverse incision with exposure of the prosthetic graft
C. Endovascular balloon occlusion of the graft via contralateral femoral artery/graft
D. Balloon occlusion using left brachial artery approach

Correct answer: B

Question 3

A 79-year-old man presents with a 3.8 cm femoral artery aneurysm with local discomfort. He has chronic occlusion of the superficial femoral artery on CTA but without symptoms of intermittent claudication. Repair of the aneurysm is best performed by excision of the aneurysm and interposition grafting:

A. With simultaneous femoral-popliteal bypass graft
B. To the deep femoral artery
C. Hybrid approach with excision of the aneurysm and retrograde recanalization of the superficial femoral artery
D. Distal anastomosis to superficial femoral artery after local endarterectomy and reimplantation of deep femoral artery into the interposition prosthetic graft

Correct answer: B

Chapter 13: Popliteal Artery Aneurysm Repair: Primary and Recurrent

Question 1

During repair of a popliteal aneurysm using a posterior approach, the dissection proceeds between the two heads of the gastrocnemii. The nerve encountered in the dissection plane in addition to the nerve to the medial head of gastrocnemius is:

A. Saphenous nerve
B. Common peroneal nerve
C. Sural nerve
D. Nerve to the lateral head of gastrocnemius

Correct answer: C

Question 2

During the repair of a popliteal aneurysm using medial approach, which superficial nerve is encountered in the proximal part of the dissection near the adductor hiatus?

A. Sural
B. Saphenous
C. Posterior tibial
D. Common peroneal

Correct answer: B

Question 3

A 60-year-old man has a 3.5 cm Tr/AP diameter popliteal artery aneurysm present behind the knee extending 2 cm above the knee joint and 1 cm below, with extrinsic compression of the popliteal vein. The best management option is:

A. Medial approach for exclusion of the aneurysm and bypass using GSV

B. Posterior approach for complete excision and bypass using lesser saphenous vein
C. Posterior approach for complete excision of the aneurysm and bypass using greater saphenous vein
D. Endovascular exclusion using covered stent

Correct answer: C

Chapter 14: Extracranial Carotid Aneurysm

Question 1

During repair of an extracranial carotid aneurysm, the stylohyoid muscle was transected and styloid process needs to be removed in order to gain distal exposure of the internal carotid artery. The commonest nerve to be injured during this maneuver is:

A. Spinal accessory
B. Hypoglossal
C. Sympathetic chain
D. Glossopharyngeal

Correct answer: D

Question 2

During repair of a giant internal carotid aneurysm in the neck extending to the base of the skull, the cephalad portion of the ICA above the aneurysm cannot be visualized despite all the techniques used to gain high exposure of ICA. The mean ICA stump (back) pressure is 52 mmHg. The best option in managing this aneurysm is:

A. EC-IC bypass by a vascular neurosurgeon and ligation of ICA
B. Ligation of ICA near its origin
C. Transcranial Doppler assessment of MCA velocity
D. OR consult with interventional neuroradiology? Neurosurgery

Correct answer: B

Question 3

During repair of 2 cm diameter ICA aneurysm arising 1.5 cm distal to the origin of ICA, with significant redundancy of the ICA, the continuity of ICA following excision of the aneurysm is best achieved by:

A. End-to-end anastomosis behind the hypoglossal nerve
B. End-to-end anastomosis with transposition of ICA in front of hypoglossal nerve
C. Interposition vein graft
D. Interposition prosthetic graft

Correct answer: B

Question 4
The commonest complication following repair of an ICA aneurysm is:

A. Myocardial infarction
B. Lymph leak
C. Cranial nerve injury
D. Perioperative stroke

Correct answer: C

Question 5
In managing a large post-endarterectomy pseudoaneurysm of the carotid artery, which was patched with Dacron, the best repair technique is:

A. Ligation proximally and distally
B. Repatching the artery with bovine pericardium
C. Interposition grafting from the common carotid artery to the internal carotid artery with PTFE
D. Interposition grafting from the common carotid artery to the internal carotid artery with autologous vein

Correct answer: D

Chapter 15: Subclavian Artery Aneurysm
Question 1
Aneurysm associated with aberrant right subclavian artery causing dysphagia is best managed by:

A. Transthoracic repair
B. Right carotid-subclavian artery bypass or transposition followed by thoracic aortic stent grafting
C. Medical management only
D. Endoscopic dilatation of the esophagus prior to hybrid repair

Correct answer: B

Question 2
Which nerve courses lateral to medially in the neck over the anterior surface of the anterior scalene muscle?

A. Phrenic
B. Spinal accessory
C. Vagus
D. Recurrent laryngeal

Correct answer: A

Question 3

A 30-year-old female has right thoracic outlet syndrome with a 2.2 cm axillo-subclavian artery aneurysm. This is best managed by a:

A. Covered stent
B. Transaxillary approach
C. Supraclavicular approach
D. Supraclavicular and infraclavicular exposure

Correct answer: D

Chapter 16: Axillary and Brachial Artery Aneurysms

Question 1

The incidence of axillary and brachial artery aneurysms among peripheral artery aneurysm is:

A. Less than 1%
B. 1–3%
C. Greater than 3% but less than 5%
D. 5%

Correct answer: A

Question 2

The most common cause of mycotic brachial artery aneurysm is:

A. Brachial artery access for coronary intervention
B. Cocaine abuse
C. Intravenous drug abuse
D. Open supracondylar fracture

Correct answer: C

Question 3

Repair of axillary and brachial artery aneurysm is recommended for aneurysm size of:

A. 0.5–1 cm
B. Greater than 1–1.5 cm
C. Greater than 1.5 cm–less than 2.0 cm
D. Greater than 2 cm

Correct answer: D

Chapter 17: Carotid Endarterectomy

Question 1

Superior thyroid artery is intimately related to:

A. Internal laryngeal nerve
B. External laryngeal nerve
C. Lingual nerve
D. Recurrent laryngeal nerve

Correct answer: B

Question 2
Six hours following carotid endarterectomy, the patient has a large neck hematoma with stridor.
The patient is taken to OR for evacuation of the hematoma. Anesthetic considerations for safer outcome are:

A. Attempt of standard orotracheal intubation
B. Tracheostomy
C. Intubation aided with glidescope
D. Removal of staples and sutures under local anesthesia, evacuation of the hematoma, and consideration of intubation if stridor is not relieved

Correct answer: D

Question 3
The most common nerve injured during carotid endarterectomy is:

A. Vagus
B. Ramus mandibularis
C. Hypoglossal
D. Glossopharyngeal

Correct answer: C

Question 4
Perioperative stroke rate for carotid endarterectomy is:

A. Less than 1%
B. 1–4%
C. 5–6%
D. Greater than 6%

Correct answer: B

Chapter 18: Carotid Endarterectomy for High Plaque
Question 1
A necessary maneuver for exposure of the internal carotid artery during carotid endarterectomy for high plaque is:

A. Cephalad mobilization and retraction with or without division of post-belly of digastric

B. Division of inferior belly of omohyoid
C. Removal of tip of mastoid process
D. Mandibular osteotomy

Correct answer: A

Question 2
Cephalad mobilization of hypoglossal nerve is facilitated by division of:

A. Sternocleidomastoid branch of occipital artery and if necessary occipital artery itself
B. Facial artery
C. External carotid artery
D. Transecting internal carotid artery at its origin and mobilization of hypoglossal nerve cephalad and transposition of internal carotid artery anterior to the nerve followed by reanastomosis of the divided internal carotid artery

Correct answer: A

Question 3
During performance of eversion carotid endarterectomy, the distal end of the plaque could not be well visualized. The best option is:

A. Interposition graft between distal CCA and ICA
B. Convert to standard CEA with patch graft
C. Intraoperative carotid stenting
D. Transection of ICA at its origin and extending the arteriotomy cephalad to reach the end point and transposition of ICA anterior to hypoglossal nerve with reanastomosis of ICA at the carotid bifurcation

Correct answer: D

Question 4
During CEA for high plaque, the surgeon is uncertain about the end point of the plaque. The next best option is:

A. Intraoperative carotid duplex imaging
B. Obtain CTA neck
C. Closure of endarterectomy with patch graft and perform intraoperative carotid arteriogram
D. Closure of endarterectomy with patch graft and obtain transcranial Doppler study

Correct answer: C

Question 5
Intraoperative carotid arteriogram in aforementioned patient shows no flow in the internal carotid artery. The optimal management consists of:

A. Open the endarterectomy site and place tacking sutures in the arterial wall at the cephalad end
B. CCA-to-ICA interposition graft
C. Ligate the ICA if stump pressure is greater than 40 mmHg and postoperative unfractionated heparin
D. Intraoperative carotid stenting

Correct answer: D

Chapter 19: Carotid Interposition Graft
Question 1
Four months following CEA with a knitted Dacron patch graft, the patient develops sinus in the neck and undergoes unsuccessful local exploration of the neck. CTA neck shows a small mass around the origin of ICA. Optimal management besides antibiotics and debridement consists of:

A. Removal of Dacron patch and its replacement with bovine pericardial patch
B. Removal of Dacron patch and placement of vein patch
C. Resection of proximal ICA including patch and interposition PTFE graft
D. Resection of proximal ICA with interposition greater saphenous vein bypass graft from mid-CCA to mid-ICA

Correct answer: D

Question 2
During radical neck dissection for squamous cell carcinoma of oral cavity, tumor is firmly adherent to the common carotid artery. Tumor is removed en bloc with a 3 cm segment of the common carotid artery. Arterial reconstruction is best performed by:

A. PTFE interposition graft
B. Interposition lesser saphenous vein graft
C. Cryopreserved arterial homograft
D. Interposition with superficial femoral artery graft

Correct answer: D

Question 3
Six months following carotid stenting, the patient develops carotid in-stent restenosis with a densely calcified plaque at the superior end of the stent, which is at the level of the C2 vertebral body. Carotid interposition graft with removal of the stent is planned. Distal control of the ICA is best obtained by:

A. Mandibular subluxation
B. Mandibular osteotomy
C. Standard exposure of ICA and application of distal clamp to ICA

D. Placement of number 3 Fogarty balloon catheter over a .014 wire placed through a sheath placed in the CCA above the clavicle

Correct answer: D

Chapter 20: Redo Carotid Endarterectomy

Question 1

Eighteen months following carotid endarterectomy, a 64-year-old woman develops a focal smooth transverse high-grade stenosis in the mid-common carotid artery. This lesion is most likely caused by:

A. Recurrent atherosclerotic plaque
B. Residual plaque
C. Lesion as a result of clamp injury
D. Result of dissection during placement of shunt during CEA

Correct answer: C

Question 2

Which of the following statements best reflects the complications of symptomatic redo CEA for atherosclerotic lesion?

A. Incidence of perioperative stroke is higher than primary CEA.
B. Incidence of cranial nerve injury is same as in primary CEA.
C. Incidence of neck hematoma is greater than primary CEA.
D. Incidence of perioperative stroke is same, but incidence of cranial nerve palsy is greater in patients undergoing redo CEA as compared to primary CEA.

Correct answer: D

Question 3

During redo CEA, the incision is extended proximally to aid in obtaining proximal control by dissecting and passing the silastic vessel loop around the common carotid artery proximal to previous arteriotomy. The cranial nerve most likely to be injured during this part of the procedure is:

A. Hypoglossal
B. Sympathetic chain
C. Vagus
D. Ansa hypoglossi

Correct answer: C

Question 4

A 74-year-old man presents to the hospital with left middle cerebral infarct with aphasia, right supranuclear facial palsy, flaccid paralysis of right upper extremity, and grade 3 motor weakness of right lower extremity. His NIH stroke scale is

18. Imaging studies show high-grade stenosis (>70%) at the origin of left ICA. He had left CEA performed 8 years ago.

Best management option is:

A. Urgent carotid stenting.
B. Urgent left CEA.
C. PT, OT, and speech therapy and continue medical management only.
D. PT, OT, and speech therapy. Revaluation of neuro-deficit. If improved with NIH stroke scale less than 15, consider left carotid intervention in 10–14 days after medical optimization.

Correct answer: D

Chapter 21: Vertebral Artery Transposition

Question 1

Posterior circulation territory strokes constitute what percentage of all ischemic strokes?

A. 5–10%
B. 11–15%
C. 16–20%
D. Just over 20%

Correct answer: D

Question 2

First portion of vertebral artery courses between:

A. Scalenus anticus and medius muscle
B. Longus coli and scalenus anticus muscle
C. Longus coli and scalenus medius muscle
D. Scalenus medius and scalenus tertius

Correct answer: B

Question 3

A 76-year-old male presents to ER with dizziness and presyncope. The patient is in atrial fibrillation with a heart rate of 110 per minute. CTA neck showed less than 50% stenosis of bilateral ICA. Right vertebral artery is hypoplastic, and left vertebral artery has 50% stenosis at its origin. CT head shows chronic white matter changes. The optimal management consists of:

A. Vertebral artery transposition into the CCA
B. Urgent cardiology consult
C. Urgent ENT consult
D. Discharge patient on antiplatelet medication and beta-blockers

Correct answer: B

Question 4
Two days following vertebral artery-to-CCA transposition, the patient develops 70 cc of milky fluid in 24 h. Initial management consists of:

A. Thoracic duct embolization
B. Immediate exploration of the neck and ligation of the site of the leak
C. Dietary modification, local compression, and octreotide
D. Total parental nutrition with minimal calories from fat

Correct answer: C

Chapter 22: Carotid-Subclavian Artery Bypass
Question 1
In contemporary vascular practice, the most common indication for carotid-subclavian bypass is:

A. Left arm ischemia secondary to proximal left subclavian artery stenosis
B. Following repair of subclavian artery aneurysm in association with thoracic outlet syndrome
C. Ischemic symptoms in vertebral-basilar territory
D. Prior to TEVAR in a patient with absent right vertebral artery

Correct answer: D

Question 2
Carotid-subclavian artery bypass in association with TEVAR is usually performed:

A. Simultaneously with TEVAR
B. Few days prior to TEVAR
C. Following TEVAR if the patient develops spinal cord ischemia
D. Through subclavian-to-carotid transposition, which is more effective in reducing the incidence of spinal cord ischemia as compared to carotid-subclavian bypass

Correct answer: B

Question 3
Carotid-subclavian artery is preferably performed with a synthetic conduit. The usual length of the bypass graft is:

A. 2 cm
B. 3 cm
C. 5 cm
D. 6 cm

Correct answer: B

Question 4
The most common nerve injury during exposure of subclavian artery for carotid-subclavian bypass is:

A. Vagus
B. Recurrent laryngeal
C. Phrenic
D. Internal laryngeal

Correct answer: C

Question 5
Thoracic duct fistula develops 6 days following carotid-subclavian artery bypass draining 400 cc of milky fluid in 24 h. The best strategy to control chyle leak is:

A. Medical management
B. Thoracotomy and ligation of thoracic duct
C. Coil embolization of thoracic duct
D. Re-exploration of the neck and ligation of thoracic duct leak

Correct answer: D

Chapter 23: De-branching Operations on Supra-aortic Trunks
Question 1
Carotid-carotid bypass is planned to extend the landing zone of TEVAR. Which of these statements describe the most optimal technique of reconstruction?

A. Arteriotomy in the Rt CCA at 12 o'clock with graft tunneled in the subcutaneous location with arteriotomy in the left CCA at 12 o'clock position
B. Arteriotomy in the Rt CCA at 12 o'clock with graft tunneled in the retropharyngeal position at 12 o'clock position in the left CCA
C. Arteriotomy at 11 o'clock position in the Rt CCA with the graft in the retropharyngeal position with arteriotomy at 11 o'clock position in the left CCA
D. Arteriotomy at 1–2 o'clock position in the Rt CCA with graft in the retropharyngeal position with arteriotomy in the left CCA at 10–11 o'clock position

Correct answer: D

Question 2
The commonest nerve injured during carotid-carotid bypass is:

A. Recurrent laryngeal nerve
B. Vagus nerve
C. Phrenic nerve
D. External laryngeal nerve

Correct answer: B

Question 3
The incidence of stroke following ascending aorta to carotid/subclavian bypass is:

A. Less than 3%
B. 3–5%
C. 6–8%
D. 9–10%

Correct answer: B

Chapter 24: Brachiocephalic Reconstruction
Question 1
A 61-year-old man, with a history of stable angina, is scheduled to undergo aorto-innominate bypass for near occlusion of innominate artery (brachiocephalic) with a history of amaurosis fugax. The most important preoperative assessment should include:

A. Pulmonary function tests
B. Stress echocardiogram
C. Cardiac CTA for calcium score
D. Coronary angiogram

Correct answer: D

Question 2
The origin of right subclavian artery is related to:

A. Recurrent laryngeal nerve
B. Superior laryngeal nerve
C. Phrenic nerve
D. Vagus nerve

Correct answer: A

Question 3
One of the absolute contraindications for aorto-innominate bypass is:

A. Contralateral ICA occlusion
B. Severe bilateral vertebral artery stenosis
C. Severe stenosis right subclavian artery origin
D. Severe calcification of ascending aorta

Correct answer: D

Chapter 25: Aortobifemoral Bypass Graft
Question 1
During a redo aortofemoral bypass, exposure can most easily be achieved using a:

A. Midline celiotomy with an infra-mesocolic approach
B. Midline celiotomy with right medial visceral rotation
C. Left flank retroperitoneal approach
D. Transverse celiotomy through an infraumbilical "smile" incision

Correct answer: C

Question 2
In a patient with a juxtarenal aortic occlusion requiring suprarenal aortic clamping, the left renal vein can be mobilized by ligating and dividing the:

A. Lumbar branch
B. Adrenal branch
C. Gonadal branch
D. All of the above

Correct answer: D

Question 3
When tunneling the graft limbs to the groins during aortobifemoral bypass, the limbs should pass:

A. Lateral to the ureters.
B. Posterior to the ureters.
C. Anterior to the ureters.
D. It does not matter in regard to orientation to the ureters.

Correct answer: B

Question 4
During the femoral anastomosis of an aortofemoral bypass, correction of disease at the origin of the profunda femoris artery is:

A. Unnecessary
B. Optional
C. Important to long-term graft patency
D. Desirable only if it is easy to do

Correct answer: C

Chapter 26: Thoracofemoral Bypass for Aortoiliac Occlusive Disease
Question 1
Thoracofemoral bypass graft is best indicated for:

A. Juxtarenal aortic occlusion in a 46-year-old male with hip claudication with erectile dysfunction
B. Infrarenal aortic and bilateral iliac artery occlusion with rest pain
C. 6 cm Infrarenal AAA with severe iliac artery occlusive disease

D. Failed aortobifemoral bypass graft in a 46-year-old female (graft occlusion just below the renal arteries) with a history of multiple abdominal operations presenting with ischemic rest pain

Correct answer: D

Question 2
An absolute contraindication for thoracofemoral bypass graft is:

A. Remote history of MI
B. Prior multiple laparotomy incisions
C. Left ventricle ejection fraction of 55%
D. Circumferential distal thoracic aortic calcification

Correct answer: D

Question 3
Thoracofemoral bypass graft is planned for a 62-year-old male with a prior history of suprapubic cystostomy for bladder pathology.

A. Right femoral limb of the graft should be brought behind the rectus abdominus in the space of Retzius.
B. Right axillofemoral graft should be considered with left thoracofemoral bypass graft.
C. Right femoral graft limb is brought from the left groin in the suprapubic subcutaneous tunnel and anastomosed to the right common femoral artery as in a standard crossover femoral-femoral graft.
D. Right femoral limb is brought through the obturator foramen and anastomosed to proximal right superficial femoral artery.

Correct answer: C

Chapter 27: Aortomesenteric Bypass Graft
Question 1
A 68-year-old female with a history of vague periumbilical abdominal pain for 6 months with no association to the intake of meals and without weight loss is seen in the clinic. CTA abdomen and pelvis shows 50% stenosis of celiac and SMA. Optimal management consists of:

A. SMA stenting
B. Celiac and SMA stenting
C. Med. management with follow-up CTA imaging in 1 year
D. Med. management and duplex imaging of visceral arteries in 1 year

Correct answer: D

Question 2

A 58-year-old female with classic symptoms of intestinal angina with significant weight loss has a 50% stenosis of small-diameter celiac artery, complete occlusion of proximal 6 cm SMA, and occlusion of IMA. Percutaneous revascularization of SMA was unsuccessful. Her cardiac risk is acceptable. Optimal management consists of:

A. Antegrade bypass from supraceliac aorta to SMA using a prosthetic graft
B. Retrograde bypass from infrarenal aorta to SMA using a prosthetic graft
C. Retrograde bypass from infrarenal aorta to SMA using greater saphenous vein
D. Trapdoor endarterectomy of paravisceral aorta

Correct answer: A

Question 3

A 78-year-old female with symptoms of intestinal angina with significant weight loss has occlusion of celiac artery and occlusion of proximal 5 cm SMA with patent IMA. Supraceliac aorta shows severe calcification. Infrarenal aorta is small in caliber (10 mm diameter) but has small posterior plaque. Optimal management consists of:

A. Antegrade bypass from supraceliac aorta to SMA
B. Bypass to celiac and SMA using retroperitoneal flank approach via ninth ICS
C. Retrograde bypass using ringed prosthetic graft from infrarenal aorta or right common iliac artery to SMA
D. Retrograde bypass from infrarenal aorta to SMA using greater saphenous vein

Correct answer: C

Question 4

A 76-year-old male with a history of prior CABG presents with symptoms of intestinal angina with occlusions of celiac and SMA. Endovascular management is unsuccessful. Optimal management consists of:

A. Antegrade aortoceliac and SMA bypass
B. Retrograde bypass from infrarenal aorta to SMA
C. Retrograde stenting of SMA
D. Trapdoor aortic endarterectomy

Correct answer: D

Chapter 28: Aortorenal Bypass and Renal Artery Reconstruction

Question 1

Results of CORAL study comparing medical therapy with renal artery stenting showed:

A. Benefit of stenting in improving GFR
B. Benefit of stenting in modest BP improvement

C. Benefit of stenting in control of BP as well as GFR
D. That renal stenting had high incidence of technical complications

Correct answer: B

Question 2
A 45-year-old man underwent renal artery stenting for uncontrollable BP on multiple antihypertensive medications. He has developed recurrent in-stent stenosis, which has been treated with angioplasty twice in the past, without improvement in BP with one episode of flash pulmonary edema. The optimal management option is:

A. Covered renal stent
B. Repeat angioplasty with drug-eluting balloon
C. Renal endarterectomy
D. Aortorenal bypass graft

Correct answer: D

Question 3
The best approach for isolated left aortorenal bypass is:

A. Left retroperitoneal approach
B. Medial visceral rotation
C. Infra-mesocolic approach
D. Use of splenic artery for left renal artery bypass

Correct answer: C

Chapter 29: Crossover Femoral-Femoral Bypass Graft and Iliofemoral Bypass Graft

Question 1
The optimal site for femoral anastomosis during performance of crossover fem-fem graft in the femoral artery should be:

A. Under the inguinal ligament at the junction of external iliac and common femoral artery
B. Superficial femoral artery
C. Distal common femoral artery
D. Deep femoral (profunda) artery

Correct answer: C

Question 2
A crossover femoral-femoral graft is being planned in a patient with a history of extensive scarring in the suprapubic region. The best alternative to subcutaneous suprapubic tunnel is:

A. Excision of burn scar and prosthetic graft coverage with rectus abdominis flap
B. Tunnel in prevesical space
C. Excision of burn scar and gracilis flap
D. Performing of bilateral axillofemoral graft instead of crossover femoral-femoral graft

Correct answer: B

Question 3
During performance of crossover femoral-femoral graft:

A. The distal anastomosis should always be performed on to deep femoral artery
B. Distal anastomosis should always be performed to superficial femoral artery
C. Distal anastomosis should be performed to distal common femoral artery extending to proximal superficial femoral artery
D. Always perform femoral endarterectomy with patch graft prior to distal anastomosis

Correct answer: C

Chapter 30: Axillofemoral Bypass Graft
Question 1
Factors affecting the patency of an axillary-femoral graft are:

A. Type of graft (Dacron vs. externally supported PTFE)
B. Patient's age
C. Graft performed on elective basis or as emergency
D. Presence or absence of superficial femoral disease

Correct answer: D

Question 2
5-Year patency of iliofemoral bypass graft is:

A. Greater than 90%
B. 80–90%
C. 71–89%
D. Less than 70%

Correct answer: A

Question 3
Patient presented with unilateral lymph leak 5 days after axillofemoral bypass graft. Optimal management consists of:

A. Antibiotics
B. Local care and low-fat diet

C. Vacuum-assisted closure
D. Local wound exploration and ligation of lymphatics

Correct answer: D

Question 4
Risk of graft infection following axillofemoral graft is:

A. Less than 5%
B. 5–10%
C. 11–15%
D. Greater than 15%

Correct answer: C

Chapter 31: Iliac and Femoral Endarterectomy
Question 1
During retroperitoneal exposure of common iliac artery, the dissection plane occurs:

A. Posterior to psoas major
B. Anterior to psoas major
C. Anterior to quadratus lumborum
D. Posterior to quadratus lumborum

Correct answer: B

Question 2
The most common cause of lymphocele following femoral endarterectomy is:

A. Postoperative hematoma
B. Interruption of groin lymphatics
C. Prior groin radiation
D. Vertical skin incision

Correct answer: B

Question 3
The preferred groin incision for femoral endarterectomy in a morbidly obese patient is:

A. Vertical
B. Hockey stick
C. Horizontal (transverse)
D. Common femoral atherectomy being preferred to endarterectomy

Correct answer: C

Chapter 32: Femoral-Popliteal Bypass Graft

Question 1

Using autologous saphenous vein for femoral-popliteal bypass graft, 5-year patency is:

A. 90% above knee and 70% below knee
B. 80% above knee and 60% below knee
C. 70% above knee and 50% below knee
D. 60% above knee and 40% below knee

Correct answer: C

Question 2

The origin of the profunda femoris artery is crossed by:

A. Lateral circumflex femoral vein anteriorly
B. Lateral circumflex femoral vein posteriorly
C. Medial circumflex femoral vein anteriorly
D. Medial circumflex femoral vein posteriorly

Correct answer: A

Question 3

During exposure of the common femoral artery:

A. The inguinal lymphatics and lymph nodes.
B. The lymphoadipose tissue is mobilized medially.
C. Dissection is performed through the lymphoadipose tissue.
D. Lymphoadipose tissue is only encountered in the groin of patients with morbid obesity.

Correct answer: B

Chapter 33: Femoral-Infrapopliteal (Crural and Paramalleolar) Bypass Graft

Question 1

During performance of femoral-tibial bypass with in situ technique, the proximal GSV cannot be brought to the common femoral artery with significant stenosis. The most useful adjunct is:

A. Common femoral stent using contralateral access
B. Common femoral atherectomy using contralateral access
C. Common femoral artery endarterectomy with patch graft
D. Using a composite graft from distal external iliac artery (PTFE) and in situ bypass distally

Correct answer: C

Question 2
The tourniquet occlusion technique for infrainguinal bypass graft is best utilized for:

A. Above-knee femoral-popliteal bypass graft
B. Below-knee femoral-popliteal bypass graft
C. Femoral-mid posterior tibial bypass graft
D. Femoral-popliteal bypass graft using PTFE graft with distal anastomosis behind the knee

Correct answer: C

Question 3
Anterior tibial artery in its mid-segment is exposed between:

A. Lateral border of tibia and tibialis anterior
B. Tibialis anterior and extensor digitorum longus
C. Tibialis anterior and extensor hallucis longus
D. Extensor digitorum longus and extensor hallucis longus

Correct answer: C

Question 4
The incidence of major amputation (BK/AK) following femoral-infrapopliteal bypass is:

A. Less than 1%
B. 1–1.5%
C. 1.6–2%
D. Greater than 2%

Correct answer: C

Chapter 34: Upper Extremity Bypass Graft
Question 1
Anatomically, axillary artery becomes brachial artery at the:

A. Lateral border of pectoralis minor
B. Lateral border of latissimus dorsi
C. Lateral border of teres major
D. Origin of brachialis

Correct answer: C

Question 2
Advanced ischemic changes with gangrene in the hand and fingers are most often associated with:

A. Diabetes mellitus
B. Scleroderma

C. ESRD
D. Subclavian artery aneurysm with thoracic outlet syndrome

Correct answer: C

Question 3
Following brachial artery occlusion, the most important collateral supply to forearm and hand is:

A. Anterior and posterior circumflex humeral artery
B. Deep (profunda) brachial artery
C. Radial recurrent artery
D. Palmer branch of ulnar artery

Correct answer: B

Chapter 35: Arterial Reconstructions in Hostile Groin
Question 1
A 68-year-old male presented with bleeding in the left groin. He had undergone aortobifemoral graft performed 10 years ago. Graft thrombectomy for occlusion of the left limb was required 2 years and 9 months ago. The patient was hemodynamically stable with slight erythema in the left groin. CTA of abdomen and pelvis showed normal body and right limb of the graft with peri-graft fluid around the left limb. WBC scan showed increased uptake in the left limb. The patient is at high risk for complete graft removal. The best option in this situation is:

A. Axillofemoral graft with left-side anastomosis to mid-superficial femoral artery followed by graft removal
B. Left axillopopliteal bypass with graft routed over the iliac crest
C. Reconstruction with a new graft flush from the origin of the left limb of aortobifemoral graft with distal anastomosis to left mid-superficial femoral artery via obturator canal
D. Local debridement and sartorius myoplasty

Correct answer: C

Question 2
Mid-superficial femoral artery is located:

A. Anterior to sartorius
B. Posterior to sartorius
C. Medial to vastus medialis
D. Behind the adductor magnus

Correct answer: B

Question 3

A 66-year-old male with hostile graft is scheduled to undergo iliofemoral graft with distal anastomosis to the mid-superficial femoral artery. An incision is made lateral to the sartorius. The dissection plane should be:

A. Adductor longus and vastus medialis
B. Adductor longus and adductor magnus
C. Vastus medialis and gracilis
D. Vastus medialis and rectus femoris

Correct answer: A

Question 4

During passage of graft through the obturator canal, the graft in the thigh should be:

A. Posterior to adductor longus
B. Posterior to vastus medialis
C. Anterior to adductor longus
D. Posterior to gracilis

Correct answer: C

Chapter 36: Lower Extremity Amputation

Question 1

The most common indication for below-knee amputation is:

A. Trauma
B. Failed arterial reconstruction for critical limb ischemia
C. Sarcoma involving lower leg
D. Critical limb ischemia in patients with diabetes mellitus with infected gangrene

Correct answer: D

Question 2

The risk of venous thromboembolism following below-knee amputation is:

A. Less than 5%
B. >5–<10%
C. 10–15%
D. Greater than 15%

Correct answer: C

Question 3

Conversion of below-knee amputation to above-knee amputation occurs in:

A. <10%
B. 10–20%

C. 21–25%
D. Greater than 25%

Correct answer: B

Question 4
The incidence of phantom pain following above-knee amputation is:

A. <1%
B. 1–2%
C. >2–4%
D. Approximately 5%

Correct answer: D

Question 5
The incidence of wound complications following hip disarticulation is:

A. <10%
B. 10–25%
C. >25–40%
D. >40–60%

Correct answer: D

Chapter 37: Carotid Body Tumor
Question 1
Preoperative embolization of a 6 cm carotid body tumor is planned. It is most ideal for the patient to be operated:

A. Within 24 h of embolization
B. Within 48 h of embolization
C. Within 72 h of embolization
D. Immediately after embolization

Correct answer: B

Question 2
A 4 cm Shamblin type 3 carotid body tumor adherent to carotid artery is best treated by:

A. Local excision
B. Local excision following preoperative embolization
C. Resection of the tumor and involved ICA and ECA with interposition of a greater saphenous vein graft from CCA to ICA
D. Resection of the tumor and involved artery with reconstruction using superficial femoral artery as an interposition graft

Correct answer: C

Question 3

Preoperative imaging studies show that the superior limit of a large carotid body tumor extends to the junction of C1–C2 vertebrae. Optimal anesthetic consideration consists of:

A. Excision under cervical block anesthesia
B. Excision under GA with orotracheal intubation
C. Excision under GA with nasotracheal intubation
D. Excision under GA with nasotracheal intubation and mandibular subluxation

Correct answer: D

Index

S. S. Hans et al. (eds.), *Primary and Repeat Arterial Reconstructions*,
https://doi.org/10.1007/978-3-031-13897-3

GPSR Compliance

The European Union's (EU) General Product Safety Regulation (GPSR) is a set of rules that requires consumer products to be safe and our obligations to ensure this.

If you have any concerns about our products, you can contact us on ProductSafety@springernature.com

In case Publisher is established outside the EU, the EU authorized representative is:

Springer Nature Customer Service Center GmbH
Europaplatz 3
69115 Heidelberg, Germany

Batch number: 10732076

Printed by Printforce, the Netherlands